Clinical Interviews for Children and Adolescents

The Guilford Practical Intervention in the Schools Series

Kenneth W. Merrell, Series Editor

Books in this series address the complex academic, behavioral, and social–emotional needs of children and youth at risk. School-based practitioners are provided with practical, research-based, and readily applicable tools to support students and team successfully with teachers, families, and administrators. Each volume is designed to be used directly and frequently in planning and delivering clinical services. Features include a convenient format to facilitate photocopying, step-by-step instructions for assessment and intervention, and helpful, timesaving reproducibles.

Helping Students Overcome Depression and Anxiety: A Practical Guide
Kenneth W. Merrell

Emotional and Behavioral Problems of Young Children: Effective Interventions in the Preschool and Kindergarten Years
Gretchen A. Gimpel and Melissa L. Holland

Conducting School-Based Functional Behavioral Assessments: A Practitioner's Guide
T. Steuart Watson and Mark W. Steege

Executive Skills in Children and Adolescents: A Practical Guide to Assessment and Intervention
Peg Dawson and Richard Guare

Responding to Problem Behavior in Schools: The Behavior Education Program
Deanne A. Crone, Robert H. Horner, and Leanne S. Hawken

Resilient Classrooms: Creating Healthy Environments for Learning
Beth Doll, Steven Zucker, and Katherine Brehm

Helping Schoolchildren with Chronic Health Conditions: A Practical Guide
Daniel L. Clay

Interventions for Reading Problems: Designing and Evaluating Effective Strategies
Edward J. Daly III, Sandra Chafouleas, and Christopher H. Skinner

Safe and Healthy Schools: Practical Prevention Strategies
Jeffrey R. Sprague and Hill M. Walker

School-Based Crisis Intervention: Preparing All Personnel to Assist
Melissa Allen Heath and Dawn Sheen

Assessing Culturally and Linguistically Diverse Students: A Practical Guide
Robert L. Rhodes, Salvador Hector Ochoa, and Samuel O. Ortiz

Mental Health Medications for Children: A Primer
Ronald T. Brown, Laura Arnstein Carpenter, and Emily Simerly

Clinical Interviews for Children and Adolescents: Assessment to Intervention
Stephanie H. McConaughy

Clinical Interviews for Children and Adolescents

Assessment to Intervention

STEPHANIE H. McCONAUGHY

THE GUILFORD PRESS
New York   London

© 2005 The Guilford Press
A Division of Guilford Publications, Inc.
72 Spring Street, New York, NY 10012
www.guilford.com

Printed in Canada

This book is printed on acid-free paper.

Last digit is print number: 9   8   7   6   5   4   3   2   1

Library of Congress Cataloging-in-Publication Data

McConaughy, Stephanie H.
  Clinical interviews for children and adolescents: assessment to intervention / Stephanie H. McConaughy
      p. cm.—(The Guilford practical intervention in the schools series)
  Includes bibliographical references and index.
  ISBN 1-59385-205-3
  1. Interviewing in child psychiatry.   2. Interviewing in adolescent psychiatry.   I. Title.
II. Series.
  RJ503.6.M329 2005
  618.92′89—dc22
                                                                          2005003777

To David, my son. He said, "You ask a lot of questions."
He helped me to listen.

About the Author

Stephanie H. McConaughy, PhD, is Research Professor of Psychiatry and Psychology at the University of Vermont. She specializes in research and assessment of children's learning, behavioral, and emotional problems. Dr. McConaughy is author of numerous journal articles, chapters, books, and published assessment instruments and is a licensed practicing psychologist and nationally certified school psychologist. She serves on the editorial boards of several professional journals and was an associate editor of the *School Psychology Review.* Dr. McConaughy's research has been funded by the U.S. Department of Education, the National Institute on Disability and Rehabilitation Research, the National Institute of Child Health and Human Development, the National Institute of Mental Health, the Spencer Foundation, and the W. T. Grant Foundation.

Preface

Most people, when given the opportunity, love to talk about themselves. Children are no different. Yet, without even thinking, adults often hinder children from speaking for themselves. Ask a child a question in the presence of a parent or another familiar adult and watch what happens. As the child starts to speak, the adult jumps in to explain what the child thinks or feels, and then continues with his or her own view of the matter. Other times, when children do manage to express their views, adults counteract with their versions of how things *should* be or how children *should* think or feel. This is captured poignantly in Cat Stevens's lament, "From the moment I could talk, I was ordered to listen . . ." ("Father and Son," from *Tea for the Tillerman*, released November 1970). In my practice as a psychologist and researcher, I have met many children like that son struggling to be heard. These are the ones we call "rebellious, oppositional, depressed, withdrawn, inattentive, shy, uncommunicative . . . ." Add your own words.

Learning children's viewpoints is an essential feature of good clinical assessment, especially assessment of children experiencing learning, behavioral, and emotional problems. I hope this book will enhance readers' professional skills for hearing what troubled children have to say and integrating children's perspectives with those of their parents, teachers, and other significant adults. To provide a broad focus, this book discusses clinical interviewing within the framework of multimethod assessment. Readers are encouraged to use other assessment methods along with clinical interviews to obtain comprehensive pictures of children's functioning. To illustrate interviewing strategies, I have included case examples and interview segments based on research and clinical experience with many children. All of the names used in these cases are pseudonyms and details of case material have been altered to protect confidentiality.

In my research and the creation of this book, I have benefited from the help and advice of many colleagues. I am particularly grateful for the advice of Kenneth Merrell, editor of The Guilford Practical Intervention in the Schools Series, who encouraged me to write this book and provided valuable editorial comments. I am also grateful to Chris Jennison and the editorial staff at The Guilford Press for their efforts and support. I thank my colleague Thomas Achenbach, who has been a friend and my closest collaborator in over two decades of research on empirically based assessment of children's emotional and behavioral problems. Our research to develop the Semistructured Clinical Interview for Children and Adolescents (SCICA; McConaughy &

Achenbach, 1994, 2001) provided the foundation for much of the theory and interviewing strategies described in this book. Our research efforts have been supported by the University of Vermont Research Center for Children, Youth, and Families; the National Institute of Child Health and Human Development; the National Institute of Mental Health; the National Institute on Disability and Rehabilitation Research (U.S. Department of Education); the Spencer Foundation; and the W. T. Grant Foundation.

For their insightful comments on drafts of chapters for this book, I am grateful to Thomas Achenbach, Cynthia LaRiviere, Leslie Rescorla, James Tallmadge, and Robert Volpe. I thank Rachel Berubé and Kathryn Miner for their help in creating forms for the appendices. I especially thank the hundreds of children who shared their thoughts and feelings in clinical interviews, along with the many parents, teachers, guidance counselors, principals, and special educators who contributed to my research and clinical work. This book represents what I have learned from them as a researcher, licensed psychologist, and school psychologist.

I have tried to write the text in a manner that makes theories and interviewing techniques easy to understand and apply. Research reviews in the chapters provide empirical bases for assessment and intervention planning. The appendices include reproducible formats for parent and teacher interviews and other assessment protocols. I hope that this book will meet the needs of many practitioners, including school psychologists, child and adolescent clinical psychologists, child psychiatrists, social workers, guidance counselors, special educators, behavioral specialists, and other mental health practitioners who interact with children, parents, and school staff. Graduate students in training programs for the above fields should also find this book helpful for learning the complexities of clinical interviewing.

Contents

6. Interviews with Teachers

7. Interpreting Clinical Interviews for Assessment and Intervention Planning

8. Assessing Risk for Suicide

DAVID N. MILLER *and* STEPHANIE H. MCCONAUGHY

9. Assessing Youth Violence and Threats of Violence in Schools: School-Based Risk Assessments

WILLIAM HALIKIAS

List of Figures, Tables, Boxes, and Appendices

FIGURES

TABLES

BOXES

APPENDICES

1

Clinical Interviews in the Context
of Multimethod Assessment

Clinical interviewing has long held a venerable position in psychological assessment. The importance of clinical interviews is reflected in the following quotes from several authors writing for clinical and school-based practitioners:

> Interviewing is a hallmark of assessment processes and perhaps the most common method used to obtain information to evaluate individuals. (Busse & Beaver, 2000, p. 235)

> Interviews are critical for obtaining information, appreciating children's unique perspectives, and establishing rapport. (La Greca, 1990, p. 4)

> Whether one is meeting informally with the teacher of a referred student, conducting a problem identification interview with a parent, or undertaking a diagnostic interview with a child or adolescent, interviewing is a widely used and valuable assessment method. (Merrell, 2003, p. 103)

In a survey of American Psychological Association (APA) members, clinical interviews were ranked first as the most frequently used of 38 listed assessment procedures (Watkins, Campbell, Nieberding, & Hallmark, 1995). Ninety-three percent of the 412 respondents said that they "always" or "frequently" use clinical interviews, versus only 5% who "never" use them. The respondents to this survey included clinicians who work with adults and children. (For brevity, I use the term *children* to include adolescents, unless the focus of discussion is pertinent only to adolescents.) In an earlier survey of members of the APA Division of School Psychology and the National Association of School Psychologists (NASP), clinical interviews again ranked first as the most frequently used among 19 procedures for social–emotional assessments (Prout, 1983). Ninety-one percent of the 173 respondents reported that they "always" or "frequently" use clinical interviews versus less than 1% who "never" use them. Interestingly, in the same survey, 66% of school psychologists said they had received training in clinical interviewing, versus 34% who reported little or no clinical or formal training in this area. This survey result contrasted with reports from directors of school psychology training programs, who ranked clinical interviews first in emphasis in their programs, and 81% of whom reported providing such training to students.

This book discusses clinical interviews with children, parents, and teachers for purposes of assessment and intervention planning. It is intended to be a practical guide and resource for school-based practitioners, including school psychologists, child and adolescent clinical psychologists, school mental health and social workers, guidance counselors, special educators, school behavioral specialists, and trainees in those fields. Many of the interviewing formats and strategies discussed can also be employed by child psychiatrists and other mental health practitioners who evaluate and treat children outside of schools. Appendices for specific chapters provide reproducible interview forms and other relevant materials that practitioners can copy and use.

It is assumed that practitioners who use this book and its materials will have received appropriate professional training in clinical interviewing, as well as in the theory and methodology of standardized psychological assessment. Practitioners are also expected to adhere to the ethical codes of their professional associations, such as the American Psychological Association (APA), NASP, the American Psychiatric Association, the American Counseling Association (ACA), or the National Association of Social Workers (NASW).

This chapter lays the foundation for discussing clinical interviews in the context of a multimethod approach to assessment and intervention planning. The next section provides a brief historical perspective on clinical interviewing, followed by sections discussing the nature of clinical interviews and the working assumptions that underlie the use of clinical interviews as components of multimethod assessment. Subsequent chapters focus on specific techniques for clinical interviews with children, parents, and teachers, as well as assessment procedures that can be used in conjunction with interviews.

HISTORICAL PERSPECTIVE ON CLINICAL INTERVIEWING

Clinical interviews can serve multiple educational and mental health purposes, including (1) providing initial clinical assessments of children's problems; (2) making psychiatric diagnoses; (3) designing school-based interventions and other mental health treatments; (4) evaluating the effectiveness of current services; and (5) screening for at-risk status, such as risk for suicide, risk for violence, or more general risk for emotional, behavioral, or learning problems (Sattler, 1998). School psychologists, in particular, often conduct interviews with children, parents, and teachers as part of a comprehensive assessment to determine whether a child exhibits "emotional disturbance (ED)," as defined by the Individuals with Disabilities Education Act (IDEA; 1990, 1997, 2004). The information obtained from children, parents, and teachers in interviews can be particularly helpful for assessing ED, as well as for planning appropriate school interventions and mental health services for children with ED. Clinical psychologists and psychiatrists also rely heavily on clinical interviews with parents and children to make psychiatric diagnoses, as defined by the *Diagnostic and Statistical Manual of Mental Disorders Fourth Edition, Text Revision* (DSM-IV-TR; American Psychiatric Association, 2000). Interviews with children, parents, and teachers are equally important in school-based behavioral assessment and problem-solving consultation for behavioral and academic problems (e.g., Kratochwill, Elliott, & Callan-Stoiber, 2002; Shapiro, 2004; Sheridan, Kratochwill, & Bergan, 1996; Zins & Erchul, 2002).

Historically, clinical interviews have been a central feature of what has been termed *traditional assessment* of children's emotional and behavioral problems (Hughes & Baker, 1990; Kratochwill & Shapiro, 2000; Shapiro & Kratochwill, 2000). This term has been used to encompass diverse paradigms, including medical diagnostic, psychodynamic, psychometric, and personality assessments. Early contributors to behavioral assessment made clear distinctions between their approach and what they called traditional assessment (e.g., Hartmann, Roper, & Bradford, 1979). Traditional assessment was said to focus primarily on underlying states or personality traits in the individual as causes of behavior. Medical approaches also focused on physical states, diseases, or disorders in the individual as probable causes of behavior. By contrast, *behavioral assessment* focused on observable, discreet, problem behaviors and contingent events in the environment that reinforced and maintained those behaviors, without any assumptions about underlying causes in the individual, such as personality traits or disorders.

Traditional assessment has also been described as *nomothetic*, because it compared an individual's functioning with groups of other individuals (e.g., normative samples). Behavioral assessment, by contrast, was considered to be *idiographic*, because it focused on target behaviors of individuals without comparisons to other people or groups (Stanger, 2003; Shapiro & Kratochwill, 2000). Traditional approaches to assessment relied more heavily on clinical interviewing, self-report forms, and tests, while behavioral assessment relied on direct observation of current behaviors in naturalistic settings.

As behavioral assessment developed and matured, it began to broaden its focus and assumptions to encompass diverse methods. As a result, distinctions between traditional and behavioral assessment have become less clear-cut. In fact, as Stanger (2003) pointed out, "to contrast behavioral and traditional assessment approaches [now], one must necessarily create a false dichotomy between them" (p. 4). Instead, advocates of modern behavioral assessment argue that it is more helpful to consider methods of behavioral assessment along a continuum of direct to indirect approaches (Mash & Terdal, 1997; Merrell, 2003; Shapiro & Kratochwill, 2000; Stanger, 2003). Interviews and self-reports are considered more indirect methods of assessment because, presumably, interviewees report behaviors that have occurred in the past. Observations in naturalistic settings are considered more direct methods of assessment because they focus on current behaviors.

Within the context of modern behavioral assessment, clinical interviews are now valued as much as they have been valued in traditional assessment:

> "Behavioral assessment" is no longer synonymous with the direct observation of behavior; rather it refers to the use of multiple methods to assess a greatly expanded range of person and situation variables that empirical investigators have found to be important to the development, maintenance, and treatment of childhood disorders. . . . In such a broad-based assessment scheme, parent, child, and family interviews are essential components of the behavioral assessment of childhood disorders. (Hughes & Baker, 1990, p. 108)

Later chapters of this book present formats for clinical interviews with children, parents, and teachers. These interviews combine aspects of traditional and behavioral forms of assessment in order to understand children's current functioning and to develop interventions, when needed. The interview topics include children's school functioning, social relations, family relations, home situation, and relevant developmental and educational history, as well as behavioral descriptions of children's current problems and competencies. The interview formats assume that practitioners will also use other assessment procedures, including tests, questionnaires, and standardized rating scales. Practitioners can use clinical interviews to obtain data that are not easily obtained by the other methods they plan to use. Interview formats are also tailored to the type of information that can best be provided by each particular informant: the child, the parent, and the teacher. The challenge for practitioners is to integrate interview data with other data to formulate a comprehensive picture of the child and to plan needed interventions.

THE NATURE OF CLINICAL INTERVIEWS

As we begin our discussion of clinical interviews, it is important to be clear about what they are and are not. Hughes and Baker (1990) defined clinical interviews with children as follows: "The child interview is a face-to-face interaction of bidirectional influence, entered into for the purpose of assessing aspects of the child's functioning that have relevance to planning, implementing, or evaluating treatment" (p. 4). This definition is a good one because it captures the basic elements of a clinical interview: a one-on-one interaction, with the dual goals of assessment and intervention planning. A similar definition can be applied to clinical interviews with parents and teachers.

Clinical interviews, as defined above, are different from ordinary conversation. Whereas there are many linguistic parameters for good communication, ordinary conversation is usually a relatively informal, spontaneous verbal interchange between two people on some topic of mutual interest. As Sattler (1998) pointed out, clinical interviews differ from ordinary conversation in the following ways:

- The clinical interview usually takes place during a formally arranged meeting.
- The clinical interview has a specific purpose.
- The interviewer chooses the topics or broad content of the discussion.
- The interviewer and interviewee have a defined relationship—the interviewer asks questions, the interviewee responds to the questions.
- The interviewer keeps attuned to aspects of the interaction—the interviewee's affect, behavior, and style—as well as the content of discussion.
- The interviewer uses questioning techniques and other strategies to direct the flow of conversation.
- The interviewer accepts the interviewee's expressions of feelings and factual information without casting judgment on them.
- The interviewer sometimes makes explicit what might be left unstated in ordinary conversation.
- The interviewer follows guidelines for confidentiality and disclosure of information.

Clinical interviews are also different from interviewing during psychotherapy. Sattler (1998) used the term *clinical assessment interview* to distinguish this type of interviewing from psychotherapeutic interviews. A major goal of clinical assessment interviews is to obtain information. The information is then used to evaluate an individual's emotional and behavioral functioning and to decide whether interventions are warranted, and if so, which types. The goals of psychotherapeutic interviews, by contrast, are usually to relieve emotional stress, foster insight, and promote changes in behavior or affect that can lead to improvements in an individual's life situation. This book focuses only on clinical assessment interviews, though some of the interview topics and strategies discussed may be equally applicable to psychotherapy situations.

Sattler (1998) also noted that goals of clinical assessment interviews are different from those of forensic and survey interviews. Forensic interviews are designed to investigate specific questions about an individual or family and to provide expert opinions for a legal decision. Examples are forensic interviews for child custody disputes, termination of parental rights, and investigations of child abuse and neglect. Survey interviews are designed to collect data relevant to specific questions or variables of interest to a researcher. Examples are epidemiological surveys on the prevalence of different disorders or diseases. This book does not discuss forensic or survey interviews because they are not usually performed by school-based practitioners. However, Chapters 8 and 9 discuss clinical interviews that focus specifically on two special issues faced by school-based practitioners: assessing suicide risk (danger to self) and assessing potential for violence or threats of violence (danger to others). Interviews for evaluating child sexual and physical abuse are not covered in detail because these types of interviews are more typically conducted by professionals who specialize in social service or criminal investigations.

WORKING ASSUMPTIONS FOR CLINICAL INTERVIEWS

When done well, clinical interviews can be rich sources of information about a child. However, in some forms of traditional assessment, interview data have been given more weight than data from other assessment methods. The sole use of structured diagnostic interviews for making psychiatric diagnoses is a good example of overreliance on interview data (McConaughy, 2000b, 2003). In early forms of behavioral assessment, the opposite was true: Direct observation was deemed more important than any other assessment method, including interviews (Shapiro & Kratochwill, 2000). With this history in mind, our discussion of clinical interviewing rests on several important working assumptions.

Need for Multiple Data Sources

The first assumption is: *There is no gold standard for assessing children's functioning*. Instead, it is assumed that comprehensive child assessment requires data from other sources in addition to interviews. Other data sources include direct observations in classrooms and other group situations, standardized parent and teacher rating scales, youth self-reports, background questionnaires, tests, and other procedures, as appropriate. Accordingly, it is helpful to keep in mind the following good advice from Shapiro and Kratochwill (2000):

> It is especially important to recognize that data collected from one method are not inherently better than data collected from others. That is, data obtained through an indirect method from a parent (such as a rating scale) are not "less true" than data obtained by directly observing a student within a natural setting. Likewise, data collected through interviews with the student are not inherently more accurate than those collected through direct observation. . . . The key to good assessment is to find conceptual links and relationships between methods and modalities of assessment. Each form of behavioral assessment contributes unique elements to solving the assessment puzzle. (p. 13)

Situational Variability

A second assumption is: *Children's behavior is likely to vary across situations and relationships.* In behavioral assessment endeavors, it is assumed that environmental conditions influence children's behavior (Shapiro & Kratochwill, 2000; Stanger, 2003). Because environmental conditions can vary across situations, children's behavior is likely to vary from one situation to the next. Children's relationships with different adults, such as parents versus teachers, are also likely to involve variations in behavior. Situational variations in behavior can lead to hypotheses about factors that maintain certain behaviors, for example, increased or decreased adult attention, presence or absence of peers, rewards or punishments (Stanger, 2003).

At the same time, certain patterns of children's behavior may also be consistent across different situations and relationships. Research has shown, for example, that aggressive behavior tends to be relatively stable across situations and over time (Achenbach & McConaughy, 1997). Good assessment requires identifying patterns of children's behavior that differ across situations and relationships as well as patterns that remain consistent, despite variations in situations and relationships.

Limited Cross-Informant Agreement

A third assumption is a corollary to the second: *There is likely to be only low-to-moderate agreement between informants who are in different situations or different relationships with the same child.* The limitations on agreement between different informants was demonstrated in Achenbach, McConaughy, and Howell's (1987) meta-analytic study that showed significant, but modest, correlations between reports about children's behavior from different informants under different conditions. They found that the average correlation was only .28 between ratings of children's behavior by parents versus teachers, or by parents/teachers versus mental health professionals. This figure contrasted with an average correlation of .60 between informants from similar situations or relationships with the child (e.g., pairs of parents or pairs of teachers).

Low agreement between informants does not mean that one is right and the other is wrong, or that one has a "truer" picture of a child than does the other. Parents may know more than teachers about many aspects of their child's functioning simply because parents spend more time with the child and they have a special, unique relationship with the child. Still, teachers may know more than parents about other aspects of functioning, such as the child's approach to academic tasks or ability to relate to peers, because of the special circumstances of school versus home. Mental health professionals may also learn more than parents and teachers about certain aspects of functioning, such as the child's feelings, attitudes, and coping styles, because of the special circumstances surrounding assessment or therapy.

It is possible, of course, that a particular informant may be biased or may deliberately falsify reports for personal gain. Later chapters address this issue. However, when there is no evidence of prevarication or intentional misrepresentation in informants' reports, practitioners should assume that different informants each contribute valid information that represents one part of a bigger picture of the child. Differences in people's perceptions of the child are as informative as are the similarities in perceptions. The challenge is to put all these pieces together to form a meaningful picture of the child's functioning under the given circumstances. By examining similarities and differences in perceptions, practitioners can identify important clues to factors affecting the child's behavior in different situations and relationships. In turn, these clues can lead to intervention strategies that are best suited to each of these special circumstances and relationships.

Variations in Interview Structure and Content

A fourth assumption is: *The structure and content of clinical interviews should vary in relation to the informant and the goals of the interviews.* Later chapters in this book present formats for semistructured clinical interviews with children, parents, and teachers. As indicated above, each kind of informant provides a unique perspective on the nature and circumstances affecting a child's functioning. By interviewing children, practitioners can learn children's views of their problems and competencies, their desires, fears, and coping strategies, and their reactions to the circumstances and important relationships affecting their behavior. Interviewers can also directly observe children's behavior, affect, and coping strategies. By interviewing parents, practitioners can learn parents' views of children's problems and competencies, children's developmental and medical history, family circumstances, and parents' reactions to their children's behavior. Parent interviews can also provide clues about parents' own psychological functioning and coping strategies. By interviewing teachers, practitioners can learn teachers' views of children's problems, competencies, and academic performance. They can also learn about teachers' instructional strategies, school interventions for academic and behavioral problems, and forms of special help or services that have been provided.

INTERVIEW CONTENT AND QUESTIONING STRATEGIES

Clinical interviews should be tailored to particular informants. Accordingly, the content and questioning strategies should be shaped by the kind of informant to be interviewed and the kind of information sought, as outlined in Table 1.1. Later chapters discuss the interview content and questioning strategies in detail for each kind of informant. As Table 1.1 shows, the clinical interviews presented in this book combine aspects of traditional and behavioral interviewing techniques. Practitioners can use *semistructured questions* to query children, parents, and teachers about many different aspects of children's functioning, including their activities and interests, school and social functioning, and family relations. If parents have completed questionnaires about their child's developmental and medical history prior to the interview, practitioners can examine this information and then ask questions about aspects of the child's history that are likely to affect current behavior. The format of semistructured questions is relatively open-ended and flexible to simulate a natural flow of conversation. Semistructured questions generally do not elicit "yes" or "no" answers, but instead encourage interviewees to express their views, opinions, and feelings about specific topics. Probe questions can then be used to obtain more detailed information.

Structured questions are appropriate for querying parents about symptoms and criteria for psychiatric disorders, as defined in the DSM-IV. Structured diagnostic interviews have a standardized set of questions and probes focusing on specific problems relevant for diagnoses. Several structured diagnostic interviews have been developed for research and mental health assessments. An example is the National Institute of Mental Health's Diagnostic Interview Schedule for

TABLE 1.1. Content and Questioning Strategies for Child, Parent, and Teacher Interviews

Questioning strategies	Informant and interview content		
	Child interview	Parent interview	Teacher interview

Semistructured questions	Activities and interests
	School and homework
	Friendships and peer relations
	Home situation and family relations
	Self-awareness and feelings
	Adolescent issues
	   Alcohol and drugs
	   Antisocial behavior and trouble with the law
	   Dating and romances
		Social functioning
		School functioning
		Medical and developmental history
		Family relations and home situation
		Child's strengths and interests
			Academic performance
			Teaching strategies
			Child's strengths and interests

Structured questions		Symptoms and criteria for psychiatric disorders	
Behavior-specific questions	Child's view of problems	Concerns about the child Behavioral and emotional problems	Concerns about the child School behavior problems
Problem-solving questions	Feasibility of interventions	Feasibility of interventions Initial goals and plans	Feasibility of school interventions Special help/services Initial goals and plans

Children—Version IV (NIMH DISC-IV; Shaffer, Fisher, Lucas, Dulcan, & Schwab-Stone, 2000). The DISC-IV and most other structured diagnostic interviews have formats for parents and older children. Few have formats for interviewing teachers.

Because of their length and detail, structured diagnostic interviews are usually not feasible for school-based assessments. However, school practitioners may still want to obtain information from parents to determine whether a child meets criteria for certain common psychiatric diagnoses. One example is Attention-Deficit/Hyperactivity Disorder (ADHD), which can qualify a child for special education services under IDEA, or for a Section 504 plan under the Rehabilitation Act of 1973 (Rehabilitation Act, 1973). Children with ADHD are also likely to need accommodations and interventions in the general education setting (DuPaul & Stoner, 2003). Children with diagnoses of depression or anxiety can also benefit from school-based interventions, as well as mental health treatment (Merrell, 2001). Appendix 5.3 in Chapter 5 provides a structured diagnostic interview that school practitioners can use to ask parents about symptoms of common DSM-IV childhood disorders.

Practitioners can use *behavior-specific questions* to query parents and teachers regarding their current concerns about the child. Behavior-specific questions are narrower in scope than semistructured questions because the focus is on a limited number of specific problem areas (Beaver & Busse, 2000). Behavior-specific questions comprise the initial phases of behavioral assessment and behavioral consultation, wherein the main purposes are (1) to identify and define problems of concern to parents and teachers (problem identification), and (2) to examine antecedents and consequences that surround the identified problems (problem analysis). Practitioners can also use behavior-specific questions to query children about their views of particular problems and their understanding of the circumstances around the problems.

Problem-solving questions focus on parents' and teachers' current concerns, with the goal of developing interventions for identified problems (Beaver & Busse, 2000). In behavioral consultation, problem-solving questions usually comprise later stages of plan implementation and plan evaluation. However, in initial clinical interviews, practitioners can use problem-solving questions to explore and gauge parents' and teachers' receptivity are to different kinds of interventions prior to implementing any interventions. For example, some parents or teachers may have negative feelings about certain types of interventions (e.g., medication treatments or structured behavior contracts), but may be willing to try other alternatives. Practitioners can also use problem-solving questions to explore the children's views of different interventions and to find out which approaches are acceptable to them.

INTERVIEWS AS COMPONENTS OF MULTIMETHOD ASSESSMENT

The working assumptions discussed in the previous section bring us to the following conclusion: *Interviews are best viewed as components of a multimethod approach to assessment of children's functioning.* Many authors have stressed the importance of multimethod assessment of children (e.g., Achenbach & McConaughy, 1997; Kratochwill & Shapiro, 2000; Mash & Terdal, 1997; Merrell, 2003; McConaughy & Ritter, 2002; Sattler, 1998; Shapiro & Kratochwill, 2000; Stanger, 2003). However, the need for multiple data sources cannot be overstated. Interviews, like other assessment procedures, have their advantages and disadvantages. The opportunity to establish rapport is one advantage that interviewing offers over other assessment methods. During interviews, practitioners can also explore details of children's problems and circumstances from different points of view.

A disadvantage is that interviews are vulnerable to low reliability and misinformation when they are used to assess specific problems that might be better assessed in other ways. For example, children may not report certain types of behavior, such as attention problems or aggressive behavior. Instead of using child interviews to assess the presence of these types of problems, it might be better to rely more on parent and teacher interviews, standardized parent and teacher rating scales, and direct observations. Similarly, parent and teacher interviews may not be as efficient, or as reliable, as standardized rating scales for assessing a wide range of potential problems. Parent and teacher interviews are also less efficient than questionnaires for obtaining details of the child's medical, developmental, and educational history. By contrast, parent and teacher interviews are good for clarifying concerns about specific current problems and for learning how parents and teachers react to identified problems. Parent and teacher interviews can also provide insights into children's strengths and competencies and the feasibility of different intervention options.

To reap the benefits of clinical interviews while avoiding their disadvantages, practitioners are encouraged to combine interviews routinely with other assessment procedures (McConaughy, 2000a, 2000b, 2003). To illustrate such a multimethod approach, Table 1.2 outlines examples of data sources for five different assessment axes described by Achenbach and McConaughy (1997): I. Parent Reports; II. Teacher Reports; III. Cognitive Assessment; IV. Physical Assessment; and V. Direct Assessment of the Child. Axes I and II include parent and teacher interviews, along with

TABLE 1.2. Data Sources for Multimethod Assessment

I. Parent reports	II. Teacher reports	III. Cognitive assessment	IV. Physical assessment	V. Direct assessment of the child
Parent interview	Teacher interview	Standardized ability and intelligence tests	Medical exams	Child clinical interview
Standardized parent rating scales	Standardized teacher rating scales	Standardized achievement tests	Neurological exams	Observations during child clinical interview
Background questionnaires	Background questionnaires	Observations during test sessions	Illnesses, injuries and disabilities	Standardized self-reports
Historical records	Educational records	Curriculum-based assessment	Hospitalizations	Direct observations in classroom, playground, and other settings
		Perceptual–motor tests Speech and language tests	Medications	Personality tests

standardized rating scales, background questionnaires, and historical and educational records. Axis V includes the child clinical interview, along with standardized self-reports, direct observations in settings such as classrooms and playgrounds, standardized personality tests, and other direct assessment procedures. Axis III covers cognitive assessment, including standardized ability and intelligence tests, standardized achievement tests, curriculum-based assessment, and tests of perceptual–motor skills and speech and language. Practitioners' observations during test sessions are also important Axis III data sources. Axis IV covers aspects of physical assessment, such as medical and neurological exams, illnesses, injuries, disabilities, hospitalizations, and medications. For comprehensive assessment, information relevant to all five axes in Table 1.2 should be considered. However, practitioners may not need to obtain data from all five axes for all children.

The Achenbach System of Empirically Based Assessment (ASEBA) is an example of a family of standardized instruments specifically designed to fit the multimethod model outlined in Table 1.2. For school-age children, the ASEBA includes the Child Behavior Checklist for Ages 6 to 18 (CBCL/6–18) for obtaining parents' ratings of their children's competencies and problems; the Teacher's Report Form (TRF) for obtaining teachers' ratings of academic performance, adaptive functioning, and school problems; and the Youth Self-Report (YSR) for obtaining youths' self-ratings of their competencies and problems (Achenbach & Rescorla, 2001). The ASEBA also includes the Semistructured Clinical Interview for Children and Adolescents (SCICA; McConaughy & Achenbach, 2001) for interviewing children ages 6–18; the Test Observation Form (TOF; McConaughy & Achenbach, 2004b) for obtaining test examiners' ratings of children's problems during test sessions; and the Direct Observation Form (DOF; Achenbach, 1986) for conducting observations of children in group settings, such as classrooms. Other ASEBA instruments are designed for preschool children (Achenbach & Rescorla, 2000), adults ages 18–59 (Achenbach & Rescorla, 2003), and older adults ages 60–90+ (Achenbach, Newhouse, & Rescorla, 2004).

The Behavior Assessment System for Children—Second Edition (BASC-2; Reynolds & Kamphaus, 2004) is another example of a family of standardized instruments for multimethod assessment of school-age children and college students. The BASC-2 includes instruments for obtaining parent and teacher ratings of children's problems and adaptive skills, youth self-reports, and structured observations in school settings. It also provides a structured questionnaire for obtaining parents' reports of children's developmental histories. Subsequent chapters discuss how practitioners can conduct child, parent, and teacher clinical interviews in ways that dovetail with other data sources so as to maximize the best of what interviews have to offer.

CASE EXAMPLES

Throughout this book, we will visit and revisit case examples that illustrate the kind of information that can be derived from clinical interviews with children, parents, and teachers. As indicated in the preface, the cases are based on research and clinical experience with many children. and names of the children, parents, and teachers are all pseudonyms. The following synopses introduce these cases.

Andy Lockwood, Age 7

Andy Lockwood was repeating first grade because of social immaturity and below-grade-level academic performance. His previous first-grade teacher had complained that he was boisterous and noisy and took forever to get anything done. At the end of that year, Andy was far behind other children in basic reading and math skills. Andy's current first-grade teacher voiced similar concerns. She said he was disruptive in class, failed to complete assigned work, and was still achieving far below other children in her class. Andy's mother agreed that he was an active child, but thought that he was typical of boys his age. She suspected that the teachers did not like Andy and were too rigid in their expectations about behavior. Ms. Lockwood also questioned whether Andy understood directions for assignments, because her attempts to help him with homework often led to tears and arguments. After several phone calls from the current teacher, Andy's mother started to worry that his second year in first grade would be no better than his first year. So she agreed to an evaluation of his learning, behavioral, and emotional functioning. The evaluation was carried out by the school psychologist and special education staff.

Bruce Garcia, Age 9

Bruce Garcia had been receiving speech and language services since age 4. When he was in third grade, the school multidisciplinary team requested a psychological evaluation as part of his 3-year reevaluation. Bruce's teacher complained that his school performance was erratic, and he seemed disorganized and confused. She also worried that Bruce had trouble fitting into peer groups because of his "odd" behavior. Bruce's mother was concerned that he seemed socially withdrawn at home and had difficulty paying attention to schoolwork. Bruce's school district had a contract with a nearby psychiatric outpatient clinic for school-based mental health and consultation services. The school multidisciplinary team referred Bruce to the clinic for a psychological evaluation of his social–emotional functioning and cognitive ability.

Catherine Holcomb, Age 11

Catherine was the younger of two children living with her mother. Catherine's father had died when she was 7 years old, and her mother had not remarried. Catherine's fifth-grade teacher was concerned because she seemed inattentive in class, was erratic in completing assignments, and was having difficulty in reading and written work. Catherine also seemed socially withdrawn and had few friends in school. Catherine's teacher voiced her concerns to Ms. Holcomb and the school psychologist. Ms. Holcomb then agreed to a school-based evaluation of Catherine's emotional functioning and possible learning disabilities.

Karl Bryant, Age 12

Karl's sixth-grade teacher referred him for an evaluation because of behavior problems in school. She reported that Karl got into fights, had problems getting along with other students, and frequently violated school rules. Because Karl failed to complete assignments, he was failing in several subjects. With permission from Karl's mother, the school multidisciplinary team conducted an evaluation to determine whether Karl qualified for special education services due to a learning disability and/or emotional disturbance. Karl's mother also wanted advice on how to manage his behavior at home.

Kelsey Watson, Age 14

Kelsey was in the custody of the state social service agency due to unmanageable behavior at home and episodes of running away. She lived in a residential group home and was enrolled in eighth grade in the local school district. She continued to have occasional home visits with her mother, who lived in a different town. Despite a history of behavioral and emotional problems and underachievement, Kelsey had never received any special services in school. Therefore, the multidisciplinary team in her new school referred her for an evaluation to determine if she were eligible for services. They also wanted recommendations for coping with potential behavior problems at school.

In each of the above cases, clinical interviews were conducted with the child and the child's parents or guardians and teachers. Parents or guardians and teachers completed standardized rating scales to evaluate the child's competencies and behavioral and emotional functioning. Catherine, Karl, and Kelsey completed standardized self-reports of their competencies and behavioral and emotional functioning. Standardized tests of cognitive ability, achievement, speech/language, and perceptual–motor functioning were also administered, as needed.

STRUCTURE OF THIS BOOK

After we discuss interviewing strategies in Chapter 2, you will learn more about each of the five children in subsequent chapters. Chapters 3 and 4 cover topics to be included in child clinical interviews. These chapters include segments of clinical interviews with one or more of the five children. Chapter 5 discusses semistructured parent interviews and a brief structured diagnostic interview for parents. Appendices for Chapter 5 provide reproducible protocols for both types of parent interviews, plus a reproducible background questionnaire concerning the child's developmental history and family circumstances. Chapter 6 discusses semistructured interviews with teachers and provides a reproducible protocol for the teacher interview in its appendix. Chapter 7 discusses interpretations of clinical interviews for intervention planning, returning to the five case examples to illustrate how practitioners can integrate interview results with other assessment data to develop intervention plans.

Chapters 8 and 9 address two special issues for clinical interviewing. In Chapter 8, David Miller (with Stephanie McConaughy) describes procedures for assessing risk for suicide (danger to self). In Chapter 9, William Halikias describes school-based risk assessments of violence or threats of violence (danger to others). As scholars and licensed practicing psychologists, Drs. Miller and Halikias have special expertise in each of these topic areas.

2

Strategies for
Child Clinical Interviews

As indicated in Chapter 1, most experts agree that interviewing the child is an essential component of multimethod clinical assessment (e.g., Merrell, 2001, 2003; Sattler, 1998; Hughes & Baker, 1990). This chapter discusses strategies for conducting child clinical interviews, with an emphasis on semistructured interviewing. Practitioners can use semistructured questions to cover a wide variety of topics, while adapting questioning strategies to fit children's developmental levels and interaction styles. Practitioners can also use behavior-specific questions to assess children's understanding of antecedents and consequences for specific problems, as well as problem-solving questions to explore children's views of potential interventions.

PURPOSES FOR CHILD CLINICAL INTERVIEWS

Within the context of multimethod assessment, child clinical interviews are especially useful for the following purposes:

- To establish rapport and mutual respect between the interviewer and the child.
- To learn the child's perspective on his/her functioning.
- To identify which of the child's current problems would be appropriate potential targets for interventions.
- To identify the child's strengths and competencies that can be marshaled to bolster interventions.
- To assess the child's view of different intervention options.
- To directly observe the child's behavior, affect, and interaction style.

Although clinical interviews differ from ordinary conversations, you can still use strategies that make interviews seem more conversational and comfortable for interviewees. For example, you can ask questions in ways that encourage interviewees to express their opinions and feelings without fear of negative reactions or challenges to their viewpoints. You can also pace the flow of

14

questions and answers in ways that encourage more talk from the interviewee than from the interviewer. These strategies are especially important when interviewing children. Many children will shut down if they feel they are being interrogated or lectured. Children can also lose interest if they have to listen more than talk and if the interview feels like a drill session or fact-finding investigation. Using professional jargon can also undermine your clinical interviews, because children may not understand it.

Good clinical interviewing requires focusing on key areas of concern, while also remaining sensitive to interviewees' reactions to the interview process. As Sattler (1998) stated, "Clinical assessment interviewing . . . even more than other assessment techniques . . . places a premium on your personal skills, such as your ability to communicate effectively and your ability to establish a meaningful relationship" (p. 3). At first, clinical interviewing may seem more like a mysterious art than an acquired skill. As Merrell (2003) pointed out, the popular media and public beliefs have fostered distorted impressions of the power of clinical interviewing. As an example, Merrell cited the frequent experience of having complete strangers suspect that psychologists or psychiatrists are "analyzing" them or reading their minds when they are simply making ordinary conversation. Although clinical interviewing is not, as Merrell noted, "a mystical conduit to the inner life of the person being interviewed," you can use various interviewing strategies to facilitate good communication and good assessment.

The guidelines in this chapter draw from other authors who have discussed techniques for interviewing children (Garbarino & Scott, 1989; Hughes & Baker, 1990; La Greca, 1990; Merrell, 2001, 2003; Sattler, 1998), as well as from my own work (McConaughy, 2000a, 2000b, 2003; McConaughy & Achenbach, 1994, 2001). The first sections are devoted to general issues concerning the setting, interviewer appearance, and limits of confidentiality. The next sections discuss considerations and questioning strategies for interviewing children at three broad developmental levels. Although it is beyond the scope of this book to provide in-depth discussions of children's cognitive and social–emotional development, these sections highlight key issues relevant to conducting developmentally sensitive clinical interviews. Additional sections cover ethnic and cultural considerations, alternating verbal and nonverbal communication, dealing with lying, and concluding the interview.

SETTING AND INTERVIEWER APPEARANCE

Child clinical interviews should be conducted in a private location with only the child and interviewer present, unless there is a good reason for another person to be there. Finding an appropriate space can sometimes be a challenge for school-based practitioners who do not have their own offices. Nevertheless, it is important to insist on a place that affords privacy for the interview.

Before interviewing young children, or overactive or aggressive children, it is important to child-proof the room by clearing desks and tables of loose items that are not needed for the interview, as well as potentially risky items, such as letter openers, scissors, pins, and electric pencil sharpeners. Toys and other props for the interview should be kept out of sight or out of reach until they are needed. It is also good to remove family pictures and personal mementos because they may distract children who are curious about the interviewer's personal life.

If possible, the room should have a relaxed, neutral atmosphere, with comfortable chairs and a table. Children under age 6 may be more comfortable sitting on cushions or mats on the floor, with the interviewer more or less on the same level. Older children can usually sit in a comfortable chair for their size, with the interviewer sitting in a similar chair. As a general rule, avoid sitting behind a desk or table across from the child, because this arrangement makes the interviewer look too much like an authority figure and creates a test-like atmosphere. Instead, you can sit at a diagonal corner of a table near the child. This arrangement allows you to take notes easily, while not creating a barrier between you and the child. The child can also use the table for writing or drawing, and can leave the chair occasionally, if needed. Adolescents should also be interviewed in a relaxed, neutral setting—preferably one without a childish decor. Whenever possible, avoid conducting child clinical interviews in offices of authority figures, such as the principal's office, or in spaces where discipline procedures are carried out, such as detention or time-out rooms.

Interviewers also need to be mindful of how their personal appearance may affect rapport with children. As a general rule, dress in professional attire congruent with community standards and the local environment. Dressing too casually may create the false impression that the interview is to be a play session or an informal conversation. Very casual dress can also undermine your "professional authority" to ask sensitive questions. On the other hand, if you dress in very formal business-type attire, children might view you as unapproachable or too stiff. In clinic settings, you should avoid wearing a white coat or other attire that makes you look like a medical doctor, because this can raise fears in children. If you use the term "doctor" in your title, tell young children that you are a "talking doctor" and that you do not give shots. Depending on the referral complaints, matching the gender of the interviewer and the child may facilitate communication, especially for assessing sensitive issues such as sexual abuse or sexual orientation.

DISCUSSING PURPOSE AND CONFIDENTIALITY WITH CHILDREN

After personal introductions, explain the purpose of the interview and the limits of confidentiality. A good way to start is to ask children why they think they are being interviewed. Young children may have been told that they are going to play games. Other children may think that they are going to be tested. Some older children may think that they are being interviewed because certain adults think that they are crazy or stupid. Others may think that they will be punished for some wrongdoing. It is important to clear up any such misconceptions at the beginning of the interview.

Next, explain the limits of confidentiality in a clear and succinct manner, using language appropriate for the child's developmental level. An example is the following standard introduction to the SCICA (McConaughy & Achenbach, 2001):

"We are going to spend some time talking and doing things together, so that I can get to know you and learn about what you like and don't like. This is a private talk. I won't tell your parents or your teachers what you say unless you tell me it is OK. The only thing I would have to tell is if you said you were going to hurt yourself, hurt someone else, or someone has hurt you."

The SCICA introduction clearly states the standard limits of confidentiality in language that most children should understand. In particular, confidentiality may be breached if you suspect that the child may be a danger to himself/herself or a danger to others, or if you suspect that the child has been abused or is in danger of being abused. After such an introduction, you can ask children if they understood what you said or have any questions. You should also inform children of other circumstances that might limit guarantees of strict confidentiality. For example, inform children of follow-up discussions that will occur with parents and/or teachers, or written reports that will include interview information. To alleviate concerns about reports to other parties, you can tell children that at the end of the interview, you will talk with them about what to say to other people. For example, you might say:

> "I am going to write a report about what I learn in our talk today. I will also be meeting with your parents and teachers on another day to talk about what I learned about you. At the end of this talk, we can discuss what I will say and how to say it. Do you understand?"

Sometimes you may want to tape-record the interview. When this is the case, you can say, "We are going to record our talk on this tape recorder to help remember our time together." The audiotape should be stored in a safe location and erased after you have finished your written reports or have finished your clinical work with the child. Keep all introductory remarks, including reviews of confidentiality issues, as nontechnical and brief as possible. At the end of the interview, you can summarize key issues and talk about what will be disclosed to others, as discussed in a later section.

DEVELOPMENTAL CONSIDERATIONS FOR CHILD INTERVIEWS

Good clinical interviews with children require sensitivity to their communication skills and their levels of cognitive and social–emotional development. Although many interview topics may be appropriate for children of all ages, interviewers will still need to adapt their style of questioning to fit the child's developmental level. Table 2.1 presents some basic considerations for interviewing children who are 3–5 years old (early childhood), 6–11 years old (middle childhood), and 12–18 years old (adolescence). These ages approximate broad developmental levels. Appropriate adjustments are also needed for children who are below or above the average range of cognitive functioning. Table 2.1 outlines aspects of cognitive functioning, social–emotional functioning, and peer interactions that you can consider when framing questions and interpreting responses for children at each developmental level.

Table 2.2 outlines general "dos" and "don'ts" for interviewing children at each of the three developmental levels summarized in Table 2.1. Table 2.2 is organized in a hierarchical fashion, such that interviewing strategies listed for one level of development may also be appropriate for the next higher level of development. For example, open-ended questions can be used with children in early childhood as well as middle childhood and adolescence. Following the child's lead in conversation is a good strategy for all ages. The next sections discuss these developmental considerations and interviewing strategies in more detail.

Developmental Characteristics of Early Childhood

Young children can be particularly difficult to interview because of their limited communication and cognitive skills, as summarized in the second column of Table 2.1. Piaget (1983) and other developmental psychologists have characterized early childhood as "preoperational" because 3- to

TABLE 2.1. Developmental Considerations for Interviewing Children

Period	Cognitive functioning	Social–emotional functioning	Typical peer interactions
Early childhood (ages 3–5)	Focus on only one feature at a time (preoperational stage) Easily confused between appearance and reality Difficulty recalling specific information accurately (limited memory development) Difficulty sustaining conversation	Difficulty understanding the viewpoint of another person (egocentric) Right or wrong based on consequences (preconventional moral reasoning) Limited verbal ability to describe emotions Can sustain a play task Can engage in reciprocal play sequences	Shared play activities Fantasy play Short interactions Frequent squabbles Unstable friendships Rough-and-tumble play Aggressive peers are generally disliked Reciprocal peers are generally liked
Middle childhood (ages 6–11)	Able to reason logically about tangible objects and actual events (concrete operations stage) Increased capacity for verbal communication	Can think about what another person is thinking (recursive thinking) Right or wrong based on rules and social conventions (conventional moral reasoning) Understands and complies with rules of a game Develops a sense of self-competence Can regulate affect in competition	Structured board games, group games, and team sports with complex rules Squabbles about rules Stable best friendships, usually with same-sex peers Aggressive or socially withdrawn peers are generally disliked Friendly, helpful, and supportive peers are liked Peer status defined by classroom group or structured activities
Adolescence (ages 12–18)	Able to reason abstractly and hypothetically (formal operations stage) Can engage in systematic problem solving Additional increases in verbal communication	Can take a third-person point of view (thinking about thinking) Right or wrong based on individual principles of conscience or ideals (postconventional moral reasoning) Identity confusion and experimentation High emotional intensity and lability Social awareness and self-consciousness Peer group acceptance extremely important	"Hanging out" and communicating with peers (e.g., talking, sending notes, phone calls, e-mail) Intimate self-disclosure, especially for girls Squabbles about relationship issues (e.g., gossip, secrets, loyalty issues) Romantic partners Aggressive and antisocial peers are generally disliked Cooperative, helpful, and competent peers are generally liked Peer status defined by norms for various groups, cliques, or clubs

Note. Adapted from Merrell (2003). Copyright 2003 by Lawrence Erlbaum Associates. Adapted by permission.

TABLE 2.2. Developmentally Sensitive Interviewing Strategies

Period	Interviewing dos	Interviewing don'ts
Early childhood (ages 3–5)	Sit at the child's level (e.g., on a mat on the floor or a small chair) Limit the length and complexity of questions Use open-ended questions about specific and familiar situations Use toys, props, and manipulatives Use the child's terms and phrases Use people's names instead of pronouns Use extenders to encourage more child talk Allow ample time for the child to respond	Do not attempt to maintain total control of the interview Avoid embedded phrases or clauses Avoid questions that can be answered "yes" or "no" Do not follow every response with another question
Middle childhood (ages 6–11)	Take time to establish rapport Listen with empathy Solicit and restate feelings Follow the child's lead in conversation Use open-ended questions and probes Sometimes provide multiple choice options as probes Talk about familiar settings and activities Provide contextual cues (e.g., pictures, verbal examples) Rephrase or simplify questions when the child has misunderstood or not responded Use direct requests to transition to new topics or tasks	Refrain from making judgmental comments Avoid too many factual questions Avoid too much direct questioning Avoid constant eye contact Avoid abstract questions Avoid questions with obvious right or wrong answers Avoid rhetorical questions Avoid "why" questions about motives
Adolescence (ages 12–18)	Be clear about limits of confidentiality Show respect Solicit and listen to adolescents' points of view and feelings Be prepared for emotional lability and stress Ask for possible alternative ways to solve a problem Pursue any indications of suicidal risk	Avoid psychological terms Avoid making judgments based solely on adult norms

Note. Adapted from McConaughy and Achenbach (1994). Copyright 1994 by S. H. McConaughy and T. M. Achenbach. Adapted by permission.

5-year-olds lack the ability to perform the logical operations of the next stage. Children in the preoperational stage tend to focus on only one feature or attribute of an object or situation, and they are easily confused by distinctions between appearance and reality. Puppets and cartoon characters can facilitate communication with young children. An example is the statement of one 3-year-old girl to her father: "Put Beaver on your hand, and he will talk." She then engaged in a lively conversation with Beaver. Because of their limited memory skills, young children have difficulty recalling specific information accurately, and may provide incomplete accounts of past events. They also have difficulty sustaining long conversations.

In terms of social–emotional functioning, summarized in the third column of Table 2.1, 3- to 5-year-olds tend to be "egocentric" because they lack the capacity to understand another person's point of view or to take the perspective of another person. Egocentrism is also a classic characteristic of children with autism. Because of their inability to understand other people's perspectives, it is not useful to ask young children how they think another person felt in a problem situation or what the other person might have been thinking. Instead, it is better to ask more specific questions about what happened and how they felt themselves. It is also important to realize that, although young children experience a range of emotions, they have difficulty verbally describing their feelings, except along broad dimensions, such as happy, sad, and mad.

Young children's views of right and wrong are generally based on the consequences of their actions, which Kohlberg (1976) characterized as a "preconventional" level of moral reasoning. For example, "pushing or hitting someone is wrong because you get sent to the time-out chair." That is, an action is wrong because you get punished or scolded. In social interactions, most 3- to 5-year-olds can sustain play activity for a short period of time. They have advanced beyond parallel play and now can engage in reciprocal play sequences that involve give-and-take with other children.

The last column of Table 2.1 summarizes typical peer interactions for early childhood (based on a review by Bierman & Welsh, 1997). These developmental characteristics are important to keep in mind when interviewing children about peer relations and friendships, as discussed in Chapter 3. Three- to 5-year-old children generally enjoy shared play activities and fantasy games. Their play often mimics familiar adult activities (e.g., playing house, playing school) or involves fantasy play with toys (e.g., cars and trucks, dolls) or shared physical activities (e.g., riding bikes, playing on the beach, running and chasing). Because young children are just beginning to learn to coordinate social behavior, peer interactions are of short duration and involve frequent squabbles and friendships that come and go. Rough-and-tumble play is typical, especially for boys, which can result in squabbles. Peers who are consistently aggressive are generally disliked, whereas peers who share, have positive affect, and have an agreeable disposition are generally liked.

Questioning Strategies for Early Childhood

Interviewers can accommodate young children's developmental level in various ways, as listed as "Interviewing dos" in the top section of Table 2.2. As noted earlier, sitting at the same level as the child can help young children feel more comfortable in clinical interviews. To facilitate communication, you should limit the length and complexity of your questions and comments. Use short, simple questions that do not contain embedded clauses and phrases. Garbarino and Scott (1989) suggested limiting questions to only three to five words more than the length of the child's usual sentence. This is a good rule of thumb for interviewing children of all ages, but especially young children. That is, always try to reduce the amount of "interviewer talk" in favor of increasing the amount of "child talk."

As another general rule, try to use open-ended questions that do not require a "yes" or "no" answer. For young children, open-ended questions should focus on concrete, familiar activities and situations—for example, "What do you like best about going to [name of preschool]?"; "What don't you like about [name of preschool]?" Using props, toys, and manipulatives (especially puppets) can also provide concrete ways for children to demonstrate actions or feelings, or to act out a situation, along with verbal descriptions. Using children's own terms and phrases and people's names (not pronouns) can help to tailor interview questions to children's level of understanding. Examples include using children's words for body parts, names of friends and family members, and terms for rules and punishments at home. Frequent use of extenders ("Oh," "Um," "OK," and

"I understand") will let children know you understand them and thereby encourage more conversation. Avoid long sentences with embedded phrases or clauses. Do not follow every response with another question, because this will make the interview seem too much like a test or interrogation. Be tolerant of silences and pauses that allow children time to think of what they want to say. Too often, adults jump in with more questions or comments whenever children stop talking, which can easily cause them to shut down.

Developmental Characteristics of Middle Childhood

As children move into middle childhood, their communicative competence, cognitive skills, and social–emotional functioning advance markedly. These advances can greatly enhance their ability to participate in child clinical interviews. In terms of cognitive functioning (Table 2.1, second column), children enter Piaget's "concrete operations" stage of cognitive development at about ages 6–7 and continue in that stage until about ages 11–12. In the concrete operational stage, children can apply simple logic to tangible objects and actual event sequences. Developmental psychologists have described a variety of new logical skills. For example, 6- to 11-year-old children are able to focus on more than one attribute of an object at the same time, such as height and width (decentration). They understand that changing the appearance of a set of objects, such as a stack of 10 blocks, does not change the quantity (conservation). They have a concrete understanding of the reverse relationship of simple operations, such as addition ($2 + 2 = 4$) and subtraction ($4 - 2 = 2$) (reversibility). Elementary teachers often capitalize on these concrete reasoning skills by using manipulatives to teach abstract concepts. An example is using graduated colored blocks to teach math concepts. Middle childhood also is a time of rapid advances in vocabulary and ability to communicate with peers and adults.

In terms of social–emotional functioning (Table 2.1, third column), middle childhood is the time when most children master "recursive thinking." This type of cognition involves the ability to imagine what another person might be thinking ("I like him and I think he likes me.") This is an important social–cognitive skill because it allows children to consider another person's perspective in a social interaction—to put themselves in the other person's shoes, so to speak. Children in this stage can not only understand and answer questions about how they think or feel in certain situations, but also how others might think or feel.

Six- to 11-year-olds' views of right and wrong are generally based on rules and social conventions, which Kohlberg (1976) characterized as a "conventional" level of moral reasoning. For example, "Fighting on the playground is wrong because it is against school rules." Children at this level of moral reasoning often have "black-and-white" views of rules as absolute principles with no exceptions. This absolutist viewpoint can often lead to arguments with peers or authority figures about whether the rules were broken or whether certain rules apply in specific situations. In fact, some children adopt a very righteous attitude about rules at home and school and have great concerns about whether they and others are treated fairly according to those rules. Children's understanding of, and compliance with, rules are also prerequisites for their participation in structured games and sports.

Middle childhood is a time when children develop a clearer sense of self-competency in several arenas, including academic skills, athletics, and social interactions with peers. The ability to regulate affect, especially excitement and anger, improves in middle childhood and thereby enhances participation in competitive games and activities. Though some people may have political or religious beliefs that eschew competition, it is important to understand that desires to compete and excel are normal aspects of development in middle childhood and adolescence.

Peer interactions in middle childhood (Table 2.1, fourth column) reflect growth in cognitive and social–emotional functioning. Structured board games, group games, and team sports with complex rules are common activities with peers. Games and sports can often lead to squabbles as children negotiate the rules and try to understand them. A child's failure to comply with the rules is a typical source of complaints by other children to parents and teachers. This is the time when children struggle between appealing to authority figures for help versus trying to solve problems among themselves. Friendships in middle childhood tend to be more stable than in early childhood. Best friendships are usually between children of the same sex, though there can always be exceptions. As in early childhood, aggressive children tend to be disliked, but socially withdrawn children can also be disliked. Peers who are friendly, helpful, and supportive are usually most liked. Acceptance into the peer group becomes much more important in middle childhood. Peer groups are often shaped by classroom groupings, neighborhood contacts, and structured social activities (e.g., Girl Scouts, Boy Scouts, sports). Chapter 3 addresses peer relations and friendships in the context of specific interview questions.

Questioning Strategies for Middle Childhood

Because of their improved language skills, 6- to 11-year-olds can respond better to interview questions than they could at earlier ages (see Table 2.2). Nonetheless, it is important to take time to establish rapport early in the interview. One of the best ways to do this is to begin by asking children about their favorite activities and interests. For example, the SCICA Protocol begins by asking, "What do you like to do in your spare time, like when you're not in school?" Most children can easily talk about something they like to do. This will not only build confidence and help them feel comfortable, but also give them the sense that their views are accepted. Chapter 3 presents additional "warm-up" questions.

Another key strategy is to listen to what children say without casting judgments on their responses. For many children, the clinical interview presents a unique situation: a one-on-one discussion with an adult who is not trying to teach them something or to shape their behavior or attitudes in some way. Many children, especially those with emotional and behavioral problems, may not have had such an experience. It is, therefore, not surprising that they might be wary and reticent about sharing their feelings and opinions. When you listen without expressing judgment, you show children that you are truly interested in their perspectives. Listening without judgment includes trying to avoid both positive and negative judgmental statements. When children hear many positive statements or too much praise (e.g., "So you like reading, that's great," or "I really like your drawing"), they may begin to respond only in ways that will please the adult. In the clinical interview, your goal is not to help children feel better, as it might be in therapy, but instead to help them feel comfortable enough to share their views on important issues. When children hear comments that hint of negative judgments (e.g., "I'll bet that made your mother mad"), they may feel threatened and stop responding, or they may become more defensive and argumentative. As an alternative, you can show empathy by restating and paraphrasing the thoughts and feelings children express. If appropriate, you can then ask children to elaborate on their responses with "tell me more" statements (e.g., "Sounds like your brother really makes you mad when he gets into stuff in your room. Tell me more about that."). As with younger children, you can also use extenders ("Um," "OK," "Uh-huh") to show that you understand.

Following the child's lead in conversation is also a key strategy. This means allowing children to control the sequencing of topics and tolerating the sometimes meandering, "illogical" nature of their conversations. Using a written protocol of topics and questions, such as the SCICA Protocol (McConaughy & Achenbach, 2001), can help you keep track of what has been discussed and what remains to be covered. The SCICA Protocol is organized in a modular fashion that proceeds from less sensitive topics (e.g., activities and interests) to more specific and potentially more sensitive topics (e.g., school, peer relations, family relations, feelings). Interviewers can adjust the sequence of topics in response to cues from the child. As with younger children, you should generally phrase initial questions in an open-ended fashion (e.g., "What do you like least in school?"), and then follow these with more specific probes that encourage children to elaborate on their thoughts and feelings (e.g., "So you don't like math? What is it about math that you don't like?"). When children have trouble elaborating on their responses, you can provide multiple-choice options that cover a variety of possible experiences (e.g., "Sometimes children don't like math because it is too hard, or they don't understand it, or it is boring. How do you feel about math?").

Despite their improved language skills, many children at this stage are still unaccustomed to in-depth conversations with adults, perhaps because they lack appropriate opportunities. Parents' work schedules and children's own programmed activities outside the home may leave little time for prolonged conversations. Table 2.2 lists additional interviewing "dos" to facilitate communication with children at the middle childhood level: talk about familiar settings and activities; provide contextual cues, such as pictures and examples; and rephrase and simplify questions when the child has misunderstood or not responded. Table 2.2 also lists several interviewing "Donts": Avoid constant eye contact that may make children uncomfortable; avoid too many factual questions; avoid questions about abstract concepts; and avoid questions with obvious right or wrong answers.

Avoiding rhetorical questions is another key interviewing "don't." Rhetorical questions are implied requests or commands that are stated in the form of a question (e.g., "Would you like to . . . ?"). Because of their concrete level of reasoning, children under age 11 or 12 can easily misunderstand such questions as presenting true options for doing or not doing what is requested. When children choose not to follow the request, then you are left in a quandary of trying to persuade them to change their minds, or taking back your request. Such situations can quickly set the stage for oppositional behavior as well as undermine trust. To avoid this problem, you can give direct requests or polite "commands" as a way to transition to new topics or activities. Examples include: "Tell me about your friends. Who are some of your friends?"; "Now let's talk about your family. . . . "; "Draw a picture of your family doing something together." Such requests carry a clear message of the interviewer's expectations and can still be stated in a warm and friendly manner.

It is also good to avoid or minimize the number of "why" questions. It is a common practice of language arts teachers to instruct children about the "wh" questions: who, what, when, and why. They also add "how" to this list. Although elementary-age children are often asked "why" questions, they may have difficulty answering them when the focus is on the reasons for their own behavior or for other people's behavior. Motivation for behavior is an abstract concept that is hard for 6- to 11-year-olds to understand and articulate because they have difficulty taking a third-person point of view to explain human interactions. Instead, they tend to focus more on actions and event sequences than on the motives behind the actions. For example, in one of my studies of children's ability to summarize short stories, fifth-grade children tended to emphasize action sequences, or "what happened," more than characters' motives, or "why it happened" (McConaughy, Fitzhenry-Coor, & Howell, 1983). This does not mean that elementary-age children are incapable of understanding motives. Nevertheless, because motivation is a difficult concept, asking "why" questions in clinical interviews often leads to "I don't know" responses.

Even adolescents, who may be more capable of focusing on motivation, will sometimes become unresponsive to "why" questions if they perceive them as accusations, threats, or tests. Such reactions are especially likely from children who have had conflicts with authority figures. An alternative to "why" questions is to use the reflective technique of repeating children's phrases and then using a polite or soft command such as "Tell me more about that." You can also ask, "How did that make you feel?" or "What did you think about that?" or "What did you do when that happened?"

Developmental Characteristics of Adolescence

Adolescence generally includes ages 12–18, at least in terms of physical development, regardless of intellectual ability. As all parents and teachers know well, the early years of adolescence can be rocky as children undergo hormonal changes leading to adulthood. By age 11 or 12, children normally move into Piaget's "formal operations" stage of cognitive development (Table 2.1, second column). This stage involves the ability to reason abstractly and apply logical rules for solving problems in several arenas. Normally developing adolescents become more systematic in their approach to academic tasks and social problem solving. They enjoy applying their new reasoning skills to hypothetical situations. You might characterize this as the "what if" stage of development, because that is a frequent question adolescents pose to adults and peers. This new and growing ability for hypothetical reasoning can make many adolescents seem argumentative. At the same time, you should not assume that every adolescent is capable of formal operational thought. Adolescents with below-average intelligence or mental retardation, in particular, are unlikely to master abstract logical thinking. Therefore, it behooves interviewers to have some knowledge of adolescents' cognitive ability or to screen briefly for ability. Vocabulary and general language skills are often good indicators of intellectual ability, except for individuals with verbal learning disabilities.

In terms of social–emotional functioning (Table 2.1, third column), many adolescents can take a third-person view of what they and other people are thinking (i.e., thinking about thinking). This has been described as "metacognitive thinking," because it allows individuals to simultaneously imagine both sides of a social interaction. That is, they can understand their own perspective and the perspective of another person, as well as how both perspectives may be viewed by someone else (e.g., "She thinks that I like him and he likes me"). Although metacognitive thinking represents another advance in social reasoning, it can also lead to embarrassing complications, especially in romantic relationships. Some adolescents who are experiencing emotional and behavioral problems may not have the capacity for this type of thinking, which can be a major factor in the poor quality of their social relations with peers and adults.

Adolescence is the time when many individuals reach Kohlberg's (1976) level of "post-conventional moral reasoning," though this ability may not develop until ages 17 or 18 in some, or at all in others. At this level, judgments of right or wrong are based on individual principles of conscience or religious or philosophical ideals (e.g., "Violence is wrong because it violates principles of a safe and just society"; "Stealing is wrong because it violates people's personal property rights"; "Lying is wrong because it violates trust"). As adolescents learn to reason according to moral principles, they may also experiment with different ideals and values, which can lead to conflicts with family and peers. Many adolescents struggle with identity issues, which can lead to self-consciousness, and they often experience intense shifts in emotions. As they become more socially aware, adolescents look to peer groups for social acceptance, which is extremely important to them.

Peer interactions among adolescents (Table 2.1, fourth column) often involve "hanging out" and communicating with friends. This can take the form of talking in groups, sending notes, making phone calls, and more recently, using e-mail and participating in online chat groups. Managing phone calls and time on the computer can be a challenge with some adolescents. Along with shared activities, intimate self-disclosure often characterizes friendships, especially for girls. Squabbles and arguments at this stage often erupt over relationship issues, characterized by gossiping, betraying of secrets, and shifting loyalties. This is also the time for emerging romantic relationships, which now occur as early as ages 11 and 12. Some adolescents experience distress about their sexual identity, which can be especially painful if they are ostracized by peers or family. As in earlier stages, aggressive and antisocial peers are generally disliked, though these adolescents may be accepted into deviant peer groups and gangs. Socially withdrawn individuals, and those with odd or atypical behavior, may also be rejected and ostracized. Peers who are cooperative, helpful, attractive, and competent tend to be liked. In adolescence, peer status is generally defined by group norms, including cliques and clubs. As one adolescent, Karl Bryant, put it in his clinical interview, "You know who all the different types are in this school. We have the druggies, the alcoholics, the preppies, the jocks, the smart kids, and the geeks." (Karl's peer relations are discussed in Chapter 3.)

Questioning Strategies for Adolescence

When children enter adolescence around age 12, their improved reasoning and language abilities make it easier for them to participate in clinical interviews. However, as Merrell (2003) cautioned, you should not assume that interviewing adolescents is like interviewing adults. Many of the interviewing dos and don'ts discussed for middle childhood apply to adolescence. There are also special challenges for interviewing adolescents. Their growing social awareness, coupled with self-consciousness and an insecure sense of identity, make it doubly important to establish rapport and trust early in the interview. Try to show respect and openness to their unique points of view. When adolescents feel a lack of respect, they are likely to shut down or may become resistant or belligerent. At the same time, it is important to clearly explain the limits of confidentiality, as discussed in an earlier section, so that adolescents will not feel betrayed by reports to other persons later on. Sometimes when adolescents hear that interview information may be shared with other people, they may be unwilling to disclose certain types of information. This is a necessary risk for all clinical interviewing. Discussing exactly what will and will not be reported can help to reduce such concerns. Chapter 4 discusses confidentiality issues with adolescents in more detail.

As when interviewing younger children, it is important to solicit adolescents' thoughts and feelings without making judgmental comments. Some adolescents may enjoy the interview process and share their perspectives freely. Others may be more resistant, particularly those who have had frequent clashes with authority figures and those who associate clinical interviews with stressful experiences, such as abuse investigations and potential removal from their home. Also be prepared for emotional lability and signs of stress. As Merrell (2003) noted, adolescence has often been characterized as a time of "storm and stress." It is not unusual to see an adolescent begin a clinical interview in a cheerful, engaging manner and then quickly become agitated and angry as the interviewer broaches more sensitive topics. The interview with Karl Bryant, discussed in Chapters 3 and 4, is a good example. Other adolescents may seem anxious or depressed at different points during an interview. It is important to acknowledge such shifts in feelings and ask questions to explore feelings further, while at the same time respecting adolescents' sense of privacy and their defenses against exploring or revealing painful experiences. When discussions turn to problem situations, you can query adolescents about their perspectives on causes and motives. You should also ask about possible alternative solutions to the problems. Such questions about problem-solving strategies are especially useful for evaluating adolescents' level of social and moral reasoning.

Adolescents are at higher risk for suicide than are younger children (Reynolds & Mazza, 1994). Therefore, it is important to ask screening questions about suicide risk and to pursue any indications of suicidal ideation or attempts. When interviewees raise issues that suggest suicide risk, interviewers should ask directly about suicidal thoughts and attempts, such as whether they have made any plans and have access to methods, such as pills or weapons. Chapter 8 discusses assessing suicide risk in detail.

In addition to most of the interviewing "don'ts" listed in Table 2.2 for middle childhood, you should also avoid using psychological terms (e.g., *psychosis*, *inferiority complex*) with adolescents, even if they appear to understand them. Avoiding such terminology will help to alleviate adolescents' fears that they are being interviewed because someone thinks they are crazy or someone thinks they need a "shrink." It is better to use everyday language as much as possible to help adolescents understand normal processes of human behavior and emotions.

You should also be mindful of adolescents' developmental level when applying clinical diagnoses. A lack of normative standards for diagnoses is one of the shortcomings of the DSM-IV and its precursors. Although some adult DSM-IV diagnostic categories may be appropriate for adolescents, you should still use caution in applying such diagnoses. For example, just because an adolescent displays emotional lability in the clinical interview, you should not assume that this lability is strong evidence for a mood disorder, such as major depression or bipolar disorder. If you use standardized self-reports and parent and teacher rating scales to accompany clinical interviews, you will have a better basis for making clinical judgments about deviance than if you rely only on interview information. For example, the Adolescent Symptom Inventory—4 (ASI-4; Gadow & Sprafkin, 1998) and Youth's Inventory—4 (YI-4; Gadow & Sprafkin, 1999) provide norms for judging the level of deviance in parent and teacher reports and youth self-reports of problems consistent with DSM-IV symptoms. The ASEBA and BASC-2 also provide norms for judging deviance in parent, teacher, and youth self-reports of problems, as discussed in Chapter 7.

ETHNIC AND CULTURAL CONSIDERATIONS

Based on its 2000 population survey, the U.S. Census Bureau (2003) reported that out of the total U.S. civilian population, 13.3% (37.4 million) was of Hispanic or Latino origin; 13% (36 million) was black or African American; and 4.4% (12.5 million) was Asian or Pacific Islander. The 2000 census also showed that 11.5% (32.5 million) of the U.S. population was foreign born (i.e., not U.S. citizens at birth), and that 18% of the population speaks a primary language other than English in the home. These statistics highlight the great diversity of ethnic and cultural backgrounds in our country. With this diversity in mind, interviewers need to be sensitive to potential differences in ethnic and cultural expectations about children's behavior, in addition to considering their developmental level. Ethnic and cultural considerations are especially pertinent to judgments about whether children are exhibiting emotional or behavioral *problems*. For example, some cultures may value inhibited or cautious behavior in children as a sign of respect and self-control. Other cultures may value more outgoing, expressive modes of interaction.

Table 2.3 summarizes key behavioral characteristics and communication patterns, outlined by Nuttall, Li, Sanchez, Nuttall, and Mathisen (2003), which are common to children of different cultures compared to the "mainstream U.S." culture. Some of these behaviors may also characterize children's parents. As Nuttal et al. caution, you should not assume that the generalizations in Table 2.3 apply to everyone from the different cultures described. However, they are likely to apply to children of recent immigrants and immigrants who have settled into ethnic neighborhoods that remain faithful to cultural traditions. Rhodes, Ochoa, and Ortiz (2005) offer extensive practical guidelines for assessing culturally and linguistically diverse children.

TABLE 2.3. Behavioral Characteristics and Communication Patterns across Cultures

Behavior	Mainstream United States	Hispanics	Asians	African Americans	Native Americans
Eye contact	Direct eye contact	Direct eye contact with adults is unacceptable when reprimanded; lowering the eyes is a sign of respect	Looking down is considered a sign of respect	Direct eye contact is unacceptable when admonished	Very limited; tendency to lower eyes to show respect
Touching	Not accepted, except among intimate friends	Accepted and expected as demonstrations of love and acceptance	Discouraged, particularly with the opposite sex	Physical touching for expression is acceptable	Not shown in public
Distance	Personal, intimate, and social distance maintained according to relationship	Interaction at a close distance is accepted and expected	Maintained among strangers	Close physical distance with friends and family; initial distance with strangers	Distance with strangers is maintained; closeness is shown through sharing
Facial and emotional expressions	Controlled, not generally expressed	Very expressive; smiles; gestures; nose, eye, and hand movements when talking	Very controlled	Facial gestures to stress words and meanings and emotions	Controlled, not expressive
Tone of voice	Generally moderate	Rural children are soft spoken; urban children are verbal and vivacious	Soft speaking voice	Use of different voice tones and pitch for meaning	Soft speaking voice; valuation of silence and contemplation

Note. From Nuttall, Li, Sanchez, Nuttall, and Mathisen (2003). Copyright 2003 by PRO-ED. Reprinted by permission.

ALTERNATING VERBAL AND NONVERBAL COMMUNICATION

Too much direct questioning can make clinical interviews tedious and unpleasant for children of all ages. One way to avoid this is to alternate between verbal and nonverbal means of communication. This is a common tactic in test batteries for assessing cognitive ability. There are several ways to interject nonverbal techniques into clinical interviews. One commonly used strategy is the Kinetic Family Drawing (KFD; Burns, 1982) technique, wherein the child is asked to "draw a picture of your family doing something together." The KFD is used routinely in the SCICA for children ages 6–11, and is optional for ages 12–18. After the child completes the drawing, you can inquire about family members and relationships. Chapter 4 discusses KFD procedures in detail, with illustrative examples and interview excerpts.

"Thought bubbles" provide another way to elicit thoughts and feelings from 6- to 11-year-olds who can think about different people's perspectives (Hughes & Baker, 1990). For this technique, draw a simple cartoon that depicts two or more characters in a problem situation. Then draw an empty thought bubble over the head of each character and ask the child to fill in the bubble with what the character is thinking and feeling. You can write children's responses into the bubbles if they have difficulty writing or do not like to write. Older children can complete their own thought bubbles. Then ask the child to tell you more about what the characters think and feel and what might happen next. Thought bubbles are good techniques for exploring children's level of social cognition and their understanding of the causal relations between thoughts, feelings, and behaviors. However, you should not assume that what children say in the thought bubbles for cartoon characters necessarily represents their own thoughts and feelings. Instead, you can ask children directly how they might think or feel in a similar situation.

Incomplete sentences offer another alternative to direct questioning for children who can understand different perspectives. This technique involves presenting sentence stems that focus on a particular person or feeling situation and then asking the child to complete the sentences. Examples include "My mother thinks I am _____"; "My teacher thinks I am _____"; and "I feel upset when _____." Chapter 4 discusses these and other examples of incomplete sentences in more detail.

Play materials can be used with 3- to 5-year-olds and other children who are reluctant to engage in conversation. Effective play materials for clinical interviews include wooden blocks, doll family figures and additional adult and child figures, dollhouse furniture, and a dollhouse, if available. While children are playing, you can interject open-ended questions about the play events and play family relationships. As with thought bubbles, you should not assume that children's play necessarily reflects what they have experienced in their own lives. For example, for children who portray violent play with doll figures, you might comment, "There is a lot of fighting going on in that family. What happens in your house? Tell me what people do in your house." It is important to ask such questions in order to determine whether children's violent play represents their own real-life experiences or worrisome violent fantasies; after all, children can view violence from many sources, other than their homes lives, such as schools and TV, movies, and their schools and neighborhoods. Other authors (e.g., Garbarino & Scott, 1989; Greenspan, 1981; Hughes & Baker, 1990) provide more discussion of play interviews as well as other nonverbal techniques such as using puppets and dolls, feeling thermometers, emotional flash cards, and social problem-solving vignettes.

If time allows, you can incorporate brief achievement tests or fine and gross motor tasks into child clinical interviews to provide breaks from verbal questioning. Such tasks offer opportunities to observe children's responses to structured school-like tasks and motor activities, in contrast to direct questioning. For example, the SCICA Protocol includes brief achievement tests of reading and math, a writing sample, and gross motor screening (e.g., hopping, playing catch) as optional tasks for ages 6–11. If such tasks are included, they should not take more than about 15–20 minutes, so as not to turn the interview into a test situation. Some children may show more anxiety and report more school problems during achievement testing than during open-ended questioning. Others may become more resistant, restless, or manipulative, and still others may act more self-assured and enthusiastic, or start joking and clowning during testing. Such contrasts in behavior can provide valuable clinical information about children's functioning under different task demands.

DEALING WITH LYING

As indicated at the beginning of this chapter, one of the main goals of child clinical interviews is to learn children's own perspectives on their functioning. However, sometimes interviewers may be concerned that children are lying or "stretching the truth" in their interview statements. Data collected for the ASEBA forms give a good indication of how often different informants reported that children lie or cheat. (On the ASEBA forms, lying and cheating are combined into one question.) Table 2.4 shows the percents children in the ASEBA normative nonreferred samples and clinically referred samples for whom "lying or cheating" was endorsed as "sometimes or somewhat true" or "very true or often true" (Achenbach & Rescorla, 2001). You can see from Table 2.4 that 24–29% of nonreferred 11- to 18-year-olds reported on the YSR that they had lied or cheated sometime in the past 6 months. Similarly, on the CBCL/6–18, 22%–31% of parents of nonreferred children reported that their child had lied or cheated in the past 6 months. On the TRF, 2–13% of teachers reported that nonreferred children had lied or cheated in the past 2 months. These findings show that even some children who are considered to be "normal" (i.e., not having severe problems) sometimes lie or cheat.

Table 2.4 shows much higher rates of lying or cheating for children referred for mental health or special education services than for nonreferred children. Among these referred children, 43–52% of 11- to 18-year-olds reported that they had lied or cheated, and 66–71 % of parents, and 32–43% of teachers, reported that the children had lied or cheated. Statistical analyses revealed sig-

TABLE 2.4. Percentage of Children Reported to Have Lied or Cheated

	Youth self-reports on the YSR[a]	Parent reports on the CBCL/6–18[a]	Teacher reports on the TRF[b]
Nonreferred girls	24	22	2
Nonreferred boys	29	31	13
Referred girls	43	66	32
Referred boys	52	71	43

Note. Data from Achenbach and Rescorla (2001). YSR, Youth Self-Report; CBCL/6–18, Child Behavior Checklist for Ages 6 to 18; TRF, Teacher's Report Form.
[a]Time frame = past 6 months.
[b]Time frame = past 2 months.

nificantly higher scores for lying or cheating among referred than nonreferred children. Parents and teachers also reported significantly more lying or cheating among younger than older children and among boys than girls.

Because the ASEBA forms included lying and cheating in the same question, it is not clear which of the two problems was being reported for a particular child. However, the ASEBA data do indicate that it is not uncommon for children to lie or cheat, especially children who have been referred for emotional and behavioral problems. During clinical interviews, lying is more likely to occur than cheating because interviews seldom present opportunities for cheating, unless they include tasks such as achievement tests. Children might lie in clinical interviews for any number of reasons, as Hughes and Baker (1990) pointed out. They may feel threatened and afraid that their answers to certain questions will get them into trouble or lead to disapproval or reprimands. Or they may be attempting to deny memories and feelings of painful or embarrassing situations. Or they may want to impress the interviewer or gain a desired outcome or advantage.

Interviewers can reduce the potential for lying by being sensitive to situations that may inadvertently induce children to lie or "stretch the truth." One strategy is to avoid questions that might seem accusatory to a child, such as "did you" questions (e.g., "Did you take the money?"), or "why" questions (e.g., "Why did you hit him?"). You should also avoid asking leading questions about children's misbehavior when you already know the answer from another source, such as a parent or a teacher. An example is asking a child whether he stole money from a teacher's desk, knowing that the teacher reported witnessing such a theft.

Young children may also appear to lie because they have difficulty distinguishing fantasy from reality or feelings from actual behavior, or they have difficulty expressing such distinctions in words. Interviewers can deal with these situations by verbalizing such distinctions for the child. For example, when a child exaggerates or describes something that obviously could not have happened, you might say, "It sounds like you really wished it could have happened that way." Or you can restate the child's feelings and then ask about reality versus fantasy, for example, by saying, "Sounds like that was really scary when _____. Was that what really happened or was that something you wished had happened?" Statements such as these help children to understand that their feelings are acceptable, and they encourage children to talk more freely about their feelings and how they wished things might have happened differently. Such statements also make it unnecessary for children to retract their statements or to admit that what they said was not exactly true or a "lie." Confronting children directly about suspected lies or exaggerations, on the other hand, is likely to be counterproductive, because it may lead them to tell more lies to save face or to defend themselves against accusations and punishments. Confronting them about lies can also make them shut down.

CONCLUDING THE CHILD CLINICAL INTERVIEW

Interviewers should have a standard protocol for ending child clinical interviews, just as they have for beginning the interviews. To conclude the interview, you can first thank the child for participating and sharing his/her thoughts and feelings. Then review statements regarding confidentiality and discuss how interview information will be shared with other people, such as parents and teachers. If there will be a follow-up meeting to discuss the interview, tell the child that you will be meeting with parents and/or teachers to talk about what you learned in the interview. (You should also have told the child about such meetings at the beginning of the interview, as indicated earlier.) Explain briefly what information you want to share with others and how you will share it. You can also ask the child if there is anything he/she wants you to share. If you will be writing a report, explain how interview material will be summarized in the report. Such disclosures are especially important for adolescents, who are likely to be more sensitive about privacy issues than are younger children.

Concluding remarks should be brief and tailored to the developmental level of the child in the same manner as opening remarks. A good general strategy is to summarize key aspects of what you learned about the child in the interview and then tell the child what general or specific issues you want to discuss with parents, teachers, or other important parties. Most children will be comfortable with this approach, especially if you explain that discussing important issues with other people can help everyone figure out how to solve identified problems. The following is an example of a concluding discussion with a 7-year-old girl:

> I: "Well, that was a pretty long talk about a lot of different things—school, your friends, your family, what makes you happy, sad, and mad, and things that are problems for you. I really appreciate how you shared your feelings with me. Do you remember what I said about this being a private talk?"
>
> C: "Yeah, you said you wouldn't tell my mom."
>
> I: "That's right. Now, one important thing I learned was about all that fighting with your sister and how you feel you always get blamed. I think that would be important to talk about with your mom, so we can figure out better ways to deal with that. Is that OK with you?"
>
> C: "Yeah, OK . . . but don't tell Mom I called Cindy a jerk."
>
> I: "No, I won't tell Mom about the 'jerk' part. I'll just tell her about the fighting and how you get blamed."
>
> C: "OK."
>
> I: "I'm also going to talk to your mom and teachers about your problems finishing your work in school and how you would like some extra help."
>
> C: "OK. Can I go now?" (McConaughy, 2000a, p. 184)

Some children, especially adolescents, may want more specific assurance of the privacy of their interviews. When children do have concerns about confidentiality, you can reassure them that you will not quote their exact words or specific statements that they made during the interview, as illustrated above, and you can paraphrase examples of what you will say. You can also avoid directly reporting children's interview statements in reports and meetings with other informants by referring to those informants' key areas of concern and saying that similar issues were discussed in the child interview.

When there is reason to suspect that the child poses a danger to self or others, or that the child is in danger of abuse, however, you do have legal obligations to report such information to others. In such cases, you should remind the child about the limits of confidentiality stated at the beginning of the interview. (As indicated earlier, your introductory remarks should clearly state that information is not confidential if there is reason to suspect that "you were going to hurt yourself, hurt someone else, or someone has hurt you.") Then you should discuss with the child the next steps in the reporting process. Chapter 4 addresses confidentiality and reporting obligations for child abuse. Chapters 8 and 9 address confidentiality and reporting issues around danger to self and danger to others.

SUMMARY

Child clinical interviews offer rich opportunities to learn children's perspectives on their competencies and problems and to directly observe their behavior, affect, and interaction styles. To facilitate developmentally sensitive interviewing, this chapter discussed interviewing strategies for children at three developmental levels: early childhood (ages 3–5), middle childhood (ages 6–11), and adolescence (ages 12–18). Key aspects of cognitive functioning, social–emotional functioning, and peer interactions were summarized for each developmental level. The chapter also discussed potential ethnic and cultural differences in children's behavior and communication patterns, nonverbal interviewing techniques, dealing with lying, and issues regarding confidentiality.

3

Clinical Interviews with Children

Talking about Activities, School, and Friends

As a general practice, Merrell (2001, 2003) recommended that child clinical interviews cover five broad content areas: intrapersonal functioning, family relationships, peer relations, school adjustment, and community involvement. The SCICA (McConaughy & Achenbach, 2001) is a standardized clinical interview that covers these broad content areas. The SCICA Protocol lists questions and tasks for topic areas similar to those outlined in Table 1.1. It also provides space for interviewers to record notes of their observations of children's behavior and children's responses to interview questions. This chapter (and Chapter 4) uses the SCICA Protocol as a model for covering different topic areas in child clinical interviews.

As part of the ASEBA, the SCICA is designed to fit a multimethod assessment model, such as the one outlined in Table 1.2. To dovetail with other ASEBA instruments, the SCICA has structured forms on which interviewers rate their observations of children's behavior during the interview and children's own reports of their problems. Interviewers' ratings are then scored on a standardized profile of quantitative scales. Chapter 7 describes the SCICA rating forms and scoring profile in detail. The SCICA rating forms and scoring profile are modeled on scoring profiles for other ASEBA instruments, including the CBCL/6–18 (hereafter called CBCL), TRF, and YSR for school-age children. The problem scales for these ASEBA profiles were developed from data on large samples of children who were referred for mental health services and/or special services in schools. The norms for the CBCL, TRF, and YSR scoring profiles are based on large, nationally representative samples of children in the United States. The ASEBA data sets are good sources of information about many different kinds of problems as well as competencies reported by parents, teachers, and children. This chapter and subsequent chapters highlight relevant ASEBA data and review other research findings to provide an empirical basis for judging the clinical significance of problems reported by children, parents, and teachers in clinical interviews. School practitioners can learn more about the SCICA, CBCL, TRF, YSR, and other ASEBA forms by visiting www.ASEBA.org or e-mailing mail@ASEBA.org.

The rest of this chapter discusses the first three of six topic areas for child clinical interviews listed in Table 3.1: activities and interests; school and homework; and friendships and peer rela-

TABLE 3.1. Topic Areas for Semistructured Child Clinical Interviews

I. <u>Activities and interests</u> 　Favorite activities 　Sports, hobbies, organizations 　Job (ages 12–18)	V. <u>Self-awareness and feelings</u> 　Three wishes 　Future goals 　Wishes for changes at home 　Feelings (happy, sad, mad, scared) 　Worries 　Strange thoughts or experiences 　Suicidal ideation
II. <u>School and homework</u> 　Best liked things about school 　Least liked things about school 　Grades 　Attitudes toward school staff 　Worries about school 　School problems 　Homework	VI. <u>Adolescent issues (ages 12–18)</u> 　Alcohol and drugs 　Antisocial behavior and trouble with the law 　Dating and romances
III. <u>Friendships and peer relations</u> 　Number of friends 　Activities with friends 　Peers liked and disliked 　Social problems with peers (fights, being left out) 　Social coping strategies 　Dating, romances (ages 12–18)	
IV. <u>Home situation and family relations</u> 　People in the family 　Rules and punishments 　Relationships with parents 　Relationships with siblings 　How parents get along 　Kinetic Family Drawing (ages 6–11)	

Note. Adapted from McConaughy and Achenbach (2001). Copyright 2001 by S. H. McConaughy and T. M. Achenbach. Adapted by permission.

tions. Chapter 4 discusses the remaining three topic areas: home situation and family relations; self-awareness and feelings; and adolescent issues. Both chapters provide sample interview questions, adapted from the SCICA Protocol, along with case illustrations of interviews with one or more of the five children introduced in Chapter 1.

ACTIVITIES AND INTERESTS

Asking children to describe their favorite activities and interests is a good way to begin child clinical interviews. These types of questions can be used as "warm-ups" to establish rapport before addressing potentially more sensitive issues, such as school, friends, and family. Discussing children's activities and interests can also provide some insight into their perceptions of their competencies. Interviewers can then compare children's reports to similar reports from parents and teachers. Although activities and interests may seem generally benign, validity studies for the CBCL have shown that clinically referred children scored significantly lower on the Activities scale than did matched samples of nonreferred children (Achenbach & Rescorla, 2001).

Table 3.2 lists sample questions for interviewing children about their activities and interests. When interviewing older children, it is good to ask additional questions about jobs, and, if they have a job, how they feel about the job and their boss. This type of information can be helpful in evaluating children's sense of independence and responsibility. It is also good to ask children whether they receive an allowance or other forms of rewards for jobs and household responsibilities. Allowances can be especially useful as reward systems for behavioral interventions in the home setting.

SCHOOL AND HOMEWORK

Assuming the length of the average school day is about 7 hours, and at least 1 additional hour is required for homework, children devote about 50% of their waking hours each weekday to school. For children with academic, emotional, and behavioral problems, the large amount of time consumed by school can be particularly challenging. According to the 24th Annual Report to Congress on the Implementation of the Individuals with Disabilities Education Act (U.S. Department of Education, 2002), over 5 million (8%) of the 2000–2001 school population ages 6–21 experienced academic problems severe enough to warrant special education services. Of these, 4.4% had a specific learning disability, 1.7% had speech and language impairment, 0.7% had emotional disturbance, and 0.4% had other health impairment (which may include ADHD). These statistics represent only the most severe cases that require specialized instruction and an Individualized Education Program (IEP).

National surveys to develop the ASEBA school-age forms provide additional data on the prevalence of academic problems in 6- to 18-year-old children. For example, on the CBCL, parents reported "poor schoolwork" for 16–27% of nonreferred children in the normative sample and 59–72% in the clinically referred sample. Similarly, on the TRF, teachers reported "poor schoolwork" for 22–38% of nonreferred children and 62–81% of clinically referred children. Teachers also reported that 23–41% of nonreferred children and 63–78% of referred children were "underachieving, not working up to potential." These findings, coupled with the sheer amount of time spent on schoolwork, underscore the importance of addressing school experiences in child clinical interviews.

TABLE 3.2. Sample Questions about Activities and Interests

Activities
What do you like to do for fun, like when you are not in school?
Do you participate in any sports/hobbies/clubs?
What is your favorite TV show/movie/music? What do like about _____?

Job (ages 12–18)
Do you have a job? Is it a paying job? How much do you earn per week?
How do you feel about your job?
How do you feel about your boss?
Do you have any other ways to earn money besides your job?
Do you get an allowance?

Note. Reprinted from McConaughy and Achenbach (2001). Copyright 2001 by S. H. McConaughy and T. M. Achenbach. Reprinted by permission.

Table 3.3 lists sample questions that elicit children's views and attitudes toward school subjects, special activities, and school staff, as well as their worries about school and potential school problems. The open-ended format of the initial questions invites children to express both positive and negative thoughts and feelings about school. Follow-up questions can then probe for more detail, as needed, to understand children's perspectives on school issues.

For most children, homework is a necessary part of the school experience. Research studies have shown that homework has positive effects on students' academic performance and test scores (Keith & DeGraff, 1997). Research has also shown that the amount of homework completed, more than the amount of time spent on homework, is a key factor in promoting good academic achievement (Cooper, Lindsay, Nye, & Greathouse, 1998). As Lee and Pruit (1979) pointed out, homework can involve several different forms and purposes: practice assignments that review material presented in class; preparation assignments that introduce topics to be presented in future classes; extension assignments that facilitate generalization of concepts from familiar to unfamiliar contexts; and creative assignments that require integrating knowledge into new concepts or products. Homework can also help to develop children's study skills and work habits.

Despite its potential academic benefits, homework creates problems for many children. Failure to complete homework is a frequent contributor to poor or failing grades at school (Cooper et al., 1998). Homework difficulties can also create conflicts between parents and children (Daniel, Power, Karustis, & Leff, 1999) and undermine collaboration between parents and teachers (Buck et al., 1996). Problems with homework can arise for various reasons: The directions for assignments may be unclear; the assignments may be too difficult; the assignments may be too tedious, too time consuming, or boring; children may lack organizational skills for completing homework assignments on their own; or it may be hard to find the right place and time to do homework

---

TABLE 3.3. Sample Questions about School

Let's talk about school.
What do you like best in school?
What do you like about _____?

What do you like the least in school?
What don't you like about _____?

What kind of grades do you get?

Do you participate in any special/extracurricular activities at school?

How about your teachers?
Which teacher do you like best? What do you like about _____?
Which teacher do you like least? What don't you like about _____?

How do you feel about the principal?
Is there anyone at school who is especially important to you?

Do you ever worry about school?
What do you worry about?

Do you ever get in trouble in school?
What kind of trouble?

If you could change something about school, what would it be?

Note. Reprinted from McConaughy and Achenbach (2001). Copyright 2001 by S. H. McConaughy and T. M. Achenbach. Reprinted by permission.

assignments, given other competing activities in children's lives. Homework can be especially challenging for children who have ADHD and/or learning disabilities (Power, Karustis, & Habboushe, 2001) as well as for children who have behavioral and emotional problems.

Table 3.4 lists specific questions that interviewers can ask about homework. These questions elicit children's perspectives on the amount of homework, their strategies for completing homework, and any problems they might have with homework. Several additional questions explore children's attitudes about receiving help with homework and what form of help (e.g., peer tutoring) might be acceptable to them.

Case Example: Andy Lockwood

Box 3.1 shows a segment from the school psychologist's discussion about school with 7-year-old Andy Lockwood, who was introduced in Chapter 1. Despite repeating first grade, Andy was still struggling with basic skills. Andy disliked everything in school, except nonacademic activities that were fun. If he had his way, Andy would avoid school altogether and just stay home. It was clear from even this short interview segment that Andy had a negative attitude about school. The interview also raised questions as to whether a learning disability or some other problem might be impeding Andy's academic progress. Even with special help, Andy still found schoolwork hard, particularly reading. When the school psychologist probed further, Andy could not explain exactly what about the work was so hard.

The school psychologist continued the interview by querying Andy about homework, as illustrated in Box 3.2. From this interview segment, it became clearer that Andy felt overwhelmed by

---

TABLE 3.4. Sample Questions about Homework

How much homework do you usually have?
How do you feel about that amount of homework? Does that amount seem fair or unfair?

When do you usually do your homework?
Where do you usually do your homework?
How long does it usually take?

Do you usually get homework done on time?
What happens when you (or other kids) don't get homework done on time?

Do you have any trouble with homework? (*If yes, probe further.*)
What kind of trouble do you have?

Does anyone help you with homework or schoolwork?
How does that work out, having _____ help you?
What would be most helpful, if you had it your way?

How would you feel about having another kid/student help you?
How would you feel about having a teacher or some other adult help you?

Where would you like to have help with homework/schoolwork (e.g., in class, in study hall, in a more private place, at home)?

When would be the best times for getting help with homework/schoolwork?
How would you feel about getting help after school or on weekends?

Note. Reprinted from McConaughy (2005). Copyright 2005 by S. H. McConaughy. Reprinted by permission.

BOX 3.1. Talking with Andy about School

INTERVIEWER: Let's talk about school. What do you like best in school?

ANDY: I don't know. I like the . . . ah, what are those? . . . I like the holidays.

I: Oh, the holidays? The holidays are the times you're not in school.

A: Yeah. We have parties. (*Smiles, squirms in seat a little.*)

I: Uh-huh. Oh, that's what you mean. You're in school, but you have parties.

A: Yeah.

I: Do you mean Halloween and stuff?

A: Yeah.

I: So you like holidays, you like the parties and stuff. What about the regular school stuff like math, reading, recess?

A: Recess.

I: Uh-huh. OK.

A: You get to go out and play a lot.

I: So you like going out and playing.

A: Yeah. You know those little miniature ATVs for kids my size?

I: Hmm.

A: Those things that are all plastic, and they have a battery that goes inside.

I: You mean the kind you can ride on?

A: Yeah.

I: All-terrain vehicles, is that what you mean?

A: Yeah. Like those Bigfoots, and they're old-fashioned and car-like. I want one of the ATVs a lot, or a Bigfoot.

I: Do you have one?

A: No. (*Frowns.*) All I have is a bike.

I: What made you think about that? We were talking about recess.

A: I don't know.

I: You were just thinking of something you like.

A: Yeah. (*Squirms in seat, fidgets with clothing a bit.*)

I: Those sound pretty neat. Well, what are some things you *don't* like in school?

A: Oh. There are lots of things. (*Smiles.*)

I: Okay. What are they?

A: School.

I: (*Chuckles.*) School. School in general, huh? Sounds like you're not too wild about school.

A: No. I like staying home.

I: Oh. Well, what don't you like about school?

A: Mmm . . . it's just no fun! I don't like to have to do all that work and stuff. I just want to get up and play with my friends a lot and have them be home so I can be home and be with them.

(continued)

I: So you think that you have a lot of work to do?

A: A lot!

I: Did you have more work this year than last year? Or did you always have a lot of work?

A: Alllways! (*Draws out word for emphasis.*)

I: Always a lot, huh? Mmm. Is the work easy or hard?

A: Hard.

I: Mmm. Tell me what's hard.

A: (*Shrugs, pauses.*) But one of the things that is easy is 100 + 100. It's 200. (*Smiles.*)

I: So 100 + 100 is easy. How about other plusses and take-aways?

A: Easy. Math is easy.

I: All of math is easy?

A: Yeah. I said math is easy.

I: OK. I wasn't sure.

A: Most of it.

I: Uh-huh. So math is easy. So what is hard for you then?

A: Hard for me . . . ? (*Looks confused.*)

I: You said some things were hard . . . I was wondering what was hard.

A: Oh. Lots of things. (*Looks around room, swings feet.*)

I: Can you give me an example?

A: Mmm . . . I don't know. There's things that are hard.

I: How about reading? Is that easy or hard?

A: Kind of hard and kind of easy. (*Pauses.*) Half easy, half hard.

I: OK, so reading is sort of half and half. Sounds like just doing all the work is hard.

A: Yeah.

schoolwork. He said, at one point, he even had homework in the summer that was left over from his last year in first grade. The interview also revealed that, at least from Andy's perspective, there were no consequences when he failed to complete his schoolwork. Instead, Andy said that his mother threw away last year's homework and that his current teacher forgets about homework. Obviously, the school psychologist will need more information from other sources to clarify the nature of Andy's academic problems. Nonetheless, these interview segments suggest that school interventions for Andy might include a restructuring of assignments and the amount of work required as well as provision of supports and incentives to improve his motivation and productivity.

FRIENDSHIPS AND PEER RELATIONS

Friendships and peer relations play critical roles in children's social–emotional development (Bierman, 2004; Bierman & Welsh, 1997; Parker, Rubin, Price, & DeRosier, 1995). Friendships involve mutual, dyadic relationships that are not the same as mere acceptance in the peer group.

BOX 3.2. Talking with Andy about Homework

INTERVIEWER: How about homework? Do you get homework?

ANDY: Yes.

I: How much homework do you usually have?

A: A lot!

I: A lot. How much is a lot?

A: I still have homework from last year when I was in school that started that year. (*Makes face.*)

I: I don't understand. Do you mean you still have homework from last year when you were in school?

A: Yeah, for last year when we were in school with my other teacher. You know, like near the end of the year, last year, when we were in school.

I: Did you do that homework?

A: No, we threw that away.

I: Oh?

A: Because my mom didn't want me to do it. It was too far back.

I: Oh, so you threw that homework away. What about this year? Do you have homework this year that you have to finish at home?

A: Yes. (*Squirms restlessly in seat.*)

I: Do you get it done?

A: No. Not very much.

I: Uh-huh. OK. What happens when you don't get it done?

A: Nothing.

I: You don't get into trouble or anything?

A: No.

I: Oh, okay. Tell me more about that.

A: She just forgets about it. (*Squirms in seat.*)

I: The teacher forgets about it?

A: Yeah.

I: What about your mom? What does she say about the homework?

A: She says try . . . (*pause*) . . . but I don't have to do it.

I: OK. So nothing happens when you don't do your homework.

A: Yeah.

I: OK. Now, were you in first grade last year?

A: I stayed back.

I: Oh, you stayed back . . . you mean, in first grade this year. How do you feel about that?

A: She was mean, the teacher from last year. She was mean.

I: What was mean about her?

A: I don't know. She was just mean. (*Looks slightly unhappy.*)

I: So now you have a new teacher. What do you think about her? I won't tell her what you say.

(*continued*)

A: She's nice. (*Smiles.*)

I: Oh, OK. What makes her nice?

A: I don't know . . . she doesn't yell.

I: Anything else about her?

A: I don't know.

I: You told me you stayed back this year. I was wondering what you thought about staying back. Did you think that was a good idea or not a good idea?

A: I didn't mind. (*Looks around room.*)

I: Hmm. Was it easier for you?

A: (*Brightens.*) Yeah, *much* easier. And I have a good chance of passing this year.

I: Oh, you do? OK.

Popular children tend to have more close friends than rejected children. However, some popular children may not have any close friends, and some rejected children may have one or more close friends (Parker & Asher, 1993).

Bierman and Welsh (1997) cited three qualities that distinguish friendships from mere peer-group status: similarity, reciprocity, and commitment. Friends are often similar in age, gender, and socioeconomic status, though there can be exceptions to any of these characteristics. Reciprocity involves the give-and-take of friendships. For young children, reciprocity is concrete: Friends like the same things, play games together, share toys, take turns, and do not hit or call names. For adolescents, reciprocity becomes more abstract and psychological: Friends share their intimate thoughts and feelings as well as interests and activities, and are loyal, trustworthy, and sincere.

As children get older, peer groups become increasingly important influences on the way they behave, think, and feel in social situations. On the positive side of the picture, developmental research has shown significant associations between positive peer relations and good social adjustment (Bierman, 2004). Social interactions with peers provide an arena for development of many important social skills. For elementary-age children, peer interactions offer opportunities to learn reciprocity and perspective taking, cooperation and negotiation, and social norms, conventions, and problem solving. For adolescents, good peer relations can support the development of self identity and autonomy.

On the negative side of the picture, poor peer relations can be a strong predictor of concurrent and future social maladjustment (Bierman, 2004; Bierman & Welsh, 1997; Parker et al., 1995). In addition, poor peer relations can contribute to stress, feelings of loneliness, poor self-worth, anxiety, depression, and antisocial behavior. Research has also shown a strong association between social maladjustment and hostile attributional biases (Crick & Dodge, 1994). That is, socially rejected and aggressive children tend to attribute hostile intent to peers (e.g., "He bumped into me on purpose"), which often leads to fights and other negative social interactions.

Although poor peer relations are potent "markers" for maladaptive social–emotional development, Bierman and Welsh (1997) caution that "it has not been clear whether poor peer relations are simply the effects of other disorders or whether they play an active role in exacerbating negative developmental trajectories" (p. 329). For example, Bierman and colleagues found that aggressive children who were rejected by peers demonstrated severe attention deficits, emotional dysregulation, and internalizing problems more often than did aggressive, nonrejected children (Bierman, Smoot, & Aumiller, 1993). Other problems may thus contribute to peers' rejection of some aggressive children, but not others. Coie (1990) has also argued that being deprived of positive peer relations may inhibit the development of the prosocial skills and empathy that promote good social adjustment.

Risk Factors for Peer Rejection

The findings from clinical and developmental research underscore the importance of focusing on children's friendships and peer relations in clinical assessments. Peer rejection is particularly important to assess, as are prosocial skills that lead to peer acceptance. Research has shown a strong association between peer rejection and aggressive behavior among children of all ages (Coie, Dodge, & Kupersmidt, 1990). However, not all aggressive children are rejected by their peers. To evaluate whether an aggressive child is also likely to be rejected by peers, Bierman and Welsh (1997) advise focusing on the following key risk factors:

- Does the child exhibit a wide range of conduct problems, including disruptive or hyperactive behavior or attention problems, as well as physical aggression?
- Does the child have deficits in positive social skills?
- Is the child ostracized by peers?
- Does the child have opportunities for positive peer interactions?
- Is the child a member of a deviant peer group, such as a gang, or does the child act aggressively alone, perhaps driven by feelings of injustice and/or need for revenge?
- Is the child's aggressive behavior physical and "instrumental" (i.e., done for a purpose; e.g., demonstrating physical superiority or warding off a fight), or is the child's aggressive behavior "reactive" (i.e., arises from poor control of emotional arousal and anger)?

Other risk factors appear to be associated with peer rejection combined with social withdrawal. Furthermore, some socially withdrawn or socially isolated children may be neglected by their peers, but not outrightly rejected. Neglected children may simply prefer solitary play or constructive and manipulative play that does not require social interaction. Children who are neglected by peers at one age may improve their status later, as they move into new peer groups or expand their interests. However, children who are socially withdrawn *and* rejected are less likely to improve their peer status (Coie & Kupersmidt, 1983). To evaluate whether a socially withdrawn child is also likely to be rejected, Bierman and Welsh (1997) advise focusing on the following risk factors:

- Does the child tend to be reticent, anxious, and/or avoidant in social interactions (e.g., "hovering" on the edge of peer groups because he/she does not know how to enter into a group)?
- Does the child have low levels of positive social skills?
- Is the child ostracized for "odd" appearance, disabilities, or "atypical" social behavior?
- Is the child lonely or depressed, or does he/she have a negative perception of his/her social competence?
- Is the child a victim of teasing, harassment, or bullying by peers?

Interviewing about Friendships and Peer Relations

Child clinical interviews offer good opportunities to assess children's perspectives on their friendships and peer relations. As discussed in Chapter 2, the nature of children's reports about social interactions will vary depending on their developmental level. Children's perspectives on their social relations may also be quite different from what their parents and teachers report. Differences in perspectives may indicate a lack of awareness of social problems by one or other informant, which should be considered when planning interventions. Even when different informants agree that children have social problems, child clinical interviews can provide important insights into possibilities for addressing the problems.

Table 3.5 lists sample questions about friendships and peer relations for child clinical interviews. Initial questions solicit children's reports about activities with friends and their perceptions of liked and disliked peers. Later questions address social problems, including social isolation and fighting. The open-ended format of most questions encourages children to freely express their feelings and opinions about potentially sensitive issues. Interviewers can then follow up

---

TABLE 3.5. Sample Questions about Friendships and Peer Relations

Friends

How many friends do you have?
Do you think that is enough friends?
Are your friends boys or girls?
How old are your friends?

What do you do with your friends?
Do they come to your house?
Do you go to their house?
How often?

Tell me about someone you like.
What do you like about _____?

Tell me about someone you don't like.
What don't you like about _____?

Social problems

Do you have problems getting along with other kids?
What kinds of problems do you have?
What do you try to do about _____?

Do you ever feel lonely or left out of things?
What do you do when that happens?

Do you ever get into fights or arguments with other kids?
(*If yes*) Tell me more about that.
Are they yelling fights or hitting fights?
Does that happen with only one other kid or with a group of kids?
What usually starts the fights?
How do they usually end?
What are some ways you could solve that problem, besides fighting?

Do you have trouble controlling your temper?

Note. Reprinted from McConaughy and Achenbach (2001). Copyright 2001 by S. H. McConaughy and T. M. Achenbach. Reprinted by permission.

with probe questions to explore risk factors for poor peer relations or rejection, including physical aggression, limited social problem-solving skills, social anxiety, depression, or poor control of anger.

Case Example: Bruce Garcia

Box 3.3 illustrates how 9-year-old Bruce Garcia responded to some of the interviewer's questions about his social interactions. Although Bruce was cooperative throughout the interview, he had difficulty expressing his ideas, and his conversation was sometimes loose and tangential. In response to initial questions about peer relations, Bruce expressed considerable distress about other children's refusal to follow the rules of a game—a typical response for his age. However, it soon became apparent that Bruce's arguments during play situations sometimes deteriorated into physical fighting. His responses to follow-up questions about fighting painted a vivid picture of a child who was a victim of teasing and physical harassment by peers.

Unfortunately, Bruce also appeared to have limited social skills for coping with peer-related problems. The only solution he could imagine for the teasing he received at the bus stop was to ask an adult to intervene by giving the offenders a detention. However, Bruce did not think that would work very well. Bruce also appeared to have few, if any, positive friends in school. The one child he liked may have been a bad influence (Jamie, who sneaks around like a robber). Bruce could not name any other children who were friends. Coupled with poor social problem-solving skills, Bruce's confusion and odd mannerisms exhibited during the interview (indicated in italics) would put him at further risk for peer rejection and victimization.

BOX 3.3. Talking with Bruce about Peer Relations

INTERVIEWER: Tell me what you like to do for fun.

BRUCE: Play games. (*Makes odd movements, twitches, fidgets with clothes.*)

I: What kind of games do you like to play?

B: Marbles.

I: Tell me a little more about marbles.

B: I was playing . . . playing with Jason. He went first. He played a big marble. It has little designs on it. And I played my little one. It had blue on it. I played him, and I won. On the last game, I said "Keeps" . . . because there's no take-outs. Do you know what "take-outs" means? (*Gets up and wanders about the room while talking.*)

I: I'm not sure. What does it mean?

B: You can't take out the marble. If somebody wins, you can't take out the marble. You just can't keep your marble, because they've won it. That's what Jason did. (*Still standing, facing interviewer.*)

I: He took out his marble?

B: Yeah, and he wouldn't even give it. Because I won. (*Looks away.*)

I: Then what happened?

B: He got mad at me. He said, "It was funs," and I said, "It was keeps." We both said it was "keeps," and then at the end of the game, he said it was "funs." (*Sits down in chair.*)

I: What did you think about that?

(continued)

B: I thought he was out of his mind, because I won, and he just didn't want to lose that game. (*Looks intensely at interviewer, then looks away*.)

I: What did you do about it when Jason took his marble and said it was "funs" instead?

B: I got mad at him, and he was irked. (*Gets up and paces around the room*.)

I: You got mad at him? What happens when you're mad?

B: Well, he got mad at me first, because he thought it was "funs," and I thought it was "keeps," and he got so mad at me. It happened before when I let him have some of my marbles. I had to because I gave him the last marble, and he tried to steal my marbles. (*Still pacing while talking*.)

I: Did he get them?

B: Nope.

I: What did you do to keep him from getting them?

B: I told him you shouldn't. After that, I tried to get away from him. Get him away from me. (*Long pause*.) Sort of like a little fight . . . so I could get away from him.

I: What kind of little fight?

B: I mean, trying to get the kid away from me. I just had to fight him so he wouldn't get my marbles. I stuffed them away like this. (*Shows interviewer how he stuffed marbles into his pocket*.) And then after the fight was done, I yelled that he's a stealer, because he tried to steal my marbles. If I'd let him, he would've stolen my marbles. (*Comes back to chair and sits down; does not look at interviewer*.)

I: Sounds like you didn't let him. What kind of a fight was it? A yelling fight? A hitting fight?

B: A punch fight and a yelling fight. Both. (*Grimaces and makes odd face*.)

I: Did anybody get hurt?

B: No. Definitely not. He's more than I am in pounds. (*Fidgets with string on pants*.)

I: But you fought anyway.

B: (*Long pause before answering*.) Yeah.

I: Do you get into fights with other kids?

B: Sometimes.

I: How much do you get into fights?

B: Not very often.

I: Like would you say every day?

B: No way! (*Looks around the room*.)

I: What do you mean "No way?" Do you mean, more than that or not as much as that?

B: Not as much as that.

I: Do you get into fights with kids other than Jason?

B: Yeah, sometimes. In the winter, I got into one. This one I think was a couple of days ago. I didn't start the fight. He just wanted to . . . (*pauses a long time to think*)—there were all kinds of kids *ganging up* on me because they didn't like me a lot. So Chuck thought I was real wimpy and then he jumped . . . *everyone* jumped on me and threw me to the ground. I was like this. (*Lies on floor, covers head, goes limp, then sits up*.)

I: So you were down like that? Then what happened?

B: And then Sam tried to kick me (*pauses, grimaces*) . . . tried to kick me in the stomach. And the second time, he did. And then they thought I would cry, and I didn't.

I: Does that happen? Do kids pick on you or gang up on you?

(*continued*)

B: Not very often. Well, yeah, they pick on me. (*Looks sad.*)

I: Do you get teased?

B: No . . . yes. They pick on me . . . tease me . . . for no reason.

I: How do you feel when they gang up on you or tease you?

B: I felt that it wasn't very fair, because I didn't do anything to them to deserve it. (*Looks mad.*)

I: What do you do about it if somebody is picking on you?

B: I just stand there. (*Looks away, stares off into space.*)

I: What could you do if you didn't want them to pick on you? (*Bruce continues to stare off into space.*) Did you hear my question? What could you do the next time?

B: Get on the bus . . . get on the bus. (*Looks confused, stares blankly.*)

I: Does this happen when you're waiting for the bus?

B: Yeah. Waiting on the bus . . . 3 or 4 o'clock, or something. And riding on the bus . . . all I have to do is tell all of them to get detentions. For detentions they have to stay after school probably until 4 o'clock, and their mother has to pick them up.

I: Do you mean you could say to them, "You're gonna get a detention?" Or do you mean you'd tell a teacher?

B: No. I would just try to be last in line, so everybody would be on their seats. And all I'd have to do is tell the bus driver and ask him if he thinks they deserve a detention. I'd say, "Can you give them a detention? I want them to have it."

I: Do you think that would work?

B: Probably . . . I don't think so, because some of the kids don't even *care* if they get detentions.

I: What else could you do?

B: (*Long pause*) I don't know.

I: So that's the only thing you've thought of so far? Asking the bus driver to give them a detention?

B: Yeah.

I: OK. Well let's talk more about the kids. Tell me about a kid that you like a lot. (*Long pause; Bruce does not respond.*) Is there somebody that you like a lot?

B: Uh . . . Jamie.

I: What do you like about Jamie?

B: Sometimes he does something daring. Like he tried to sneak so nobody would see him . . . what's it called—somebody who sneaks around? (*Shows facial tic, plays with hair, rocks back and forth in seat.*)

I: I'm not sure what you mean.

B: Robber. (*Rubs his arm back and forth in circles on the table.*)

I: Like a robber? Jamie sneaks around like a robber?

B: (*Continues to rub the table in circles.*) Yeah. I'm his partner and I do what he says. And he's really nice. And there's other fourth and fifth graders . . . they're both my friends too.

I: Is Jamie the one who's in fourth grade?

B: The kid that has a red jacket on I think is in fourth grade, and the one that has a blue jacket on is in fifth grade. (*Looks confused.*)

I: Do you know those kids' names?

B: No, I don't . . . (*pause*) I can't remember.

Case Example: Karl Bryant

The clinical interview with 12-year-old Karl Bryant, shown in Box 3.4, illustrates a very different pattern of poor peer relations compared to Bruce. Karl was more often the perpetrator than the victim of physical aggression. Karl engaged easily in conversation during the interview and was eager to talk about his problems. When he discussed his interests, he was happy and even charming, to the point of seeming overly confident about his abilities. Although Karl sometimes fidgeted with objects or his clothing, he was only slightly restless or distracted and showed little anxiety.

In the interview segment, Karl described physical fights at school with a sort of relish. He freely admitted that he initiated some of these battles to seek revenge for insults or to right some perceived injustice. As Karl described his fights, he became more and more agitated. He reported having a very bad temper and said that anger built up inside him until he blew up and lost control. Karl also seemed to have concerns about fairness at school that bordered on obsessional, but he did not accept any personal responsibility for his actions. An example was his story about attempting to "restrain" another child and feeling indignant when the teachers did nothing to stop other children from pushing him around. Karl also showed no remorse or guilt for fighting, or showing cruelty toward other children. In Karl's mind, everyone deserved exactly what they got from him.

The two interview segments in Boxes 3.3 and 3.4 suggest that social skills interventions might help both Bruce and Karl improve their peer relations. However, the form of such interventions would have to be different for each boy. For Bruce, the focus should be more on developing social skills and coping strategies to reduce his vulnerability to teasing and bullying. For Karl, the focus should be more on anger control, aggression-replacement training, and advancing his level of moral reasoning. Karl's statements at the end of the interview segment also suggested a need for further assessment of his risk for violence beyond the physical fighting he described in the interview. Chapter 9 discusses procedures for assessing violence threats and children's risk for violence.

BOX 3.4. Talking with Karl about Peer Relations

INTERVIEWER: Tell me a little more about how things go at school. Like, have you ever gotten into trouble at school?

KARL: Not lately.

I: In the past 6 months, have you gotten any detentions, or anything like that?

K: Just two. Maybe more, I don't remember.

I: Is it hard to remember?

K: Yeah. I don't keep track.

I: Well, what did you get two for?

K: See, that's another thing I want to talk to you about.

I: OK.

K: Mr. Smith, our principal, he says just because I get in a fight with somebody or a kid punches me in the head and gives me a bloody nose . . .

I: Uh-huh.

(continued)

K: And I'm supposed to go and tell a teacher, and the teacher doesn't do a thing.(*Squirms in seat, looks angry.*) Well, I went back to that kid and I floored him. I threw him up against the wall. I was really furious. I was out of it. Everybody was trying to stop me, and I just wouldn't let up. And I pounded him, thinking because the teacher wouldn't do anything. So I just pounded the kid—I mean, I just lost it completely.

I: So then what happened?

K: I went into the office. They tried to sit me down, and I wouldn't—I just wanted to get him so bad. (*Voice gets louder and louder.*) The principal gave *me* a detention because he had to get one. (*Looks angry.*)

I: What do you mean "because *he* had to get one"?

K: His parents said that he needs a detention every morning, if he gets into a fight. Because he started it and everything, he got a detention, so I had to. That's baloney! (*Looks angry, loud voice.*)

I: What's baloney?

K: I mean, I get into a fight and I pound somebody, and the other person isn't so badly into it. When he just comes out and pushes me, I'll push him back. I get the worst rap. They get off easier. He says there are different punishments for different things that are done. Well, that's baloney! (*Loud voice*)

I: What do *you* think about that?

K: It's worthless. His *ways*. Everybody hates him. (*Looks intensely at interviewer; angry expression.*)

I: How do you feel about him—the principal?

K: I hate him! (*Loud voice, still angry*) Nobody likes him in the school, except the teachers.

I: Do you think . . . ?

K: (*Interrupts.*) Truthfully, I hate him. I don't like him at all.

I: Do you think he's fair or unfair?

K: He's not fair about anything! (*Looks angry.*)

I: So about this detention—was that fair or unfair?

K: Definitely unfair! And then he gave me another detention for a kid by the name of Mike. He started a fight with me in school, and he thought he was Mr. Macho because he thought he was the strongest kid. Well, I proved him wrong. (*Looks smug, gestures with hands.*)

I: What did you do?

K: Just for restraining the kid . . . just for *restraining* him . . . because he tried to ram into me. You know, he put his shoulder on me and tried to hit me in the stomach. I picked him up right off the ground and put him on the ground until the teacher got there. I didn't even touch him for it. (*Squirms in seat, changes positions several times, gestures to stress his point.*)

I: Did you hit him?

K: No. I just restrained him. I just brought him to the ground and I held him there until a teacher came. (*Calmer voice*)

I: Uh-huh. And you didn't hit him or kick him or anything?

K: I didn't *touch* him. I just picked him up. All I did is, he came running, and I moved. (*Gets up to show move.*) I picked him up right by his shirt, and I set him on the ground, and I held him there. (*Shows how he set kid down.*)

I: So how hard did you set him on the ground? Did you knock him down?

(continued)

K: No. I just grabbed him. He pushed *himself*, really, he pushed himself onto the ground. (*Calmer, quieter voice*)

I: Hmm . . . So that time, it sounds like you feel you didn't lose it like you did that first time.

K: Right.

I: So what was the difference? Why didn't you lose your temper that time like you did with the first time?

K: All I did was *restrain* him. (*Voice gets louder.*) He was trying to *hit* me, and he didn't. But the kid before had *hit* me. He'd been pushing me, throwing stuff at me—rocks, sticks. And the teacher wouldn't do *anything*. (*Loud voice*) Finally, he hit me in the head, right in the nose. (*Gestures to show punch in nose.*)

I: Oh, that's when you got that bloody nose, huh?

K: Yeah. And that's when I let loose on him.

I: What did you do then?

K: I really pounded the crap out of him.

I: So it sounds like when somebody does something to you, then you get really mad and it's hard to. . . .

K: (*Interrupts. Looks agitated.*) Not necessarily—it's just when a *teacher* won't do anything.

I: Oh. So *that's* the big thing? Is it when a teacher won't do anything?

K: Yeah—when the teacher won't do anything about it when they're pushing me. It's like, *why*? (*Gestures dramatically.*)

I: Uh-huh.

K: You know, it's like if somebody complains to them about me, or something. (*Imitates teacher's singsong squeaky voice*) "Oh, Karl, go sit up against the wall." You know. But if it's them doing something, "Oh, they won't do that again. Just leave them alone." (*Imitates teacher's voice again.*)

I: Oh, I think I get it now. So, what you think is that when you're doing stuff to other kids, the teacher will do something about it, but when they're doing it to you, the teachers don't do anything about it.

K: Exactly! Exactly! (*Sighs and looks calmer.*)

I: And you don't think that's fair?

K: Yeah. And I will prevent that!

I: You'll prevent it?

K: Right. Like I have certain friends who get into a lot of trouble. They don't care if they get in trouble. I just tell them to go at it, because I don't need them to fight my battles.

I: So how is it that you'll prevent it?

K: I don't take it. The next time that person touches me, I *flog* 'em.

I: So you flog them.

K: Yeah. For instance . . . (*pauses, looks suspicious*) . . . wait a minute, who are you going to tell all this to?

I: Tell what to?

K: What we're talking about. Are you going to tell the principal or my teachers?

(continued)

I: This is a private talk. Remember what I told you in the beginning? I won't tell your parents or teachers what we talked about, unless you say it's OK . . . unless I think you're going to hurt someone else or someone has hurt you.

K: Well, you're not going to probably believe *this*, but I pinned a kid up in a tree. (*Grins, chuckles.*)

I: You pinned a kid up in a tree.

K: Me and another kid picked him right up, and we put him in a tree—a big pine tree. We stood up on the roof and we stuck him in the tree, on a branch. (*Looks pleased, smiles.*)

I: Uh-huh.

K: He kept ramming, ramming. He kept throwing a ball and hitting us with a whiffle ball bat. So I just said, "*Get up* there," and pushed him up in the tree. (*Gestures to show how he put the boy up in the tree.*) Because he was pushing us, you know.

I: And did he get hurt?

K: No. But he looked really scared and started crying.

I: What did you do when he started crying?

K: Nothing. We just made him stay up there.

I: Did anybody see that?

K: No. Thank goodness.

I: Thank goodness?

K: Because we really would have gotten into trouble.

I: And how did you feel afterward? Like, did you feel bad for making the kid cry?

K: No way! He deserved it—I won't take it!

I: Did you feel bad that you might get in trouble, like, if the teachers saw you?

K: No. Like I said, he deserved it. He pissed me off! (*Pauses, looks for reaction from interviewer.*) Well, I mean he got me mad. (*Pauses.*) He had it coming.

I: So it sounds like *fairness* is really important to you.

K: Yeah. I mean, because I don't care if I get in trouble. But when I get mad, I won't put up with . . . when somebody's bugging me. (*Pauses, looks worried.*) And I've got all kinds of worries about other things, other things. (*Pauses, uses sing-song voice.*) Like worrying about divorces, worrying about my future life, or something. (*Pauses, moves around in seat, grabs at shirt collar and shirt tails.*)

I: Tell me about those worries.

K: Like I have problems with schoolwork and everything, and it's all built up in me, and when somebody hits me, I just lose it. All that anger comes out, and I just lose it. (*Looks agitated.*)

I: So are you trying to tell me that you're going around school worrying about divorce and your future life and stuff like that?

K: No. No! Just the *work*.

I: So it sounds like you have problems with schoolwork.

K: Right. My teacher *loads* it on, and I can't take it, and she *hollers* at me. She *screams* at me. (*Voice gets louder.*) She says *I* always do stuff, and nobody else does anything.

I: Like what kind of stuff?

(continued)

> K: Like she makes me stay after school for not doing my work, but not the other kids. So I get so much anger built up, I mean, it's like when somebody does something to me, that's it, I just lay 'em out. (*Looks agitated, angry, grabs at shirt.*)
>
> I: So you just blow up when you get all this anger built up.
>
> K: Yeah.
>
> I: Well, how often do you feel that way, with all that anger?
>
> K: Pretty often.
>
> I: Would you say it's every day or every week?
>
> K: I don't know.
>
> I: Can you give me an idea?
>
> K: It's just that it gets built up in me. I guess every week. Well *usually* every day. I mean, I think about things, and I can't take it. I've got to *shut my mouth* or else I get in trouble. (*Pauses, looks directly at interviewer.*) You know, by just firing right back. It's like my teacher is the bullet and I've got the trigger. (*Gestures with hand, as if holding a gun at interviewer; looks angry.*)

SUMMARY

Child clinical interviews are essential components of most assessments of children's behavioral and emotional functioning. The flexibility of semistructured clinical interviews makes them well suited for obtaining children's views of their behavior, feelings, and life circumstances. This chapter began with sample questions covering children's activities and interests, school and homework, and friendships and peer relations. Relevant research findings were discussed to guide interviewers in addressing these topics. Segments of clinical interviews with Andy Lockwood, Bruce Garcia, and Karl Bryant (all pseudonyms) illustrated the give-and-take of semistructured clinical interviews with children. Chapter 4 presents additional interview segments on other topics, and subsequent chapters discuss interviews with parents and teachers, along with other assessment data.

4

Clinical Interviews with Children

Talking about Family Relations, Self-Awareness,
Feelings, and Adolescent Issues

Chapter 3 discussed interviewing children about their activities and interests, school, and friends. These are familiar topics for most children and thus may be relatively easy to talk about, even when children have problems in these areas. This chapter moves into topics that are often more sensitive and may be harder for children to talk about: home situation and family relations, self-awareness and feelings, and issues more specific to adolescents, including alcohol and drug use, antisocial behavior and trouble with the law, and dating and romances. Although these topics are presented in a certain sequence, you should feel free to change the sequence, as needed, to follow a child's lead in conversation. If a child seems reluctant to discuss certain topics you can switch to other topics, and then return to the sensitive topics when the child seems more comfortable or more willing to discuss them. You can also save topics that are likely to be most sensitive for the end of your interview, so as not to jeopardize rapport for less sensitive topics.

HOME SITUATION AND FAMILY RELATIONS

Interactions between parents and children lay the foundations for children's social and emotional development. Consequently, no clinical interview would be complete without talking about the home situation and family relations. At the same time, school-based practitioners should remain sensitive to privacy issues around home and family. Some parents may not want school staff to know details about their home situation and their family affairs, including their financial situation and family conflicts. In such cases, asking children about sensitive family issues may make them uncomfortable and may also get them into trouble at home if they tell parents what they talked about during the interview. It is important, therefore, to explain to parents ahead of time that you want to talk with their child about home and family. It is also important to assure children that you will respect the privacy of what they say about home and family, within the bounds of confidentiality discussed at the beginning of the interview.

Conflicts between parents and children naturally occur through all stages of development. Some parent–child conflicts and arguments are normal features of children's gradual movement into independence as adults. However, some families experience what Foster and Robin (1997) defined as "clinically significant conflict," especially as children transition into adolescence. This more severe form of parent–child conflict has the following features: (1) repeated, predominantly verbal disputes about a variety of issues; (2) failure to produce satisfactory solutions to disagreements; (3) unpleasant or angry interactions about problem issues; and (4) pervasive negative feelings (e.g., anger, hopelessness, distrust) in the child and/or parent. Conflicts of this sort can also occur between children and other adult family members, such as stepparents, a single parent's partner, or other adults, such as grandparents, who live in the child's home.

Ample research has shown strong associations between family conflict and emotional and behavioral disorders in children, especially DSM-IV diagnoses of Attention-Deficit/Hyperactivity Disorder (ADHD), Oppositional Defiant Disorder (ODD), and Conduct Disorder (CD; Foster & Robin, 1997). In fact, symptoms for ODD include a variety of negative adult–child interactions, such as "often argues with adults" and "often actively defies or refuses to comply with adults' requests or rules." In particular, research has linked inconsistent, harsh, and punitive parental discipline to escalating cycles of negative parent–child interactions and aggressive behavior in children (McMahon & Forehand, 2003; McMahon & Estes, 1997; Patterson, 1986). Low levels of parental monitoring have also been linked to aggressive and antisocial behavior. Clinically significant conflicts can also occur between family members and children who have internalizing disorders characterized by depression or anxiety. Parents of internalizing children may be overprotective and use discipline practices that are overcontrolling, which can lead to anxiety and/or social withdrawal (Rubin & Stewart, 1996).

Children's reports of their interactions with parents and others in the home can provide one window on family relations, and their perceptions of rules and punishments may shed further light on discipline patterns. Asking children about chores and reward systems can also assess the responsibilities assigned in the home and children's perceptions of how family members encourage desired behavior. School-based practitioners can use this information, along with additional information obtained from parents, to decide whether there is clinically significant conflict that may warrant a family assessment. Such assessments are usually performed by mental health practitioners outside of school, but some family assessment might be done by a school social worker, school psychologist, or consulting psychologist. School-based practitioners may also decide to recommend family therapy or parent training in cases involving high family conflict.

Table 4.1 lists sample questions that you can ask children about their home situation and family relations. A good way to introduce this topic is simply to ask, "Who are the people in your family?" This open-ended question allows the child to name all people who might be considered "family," including biological or adoptive parents, a single parent's boyfriend, girlfriend, or same-sex partner, stepparents, siblings, stepsiblings, foster children, and members of the extended family. If the family constellation becomes too complicated or hard to follow, then you can ask "Who lives in your home?" This question helps to clarify living situations for children who have experienced divorce or other changes in their home situation.

TABLE 4.1. Sample Questions about Home Situation and Family Relations

Home situation

Let's talk about your family.
Who are the people in your family? Who lives in your home?
In your home, do kids have separate bedrooms? How do you like having separate
          bedrooms/sharing a room with _____?

Rules, punishments

What are the rules in your home?
Who makes the rules?
What happens when kids break the rules?
How do you feel about the rules? Are they fair or unfair?
What are the punishments in your home?
Do kids ever get spanked/physically punished for bad behavior?
Who usually gives the punishments?
How do you feel about the punishments? Are they fair or unfair?

Chores, rewards

Do you have any special chores/jobs at home?
Do you get an allowance? (*If yes*) What do you have to do for it?
Do you have other ways to earn money?
What happens when a kid does something really good or special?
Do kids get any special rewards or treats for doing something good?
Does this ever happen for you?

Family relations

How do you get along with the people in your family/home?
Who do you get along with best?
Who do you get along with least?

*Ask about the child's relationship with each member of the family, as appropriate: father,
          mother, stepparents, other adults in home, other caregivers, siblings, stepsiblings.*

How do your parents get along?
Do they have arguments? (*If yes*) What kind of arguments?
How does that make you feel when they argue?

Note. Reprinted from McConaughy and Achenbach (2001). Copyright 2001 by S. H. McConaughy and T. M. Achenbach. Reprinted by permission.

Kinetic Family Drawing

As a supplement to verbal queries about the family, you can ask children to provide a Kinetic Family Drawing (KFD). To do this, hand the child a piece of blank paper and a pencil and ask him/her to "draw a picture of your family doing something together." The KFD is a standard part of the SCICA for 6- to 11-year-olds, and is optional for 12- to 18-year-olds. Because the KFD provides a break from questions, it can be especially effective with younger children. The KFD can also be surprisingly effective with many adolescents, as long as they do not view it as a childish task. Children's descriptions of their drawings and the way they depict family interactions ("doing something together") often provide insights into their perceptions of family relations. Burns (1982) presents examples of KFDs from children in many different situations, along with his own research and clinical interpretations. His book can serve as a good reference source. However, it is not necessary to do any quantitative scoring or projective interpretations of the KFD. After the child has completed the KFD, ask him/her to describe the drawing and then tell something about each family member. As an example, the SCICA Protocol includes the following questions about the KFD:

Who are the people in your picture?
Ask the child if it is OK for you to write the name above each person in the picture.
What are they doing?
Tell me about the people in your picture. What kind of person is _____? Tell me three words to describe _____.
How does _____ feel in that picture?
What is _____ thinking?
Who do you get along with best/least?
What is going to happen next in your picture?

Case Example: Bruce Garcia

Figure 4.1 shows 9-year-old Bruce Garcia's KFD. Bruce was the middle child in a blended family of three children. Bruce drew a picture of the family having a barbecue ("barboquie") in the backyard. First he drew the house at the top of the page, rotating the paper several times as he drew. The two small rectangles attached to the house are the front and back doors. The small rectangles inside the house are bathrooms. He labeled the position of each room: den (Dn), living room (LR), kitchen (Ki), and stairs (St) to his room. He described the three wiggly ovals next to the house as "the things that prevent ants from coming in . . . [with] . . . little red stuff that looks like throw-up . . . it prevents ants from coming in." These probably depict ant poison baits. Then he drew the barbecue pit at the bottom of the page, with the cover, the "thing to clean it . . . two pieces of big wood, a newspaper, some kindling wood, some charcoal . . . and . . . the fire." Lastly he drew the family members: his mother, his stepsister Barbie, older stepbrother Sam, and himself between Barbie and Sam (all pseudonyms).

Bruce was very focused during his drawing, which took about 10 minutes to complete. He erased and redrew several parts of the picture, including changing the position of the three children in the drawing. First he drew Sam on the left side, Barbie in the middle, and himself to the right of Barbie. He drew Mom to the right of the three children. Then, as he began to describe his drawing, Bruce switched positions and erased and rewrote names to put himself in the middle of the children next to Sam. Bruce described each part of the picture as he drew. Sometimes his comments involved explanations of his drawing to the interviewer, but at other times, he seemed to be talking more to himself.

Bruce's drawing had two immediately notable features. First, his drawing of the house and the boxy shapes of the human figure drawings seemed immature for a 9-year-old, suggesting that Bruce may have some visual–motor delays. Second, his initial drawing included only the three children and his mother—which raised questions about what roles Bruce's stepfather and biological father played in his life. After Bruce completed his KFD, the interviewer asked him to talk about each family member. Box 4.1 contains a segment from this part of the interview. When the interviewer asked about his stepfather, who was missing from the drawing, Bruce added the word *Father* to the right of the barbeque. He also added the word *Grandmother* to the left of the barbeque.

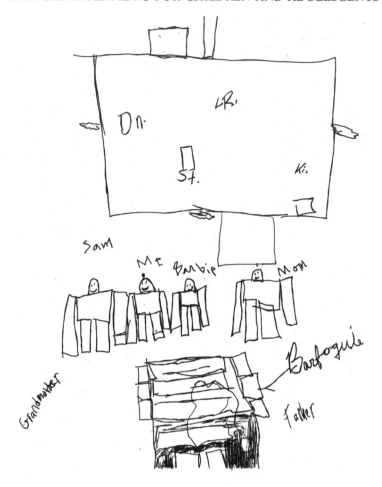

FIGURE 4.1. Kinetic Family Drawing from Bruce Garcia, age 9.

Bruce's halting speech, frequent pauses, and repetitive phrases suggested difficulty with expressive language, similar to the interview segment with Bruce about peer relations in Chapter 3. His descriptions of family members tended to focus on physical features (e.g., Sam is strong and tall; Barbie thinks she's fat) and people's actions toward him (e.g., Sam lets him use his video games; Mom buys them stuff; his real dad takes them to restaurants and gives presents). Such literal descriptions of other persons are typical for children in the concrete operational stage of development.

Bruce's comments also revealed mixed feelings toward different family members. He appeared to have a positive perception of his stepbrother Sam and his stepfather, both of whom he viewed as his protectors. He had a more negative perception of his stepsister Barbie, and both positive and negative perceptions of his mother. From this interview segment, we learn that although Mom is "sometimes nice," she is also "sometimes mean." Bruce clearly felt bossed around by Mom, which aroused angry feelings in him. He reported having difficulty controlling his temper in such situations and contended that he wanted to have more "meekness" (an odd word choice for a child). Bruce seemed to have a positive perception of his biological father,

BOX 4.1. Talking with Bruce about Family Relations

INTERVIEWER: So it's all done. Tell me about the people in your picture. Who do you want to talk about first?

BRUCE: My brother, Sam. (*Writes "Sam" above figure.*)

I: What kind of a guy is Sam?

B: He's a strong and tall guy.

I: What do you think about Sam?

B: (*Taps pencil on table, scratches self, looks away.*) I think . . . I think he's pretty . . . creative . . . cause when I barely came to my last house, he was really nice to me. He let me use his video . . . his games . . . and he's (*long pause*) . . . I can't remember.

I: Is Sam your real brother?

B: No, step . . . and about Barbie . . . she thinks she's fat. (*Writes "Barbie" above figure next to Sam.*) Change names. (*Erases "Barbie" and writes it above third figure; writes "Me" above figure next to Sam.*) Barbie's over here. OK . . . Um . . . I'm here.

I: I was wondering, why are they changing?

B: Because . . . When I think about it . . . I'm more detailed.

I: Now you're next to Sam. And then Barbie.

B: OK. Now about me is . . . (*Pauses, rubs pencil on table.*) What's the question now?

I: You were telling me about the people in the picture.

B: About me . . . I'm not a very good drawer, but I'm really good in math. I'm a really good fan of the Dolphins. Barbie is . . . she thinks she's really fat, but she's not. . . . She's pretty tall for her age, but I'm going to outgrow her. (*Rubs pencil, looks away.*)

I: So Barbie thinks she's fat, but you think she isn't. What kind of a person is she?

B: She's not sure. . . . she's pretty tall, but I'm going to outgrow her.

I: What makes you think you'll outgrow her?

B: Because she's up to here. (*Gestures with hand to demonstrate height.*) If we measured her and me head to head, I'm almost to here. (*Gestures to show his height.*)

I: Do you want to outgrow her?

B: Yes. (*Picks at ear, face.*) I'm almost the shortest kid in my class. I don't think it's fair that the girls outgrow the boys.

I: Sounds like you really want to be taller.

B: I do.

I: OK. Now let's talk about Mom. What kind of a person is Mom?

B: (*Long pause*) She's nice . . . sometimes nice . . . sometimes mean.

I: How is she nice?

B: She buys us stuff . . . she buys candy . . . sometimes she buys toys.

I: So Mom's nice when she buys candy and toys. How is she sometimes mean?

B: This morning she wasn't . . . she's sort of mean . . . sort of mean.

(continued)

I: How is she mean?

B: Says do this, do that. (*Long pause*) I get sick of it . . . don't want to. (*Looks away, avoids eye contact, squirms around in seat.*)

I: Like, do what?

B: Chores. I know I'm supposed to do chores. I don't want her to remind me.

I: So she reminds you to do your chores.

B: She says, "Do it now!" (*Imitates loud, mean voice of Mom.*)

I: What do you do then?

B: Get mad.

I: What happens when you get mad?

B: I turn into a grump . . . turn into a grump.

I: How do you turn into a grump?

B: I blow my top . . . blow my top.

I: Do you have temper tantrums?

B: Yeah . . . I blow my top . . . I get so mad . . . (*Squirms in seat, looks away.*)

I: So you blow your top?

B: Yeah, I blow my top . . . I get so mad . . . I just don't have meekness in myself. Do you know what meekness means?

I: What does it mean?

B: It means you have full control. (*Rolls pencil on the table over and over.*) You feel you just don't get mad . . . like killing and stuff that.

I: You don't have meekness.

B: I have so much anger . . . I can't get it out of myself and be really calm. (*Looks away, fidgets with drawing pad.*) I feel really mad at somebody.

I: What sort of things make you mad?

B: Saying "do this" and "do that."

I: Sounds like your mom makes you really mad.

B: She bosses me around. (*Looks glum, sad; rolls pencil on the table.*)

I: Anybody else get you mad?

B: My brother is a lot nicer than Barbie. (*Continues to roll pencil on table.*) He protects me. He's stronger than me. He grabs Barbie and says "don't do that to him." (*Shows how Sam grabs Barbie by the throat.*) My brother could easily kill my sister, but he doesn't.

I: How do you get along with Barbie?

B: I don't know . . . We don't get along.

I: How do you not get along?

B: She's mean . . . says what I do is queer. (*Rolls pencil on table.*)

I: So Barbie says what you do is queer. How does that make you feel?

B: I get mad . . . she says I'm queer . . . makes fun of me. (*Looks down, grimaces.*)

(continued)

I: I can see that Barbie makes you mad. I noticed that your stepdad isn't in this picture. I was wondering about him. What kind of a person is he?

B: He's a strong guy. . . . Is this alright? One time my sister was slapped by four 18-year-olds . . . 18-year-olds. He took all of them and throwed them against the thing. He's really strong.

I: So your stepdad seems pretty strong. What else about him?

B: He works a lot, too.

I: What does he do?

B: He does a lot of work around the house. Probably two times as much as I do in the house. He's in the army. He does a lot of work in the army.

I: How do you get along with your stepdad?

B: OK . . . (*pauses to think*) . . . and he's concerned about my life, because just before a car was coming . . . it was crossing the road . . . he saved me from getting run over by a car.

I: So you know he is concerned about your life.

B: My mom, too. They both love me very much. I can't think of anything more.

I: How do you know they love you?

B: Because they show it.

I: How do they show it?

B: They show it by . . . my stepdad pushed me back so the car wouldn't run over me . . . and Mom . . . I don't know.

I: You don't know how Mom loves you.

B: She just says she loves me very truly.

I: I also noticed your real dad is not in your picture. Tell me about your real dad.

B: How do you know I have a real dad? (*Looks surprised.*)

I: Well I was guessing you have a real dad because you said you have a stepdad. Do you visit your real dad?

B: Um . . . once I saw him . . . Mom took me. It takes a lot of money to get there. We went to a restaurant . . . my favorite is spaghetti. We ordered that. I asked him if he had enough money, and he said yeah, and after he said he barely had enough money to pay everything.

I: Were you worried?

B: I didn't want him to run out of money.

I: What is he like? I mean what kind of a person is your real dad?

B: He's nice. He is a real giver.

I: How is he a real giver?

B: He gave me football cards and the Dolphins' record and a poster of the Super Bowl. (*Looks away, rolls pencil on table.*)

I: Where does he live?

B: Florida.

I: How often do you get to see him?

B: Not often. Maybe I'll see him this summer. (*Looks away, taps pencil in hand.*)

I: How do you feel about that?

B: I'm excited. I might see the Dolphins. They might even live there.

whom he had not seen often—which did not seem to bother him much. He was concerned about how much money it cost for the trip to visit his father and for dinner, which suggested there may have been financial difficulties in the family. Cost may also have been the reason his mother gave for the infrequent visits with his father in Florida.

A strikingly recurrent theme was Bruce's focus on being strong and tall and his desire to be protected. This self-perception was consistent with his earlier reports about being a victim of teasing and physical assaults by peers. Such reports suggested that Bruce viewed himself as powerless and in need of other people to defend him or to help him cope with social problems. Although Bruce described arguments between family members (Sam and Barbie; himself and Barbie; himself and Mom), more information would be needed to determine whether such arguments represent clinically significant conflict. Nonetheless, Bruce's intensely angry reactions to his mother's demands about chores were worrisome, because negative parent–child interactions such as these can easily lead to oppositional behavior in children.

Case Example: Karl Bryant

The KFD was also a good entrée for discussing family relations with 12-year-old Karl Bryant. He drew a picture of his stepfather, mother, younger sister, and himself all going out to buy ice cream cones, as shown in Figure 4.2. Karl considered himself to be a very good drawer and was very meticulous in his approach. For example, he used the edge of the paper as a ruler to make straight lines, and he added shading and details to his drawing. Karl commented on his good drawing skills several times, which he considered to one of his special talents. Even his derogatory comments about his drawing ("It's the worst drawing I have ever done") seemed boastful. In my experience, the KFD typically takes about 5–10 minutes for most children. Karl drew for at least 20 minutes, and would have continued even longer had the interviewer not intervened to ask questions.

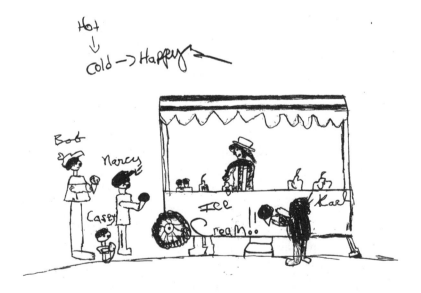

FIGURE 4.2. Kinetic Family Drawing from Karl Bryant, age 12.

Limiting the time for the KFD can be challenging with children such as Karl. The goal is to use the KFD to obtain children's perceptions of their family. However, interviewers should not allow the KFD to consume too much time or take the place of talking about the family. If a child needs extra time to do the KFD, you can begin asking questions about the family before the KFD is completed, as the interviewer did in Karl's case. Or you can set a time limit when you introduce the KFD by saying, "Now I would like you to draw a picture of your family doing something together. It should take about 5 minutes." Sometimes children are reluctant to do the KFD because they think they cannot draw well or they do not like to draw. In such cases, you can say, "I still want to see a picture of your family doing something together. You can draw it any way you want to. This is not a test." Most children will then go ahead with the drawing.

Box 4.2 presents excerpts of the interview with Karl about his perceptions of family members, using the KFD as a focal point. Karl was the older of two children in a blended family that included his biological mother (Nancy Ladd), stepfather (Robert Ladd), and 7-year-old sister (Casey; all pseudonyms).

You can see how Karl started out painting a generally positive picture of his stepfather, whom he viewed not only his "father" but also a "friend" who treated him "fairly." Fairness was a strong and recurrent theme throughout the interview with Karl. In an earlier interview segment in Chapter 3, Karl had talked a lot about how unfair he thought things were at school. In this segment, we learn that Karl's notion of fairness was typical of a conventional stage of moral reasoning. Fairness to him meant that both children, Karl and Casey, got the same things at home (e.g., a candy bar, going somewhere with Mr. Ladd), and got the same consequences for misbehavior. Later, we learn that Bob, Karl's stepfather, was "the boss of the house" and the one who gave out the punishments. It is important to note that Karl felt that he had no say in deciding the punishments ("the decision is the decision"), and apparently that lack of input was not upsetting to him.

Karl's perception of fairness at home contrasted sharply with his perception of extreme unfairness at school, where he felt singled out for undeserved punishments—usually detentions (see Chapter 3). In this context it is especially important to note Karl's responses at the end of this interview segment to questions about school and what he would do to make things fairer there. At first, Karl seemed to think there was nothing he could do to change things ("You can't give them advice. They won't take it."). The interviewer then encouraged him to pretend: "What if you were the principal of the school—what would you do to be fair?" This strategy was successful in eliciting several ideas from Karl that actually might be incorporated into a school-based intervention plan. For example, Karl wanted more of an open-door policy from the principal. And he wanted the principal to listen to a kid's side of the story. He then laid out a series of steps for disciplining kids at school, including requiring them to write a "success plan." It is a good guess that Karl had already had to do one or more of these success plans.

This section of the interview provided some good insights into behavioral interventions that might be successful with Karl at school. More information would be needed to determine whether school staff were already using discipline procedures such as the ones Karl suggested in the interview. Even so, Karl's comments about discipline at home versus what he would like at school underscored the importance of establishing clear and consistent rules and consequences that would fit Karl's conventional level of moral reasoning. It was also clear that Karl needed to feel that adults listened to his point of view. However, listening to Karl's side of a story could easily create a tricky situation for authority figures, who must also avoid getting into

BOX 4.2. Talking with Karl about Family Relations

INTERVIEWER: Let's do something a little different. Draw a picture of your family doing something together. (*Interviewer hands drawing pad and pencil to Karl.*)

KARL: OK. I am heavily into drawing. It's one of my better subjects. I'm an artist (*Smiles.*) That's what Miss Tangier told me. I've got a good knack for drawing. My stepdad was amazed when I drew the house in perfect detail . . . simply amazed . . . he could not believe it. (*Starts drawing a structure and continues talking.*)

I: How long has he been your stepdad?

K: About 6 or 7 years. He's been through a lot with me. Like when I was burned by hot water. You should go back and ask my mom about that. He's brought me through everything. He was there and comforted me.

I: You remember that.

K: I sure do. I can't emphasize enough for every child not to play around hot water.

I: What happened?

K: (*Continues drawing while telling about event, looking up periodically.*) I was jumping around in the kitchen. My grandfather liked hot water and had just started it on the stove. We were goofing around, like on a skateboard. I brought the whole thing over. The pot landed on my head, and I got a big dent in my head. I can still feel it. (*Looks at interviewer, rubs head dramatically.*) And it burned my skin.

I: When did that happen?

K: About a year ago.

I: And your stepdad was there?

K: Yeah, he helped me. (*Starts drawing again.*)

I: Was that Bob?

K: Yes. I like him a lot.

I: What do you like about him?

K: He's funny. He treats me fairly. He's not only my father, he's a friend. If he does something, he says, "do you want to come?" He takes me everywhere.

I: How does he treat you fairly?

K: Say he gives Casey a candy bar, he'll go back and get one for me. That's just an example. If he takes Casey somewhere, then the next time he takes me.

I: Oh, so if Casey gets to go one time, you get to go the next time?

K: Yeah, he's really fair.

I: Who is Casey?

K: She's my sister. I have two families. I have relatives I haven't even met. I've got my mom's side, my stepdad's side, my real dad's side, and my stepmom's side. I have four sets of family.

I: So who all lives in your home with you right now?

K: Mom, Casey, and Bob. That's about it. (*Still carefully drawing, using the edge of the paper as a ruler for straight lines.*) This is not the most accurate drawing I've ever done. (*Erases.*) You can ask my mom how much time I spend on drawing. I have some drawings I have never even finished yet. (*More than 5 minutes have passed.*) How about the people? Who do you want in it?

(continued)

I: Anyone you want.

K: OK, I'll put in them all. (*Continues drawing structure.*) What do you think this drawing is?

I: I'm waiting to see.

K: Trust me, you will not know what this drawing means. I like drawing things that are exaggerated sometimes, and sometimes I like drawing things that are truthful. (*Continues silently for several minutes, then asks if interviewer can guess what it is.*) If anybody bumps me in the class while I'm drawing, look out.

I: What happens?

K: I scream. If anyone gets me when I'm drawing, I kill.

I: (*Karl starts drawing Mom.*) While you are drawing, tell me about your mom.

K: She's a nice person. She hollers at me sometimes and usually has a pretty good reason why she does.

I: Like what?

K: Like if I go somewhere I'm not supposed to go, if I didn't hear her correctly, she's patient with me. Like last night, I wanted to see the basketball game on TV. At first she said no, but then she said OK, you can watch the game, but you have to wake right up for me tomorrow morning. And I did. She's very patient with me.

I: Does she ever get angry with you?

K: Yeah. I mean every parent gets angry with a child every now and then.

I: Yeah, so what is she like when she is angry?

K: You don't want to know (*pause*) . . . she punches me sometimes when I do something wrong (*head down, drawing*), but it's not like she truthfully kills me.

I: So tell me more about the punching.

K: (*Ignores the question.*) Bob is a tall guy. (*Draws Bob, then Casey, then himself.*) I draw much better than this, I'm just drawing cartoons, looney tunes. I just rushed this thing so quickly, it's unreal. It's the worst drawing I have ever done.

I: You think so?

K: I know it is. If I had used my compass and a ruler, it would have been a lot better. (*Tells interviewer about another drawing he did that was much better.*)

I: Tell me about this drawing.

K: Alright. Should have put our car in, but that would have taken too long. This is my dad, Bob. This is Casey. Do you know what it is?

I: Looks like an ice cream stand.

K: You're right. We went to get ice cream because it is a hot day. This is Casey down here. This is me, and this is Mom.

I: How are the people feeling in this picture?

K: (*Pause*) Cold (*laughs*) and happy. They were hot before and now they cooled down. (*Writes* Hot → Cold → Happy.)

I: What are the people thinking?

K: I wouldn't know.

I: Well, if you imagined a story about the picture.

(continued)

K: They are thinking about what the bill will be. (*Laughs*.)

I: What does this family think about bills?

K: I don't know.

I: Does this family worry about bills?

K: No.

I: Tell me more about Mom.

K: She is a smart person. Whenever I have homework . . . I hardly ever have it, because I get it all done. She helped me with geometry, the 90-degree angles.

I: Do you ever get into arguments about homework?

K: No. I used to before with my dad, but we don't anymore. I liked working with Gail.

I: Who is Gail?

K: Stepmom.

I: So it was easier doing homework with Gail?

K: Yeah.

I: How was it easier?

K: Well, when I said an answer, she would check and say it was right and I knew it was right. My dad would say it was wrong.

I: Which dad are we talking about?

K: My real dad.

I: So you used to argue with your real dad about homework? What would happen?

K: We would just argue about it, and finally I would say "forget it" and go out in the other room.

I: What about your real mom? Do you get into arguments with her?

K: Not much anymore.

I: Does she give punishments?

K: Yeah, every kid gets punishments sometimes.

I: What are the punishments in your house?

K: No baseball—well, they can't take that away because there isn't anymore—no biking, no leaving the yard.

I: How about hitting punishments, like belts or spankings?

K: Not anymore. My mother doesn't believe in hitting anymore.

I: Did she used to?

K: Some . . . but not really. I don't really remember.

I: It's probably not fun to remember. How about Bob? Does he give punishments?

K: He's the boss of the house. He makes my mother talk to him. When she finds out what I did wrong, she talks to him and he makes the decision about the punishments. Then I get it.

I: So what are some of his punishments?

K: No TV, no going out.

I: If they say "no going out," do you stick with that?

K: Yeah, I listen to him.

(continued)

I: What if you think it's not fair?

K: I really don't have any say in that.

I: No say?

K: He says, "the decision is the decision." I don't have any say.

I: So the decision is the decision at home. What do you think about the punishments? Are they fair or unfair?

K: I have to go along with it. I have no say in whether it is fair or unfair.

I: So you have no choice in whether it is fair at home. I was wondering because earlier we were talking about school, and you said a lot of things were unfair at school, and that made you mad. (*Karl looks down and starts drawing again.*) Is home different from school?

K: Much different.

I: What makes it different?

K: The way my parents treat me compared to the school.

I: How is that?

K: (*Pause . . . drawing . . . looks down.*) They treat me more fairly. I believe it truthfully.

I: I was wondering what counts as fair to you.

K: I can't really say.

I: Well, if we wanted to give some advice to the teacher about fairness, what advice would you give?

K: You can't give them advice. They won't take it.

I: Well, let's pretend you could, what would you say?

K: Tell them to quit and get a new job. (*Laughs.*)

I: What if you were the principal of the school, what would you do to be fair?

K: For one, I would be more open. I would let kids come into my office, and I would listen to them. I would give a fair punishment. If they got into a fight, I wouldn't just go up and say "you get a detention because he has to have one." (*Looks angry.*) I wouldn't do that! If that other kid wasn't in it, he wouldn't get a punishment. Let me make it up. Say if Sam punched Mike and Mike punched Sam. Two wrongs don't make a right. So what I would do is give them both an essay, probably about 250 words, if they were sixth graders.

I: So they would both get the same amount?

K: Same amount, and the one who started the fight, which would be Sam, would be the one to get the detention, if a detention is to be given. I wouldn't give a detention. If it was his first offense, I would give him a warning. If it was his second offense, I would give him a success plan that had to be signed by his parents.

I: What is a success plan?

K: It's a plan where you ask yourself questions, like what are you going to do the next time? What is your success going to be?

I: Sounds like you really find that helpful to write down things in a success plan.

K: (*Nods yes.*)

I: Well, that's helpful to know.

endless arguments and power struggles with him. Karl's perception of fairer treatment at home further suggested that closer collaboration between home and school could be very beneficial.

This interview segment with Karl also provides a good example of how you might deal with a child's reluctance to discuss certain sensitive issues, such as Karl's relationship with his biological mother. The interviewer broached the topic of Karl's relations with his mother several times, weaving it in and out of discussion about other family members. At first, Karl tried to paint only a positive picture of his mother (e.g., she helped him with homework). He was reluctant to elaborate on his mother's reactions when she was angry with him ("you don't want to know") and would not elaborate on his statement that she punched him when he did something wrong. Later in the interview, Karl acknowledged that his mother used to give "hitting" punishments, but excused this as a normal reaction ("every kid gets punishments sometimes"). Karl reported that the hitting punishments had ended when his stepfather took on the role of disciplinarian in the home. This change appears to have been a positive turn of events in Karl's mind. After hearing Karl's perception of the home situation, it would be important to learn in the parent interview what discipline strategies Mr. and Mrs. Ladd used in the home and whether they felt they were successful. It would also be important to learn more about Karl's relations with his biological father, whom Karl hardly mentioned in the child interview.

SELF-AWARENESS AND FEELINGS

Clinical interviews provide good opportunities to assess children's self-awareness and feelings. Goleman's (1995) theory of emotional intelligence provides a useful framework for interpreting children's responses to questions about self-awareness and feelings. Goleman described five main domains of emotional intelligence, each of which builds upon the other. The first domain is *knowing your own emotions*, or *self-awareness*, which is the ability to recognize a feeling in yourself as it happens. Goleman considered self-awareness to be the keystone to emotional intelligence. The next domain is *managing emotions*, which means handling or controlling your feelings so that they are appropriate to the situation and do not become overwhelming. The third domain is *motivating yourself*, which involves marshaling your emotions to serve a specific goal. Sometimes this can take the form of "pumping yourself up" to achieve a goal, or it can mean controlling your emotions by delaying gratification or stifling impulsiveness in order to achieve a later goal. The fourth domain, *recognizing emotions in others*, involves thinking about what another person is thinking or feeling. This is often termed *empathy* and requires the ability to engage in recursive thinking, as discussed in Chapter 2. The fifth domain, *handling relationships*, involves managing emotions in other people and usually requires the metacognitive ability to take a third-party perspective on social interactions (also discussed in Chapter 2).

In clinical interviews you can routinely ask children about their feelings when discussing topics such as school, peer relations, and family relations. Interspersing questions about feelings is a good way to assess the first two domains of emotional intelligence: recognizing and managing feelings. The interviews with Bruce Garcia and Karl Bryant about family relations were good examples of this process. You can also ask children direct questions that tap into their self-awareness and feelings, as shown in Table 4.2.

TABLE 4.2. Sample Questions about Self-Awareness and Feelings

<u>Wishes</u>

If you had three wishes, what would you wish for? Reasons for each?

What would you like to be when you're older/grown up?

If you could change one thing about yourself, what would it be?

<u>Feelings</u>

Tell me about yourself.
What makes you happy?
What makes you sad? What do you do when you are sad?
What makes you mad? What do you do when you are mad?
What makes you scared? What do you do when you are scared?
What do you worry about?

How do you feel most of the time?

What do you need the most?

Have you ever had any strange experiences or things happen that you don't understand?

<u>Screening questions for anxiety, depression, suicidal risk</u>

Do you feel unusually anxious or worried about things?
(*If yes*) Tell me more about your worries.

Have you ever felt very sad or depressed for a long period of time?
(*If yes*) Tell me more about that.

Have you ever been so sad that you wished you were dead?
Have you been thinking about hurting yourself or killing yourself?
Have you ever tried to harm or kill yourself?
(*If yes, probe for suicide plans, preparations, and available methods*.)

Note. Reprinted from McConaughy and Achenbach (2001). Copyright 2001 by S. H. McConaughy and T. M. Achenbach. Reprinted by permission.

Three Wishes

Asking children to give "three wishes" is a technique that is commonly used with young children, but it can also be very effective with adolescents. Children's wishes can provide some insight into their level of imagination and desires. Asking what they want to be when they grow up and what they would change about themselves are additional questions that tap into children's goals and sense of ideal self.

In research to develop the SCICA, 6- to 11-year-olds often expressed wishes for concrete things (e.g., toys, money, pets) or fun activities (e.g., to go to Disney World). Another common response was more wishes (e.g., a lot of wishes; a million wishes). These typical wishes reflect children's desires for fun and happiness, despite problems they might have reported earlier in the interview. Other SCICA participants expressed specific wishes for improvements in their home situations or relationships (e.g., for dad to be home; to have a better, nicer sister; a mother to take care of the children). Others expressed wishes to be better at an activity, sport, or academic skill (e.g., to be good at soccer; to be a better reader). These types of wishes, coupled with other interview content, can provide insights into which issues are especially poignant for children.

Bruce Garcia's three wishes were "to be on the Dolphins' team—the last best player"; "to go to Florida" (where the Dolphins play); and "to be the tallest person in the whole world." Bruce's wishes were consistent with other interview statements reflecting his desire to be stronger and taller. They also reflected a somewhat obsessional preoccupation with his favorite football team. Karl Bryant's wishes were "to live in a mansion with a pool, Jaguars, and Porsches" and "everlasting life for the whole family—that no one would ever die." He did not give a third wish. Karl's first wish reflected his desire for a grandiose lifestyle, which was consistent with earlier statements suggesting that he wanted to be important and respected. His second wish reflected concerns about the safety of family members. In Chapter 7 we learn that Karl had witnessed episodes of violence in the home as a young child.

Questions about Basic Feelings

Direct questions about basic feelings (happy, sad, mad, scared, and worried) can assess how well children recognize their feelings and whether they can differentiate among feelings. You can then probe for the behaviors that feelings elicit by asking, "What do you do when you are sad/mad/ scared? What do you worry about?" After asking questions about basic feelings, you can query children about their most predominant mood ("How do you feel most of the time?") and what they perceive as their basic needs ("What do you need the most?").

Elementary school children can usually identify something that makes them happy. Often their responses reflect their concrete operational level of reasoning. Examples from the SCICA participants were "getting presents for my birthday"; "money"; "getting toys"; "Mom giving me treats." Some responses also revealed children's concerns about family problems and peer relations: "having Dad back home"; "getting my own way"; "kids letting me in the game." Elementary school children seemed to have more difficulty talking about sad than happy feelings, and some had trouble differentiating sad from mad. For example, the SCICA question "What makes you sad?" elicited more "don't know" responses than questions about other feelings. Other responses to the question about sadness were "when a pet dies"; "when someone dies"; "when I get punished"; "when my sister slaps me."

Children seemed to find it easier to say what makes them mad than what makes them sad. The most typical SCICA responses involved sibling conflicts: "my brother punches me"; "my brother breaks my toys"; "my brother/sister gets into fights with me"; "my sister gets more attention." Other typical responses to the mad question were "getting punished"; "not getting my own way"; "people picking on me." Sample SCICA responses to the question "What makes you scared" included "scary movies," "dragons," "Dracula," "the dark," "monsters in my room," "chicken pox," "bad dreams." Sample answers to "What do you worry about?" were "not passing a grade"; "parents not taking care of me."

Sample responses from SCICA participants give some idea of what clinically referred 6- to 11-year-olds might say about their feelings. Three additional research studies provided further insights into the types of worries reported by "normal" children who had not been referred for clinical services. Not surprisingly, Vasey and Daleiden (1994) found that children expressed different types of worries as they grew older: 5- to 6-year-olds worried most often about threats to their physical well-being, whereas 8- to 12-year-olds worried about behavioral competence, social evaluation, and psychological well-being.

Muris, Meesters, Merckelbach, Sermon, and Zwakhalen (1998) reported the following top 10 most intense worries among normal 8- to 13-year-olds: school performance; dying or illness of others; getting sick themselves; being teased; making mistakes; appearance; specific future events (e.g., a party); parents divorcing; whether other children like them; pets. Henker, Whalen, and O'Neill (1995) reported the following 10 most frequent worries in children in grades 4–8 (approximately ages 10–14): academic or school-related problems; health and safety issues; environmental degradation; social relations; death and dying; social ills; positive disposition (e.g., "Am I doing the right thing?"); family relations; environmental disasters; drugs. Knowing what worries are most typical for children of different ages can help you determine whether worries expressed by particular children are unusual compared to their peers.

Strange Thoughts and Suicidal Ideation

Though few children report strange or psychotic thoughts, it is still good practice to screen for such critical problems (e.g., "Have you ever had any strange experiences or things happen that you don't understand?"). When interviewing adolescents, you can also ask more direct questions to screen for anxiety, depression, and suicidal ideation, if you have not covered these in other sections of the interview. Table 4.2 lists the following examples of screening questions: "Do you feel unusually anxious or worried about things? [*If yes*] Tell me more about your worries. Have you ever felt very sad or depressed for a long period of time? (If yes) Tell me more about that."

Whenever children express very sad feelings and/or concerns about death, you need to probe further for suicidal ideation by asking questions such as "Have you ever been so sad that you wished you were dead? Have you been thinking about hurting yourself or killing yourself? Have you ever tried to harm or kill yourself?" If children answer such questions affirmatively, you should probe for potential suicide plans, preparations to carry out plans, available methods (e.g., pills, guns), plans regarding place or setting, and whether there are any deterrents to suicide. When you suspect that a child is seriously considering suicide, you should try to obtain a promise or written contract against any self-harm in your interview. You should also explain that his/her suicidal intents cannot be kept confidential and discuss what will happen next. After the interview is completed, you must take immediate protective action, such as notifying parents, a child protection team, or a local crisis center, depending on the circumstances and legal requirements. Chapter 8 discusses assessing suicide risk in detail and provides recommendations for protective actions.

Incomplete Sentences

Another way to explore children's self-awareness and feelings is to use the incomplete sentences technique. This involves presenting children with sentence stems that focus on particular content areas and then asking them to complete each sentence as they wish. Examples are "What I like best is _____. What I like least is _____." There are numerous versions of incomplete sentences. Appendix 4.1 is a reproducible worksheet of incomplete sentences drawn from Hughes and Baker (1990) and my own clinical work. You can pick and choose from this list, as well as add your own sentences to tap specific issues or concerns.

To introduce the incomplete sentences, you can say,

"Here are some sentences I'd like you to finish for me. It will help me to get to know you and learn how you think and feel about things. You can say whatever you think, and I will write what you say right here [point to the blank in the sentence]. There aren't any right or wrong answers—it is just what you think and feel. Here is the first one [read sentence]."

Read each sentence and record responses for young children who have limited writing skills. You can give older children the option of writing their own answers or having you write their responses for them. Try to avoid making the task seem like a test. After children finish the sentences, you can select certain ones and ask children to tell more about that thought or feeling.

Appendix 4.2 is a reproducible worksheet of additional incomplete sentences, taken from Merrell (2001), that focuses specifically on feelings. Merrell recommended using incomplete sentences about feelings in cognitive-behavioral therapy for children with anxiety or depression. He also described several other techniques for addressing feelings in therapy: a worksheet listing comfortable and uncomfortable feelings; a self-rating form for evaluating how hard it is to express certain feelings; and a self-rating inventory of hypothetical situations that evoke different feelings. You can incorporate some of these techniques into clinical interviews as well as using them in therapy. Such indirect techniques may be especially effective with children who are resistant or unresponsive to direct questioning about feelings. However, incomplete sentences and other similar techniques will probably not be very effective with children under age 8 who cannot engage in recursive thinking about their own thoughts and feelings.

Case Example: Catherine Holcomb

The interview with 11-year-old Catherine Holcomb provides a good example of asking direct questions about feelings. Catherine, who was introduced in Chapter 1, lived with her mother and one older brother. In an early part of the interview, Catherine had reported that she still felt very sad about her father's death, which had occurred when she was 7 years old. At first, Catherine was reluctant to discuss her sad feelings. However, after she became more comfortable, the interviewer reopened the topic of her father's death as an entrée to explore her experience of basic feelings.

The interviewer began by asking what Catherine remembered about her father. She then moved into assessing the frequency and pervasiveness of her sad feelings. Catherine reported that she was often sad, even during school hours, which may help to explain the inattentiveness and apathy reported by her teachers. During this conversation, the interviewer learned that Catherine had never talked with anyone, including her mother, about her sad feelings. The fact that she was willing to discuss such painful feelings in the clinical interview suggested that, at this stage of her development, Catherine might have become amenable to psychotherapy. Her negative responses to probe questions about thoughts of dying also indicated that she was not currently at risk for suicide.

The interview segment with Catherine also illustrates how she responded to questions about other basic feelings. Her reports of getting mad when her brother hit her or irritated her were typical of children her age. However, the intensity of her negative feelings still suggested that her poor relationship with her brother was an important issue for Catherine. She also reported being scared of bad dreams and being afraid to go to summer camp. These fears seemed somewhat unusual for an 11-year-old. In another part of the interview, Catherine reported that she some-

BOX 4.3. Talking with Catherine about Feelings

INTERVIEWER: Tell me a little bit about your father. You said earlier that your father died? When did that happen?

CATHERINE: Just about 4 years ago. (*Looks sad, avoids eye contact.*)

I: When you were about 6 years old?

C: No, I was about 7, and Billy was about 10.

I: What kind of a person was your father?

C: He was nice. (*Fleeting eye contact, then looks away.*)

I: Tell me a little bit about him . . . you know, what you remember.

C: Well, I remember going on a lot of camping trips with Dad. He loved going on camping trips. And we'd go canoeing a lot. We have a big canoe. He called it Thunder, because it sounds like thunder. It's a really big canoe.

I: So you remember going on camping trips and things. How do you feel about all that now?

C: Sad. (*Fidgets with pant leg, looking down.*)

I: You're still sad about it. Do you talk about that with your mother?

C: No. (*Sounds sad, looks away.*)

I: Do you talk about it with anybody?

C: No. (*Pause, looks sad, sniffs, wipes a tear.*)

I: It sounds like it's hard to talk about, and you still feel sad about it.

C: (*Long pause*) I just wish my father was still alive. (*Fidgets with clothes, looks down.*)

I: Sounds like you miss him.

C: I do. (*Chokes up, looks about to cry.*)

I: Did you cry when he died?

C: Uh-huh. (*Rocks in chair, looks down.*)

I: Does it still make you cry sometimes?

C: Uh-huh.

I: How often do you think about that?

C: I think about it a lot.

I: Do you think about it when you're in school?

C: Yeah. (*Speaks softly.*)

I: What do you think about in school?

C: (*Long pause, no reply*)

I: Is it kind of hard to talk about that?

C: (*Nods "yes"; no verbal reply.*)

I: I can see it's hard to talk about it. Let's talk about some of your other feelings. What kind of things make you happy?

C: If I got a puppy for my birthday. (*Pauses.*) Christmas is fun. I get presents.

I: So you want a puppy for your birthday. Like that puppy you told me about earlier?

C: (*Brightens, nods "yes."*)

(continued)

I: And it makes you happy to get presents at Christmas. How about what makes you sad. You told me about one thing that makes you sad. Are there some other things that make you sad?

C: (*Pauses.*) I can't think of any.

I: When you're feeling sad, do you ever feel so sad that you wish *you* weren't alive?

C: No. (*Looks down.*)

I: You don't feel that sad?

C: No.

I: Have you *ever* felt so sad that you wished *you* weren't alive?

C: No.

I: What do you think about when you're sad?

C: I really don't think about anything.

I: You don't think about anything? Just kind of being sad, huh? (*Nods "yes."*) What about *mad*? What kind of things make you mad?

C: If somebody hits me.

I: Does that ever happen to you, people hitting you?

C: Sometimes people hit me.

I: Where does that happen? At home . . . or at school?

C: At home . . . my brother hits me sometimes.

I: Sometimes?

C: Uh-huh.

I: What do you do when he hits you?

C: I get mad . . . and go to my room.

I: Do you ever hit him back?

C: Sometimes I hit him back. He can get very irritating. (*Voice gets louder and sounds annoyed.*)

I: Your brother can get very irritating, huh? How is he irritating?

C: Like he might do something . . . like he might start pounding his fist on my toes. And then when I told him to stop, he wouldn't listen to me. He'd keep on doing it. I'd say it louder, and then I'd start screaming at him. (*Squirms in seat.*)

I: So first you tell him to stop, and he keeps on doing it. Then you scream at him and get mad. Then what would happen?

C: I would leave and go to my room.

I: What kind of things make you *scared*?

C: Sometimes my brother hides, and when I walk into my room, he scares me.

I: So he hides on you and scares you. Does that *really* make you scared?

C: Yes . . . he jumps out and scares me.

I: What other kinds of things are you afraid of?

C: Sometimes I'm afraid of having bad dreams. I don't like having bad dreams. (*Looks agitated, squirms in seat, rubs clothing.*)

I: What kind of bad dreams do you have?

C: I had one where I was in my closet, and there were green hands on my shoulders. (*Pulls at shirt.*)

(continued)

I: What would the green hands do?

C: They were just sitting on my shoulder and talking.

I: Talking green hands? What was bad about that dream?

C: It was just scary.

I: What did the green hands say?

C: I don't remember. I woke up.

I: Do you ever have any good dreams?

C: Uh-huh. (*Laughs a little, giggles, smiles at interviewer.*)

I: What is a good dream you've had?

C: (*Looks happier.*) I had a big black horse.

I: A big black horse. Tell me about that one.

C: Well, I got this horse, and I kept working it and showing everybody, and I woke up before I could even get on the horse. (*Giggles.*)

I: (*Interviewer laughs too.*) So you were walking around showing him and everything, and you didn't get to get on him? The big black horse. Do you like horses?

C: Uh-huh.

I: Do you ever get to ride horses?

C: Not very much. Only when I'm down at Moose Lake.

I: Moose Lake. What is that?

C: It's a camp in the summer. They have horseback riding . . . archery. Now I don't have to be led anymore.

I: You don't have to be led?

C: I used to have to be led, and now I don't have to.

I: Does that mean you can ride by yourself?

C: Uh-huh. It's fun. (*Looks at interviewer smiles, pauses.*) One time I was riding on a horse, and he started to run.

I: How did you feel then?

C: I was scared. He was fast.

I: I remember riding a horse, and it was kind of scary when he ran.

C: (*Brightens up and looks at interviewer.*) It's fun riding horses.

I: You really like to do it. Is Moose Lake a place that you stay overnight?

C: Not when I was a kid. I'm old enough now, if I want to go. But I don't now.

I: You don't want to stay overnight?

C: (*Nods "no."*) Billy does, though.

I: Why don't you want to stay overnight?

C: It's scary. I don't want to stay by myself.

I: OK. Let me ask a different question. What would you say you *need* the most?

C: (*Pauses.*) Uh . . . food.

I: Food? What do you mean, you need food?

C: You need food to keep living. (*Looks sad again, quiet voice.*).

I: Oh. So if you're going to keep living, you need food. OK.

times would crawl into her mother's bed at night when she has a bad dream or stomachache. In this interview segment, Catherine's expression of her fears and recurrent feelings of sadness raised the possibility of a mood disorder, though more information would be needed from other sources to make such a diagnosis.

Child Abuse and Neglect

Both the United States and Canada have legislation mandating that professionals report cases of suspected abuse or neglect to official child protective service (CPS) agencies. In the United States, mandated reporting is required under the Child Abuse Prevention and Treatment Act (CAPTA; Public Law 93-247), originally passed in 1974, and reauthorized and amended many times since then. Maltreatment includes physical abuse, sexual abuse, emotional abuse, and neglect. CAPTA provides definitions of each type of maltreatment. The individual states, in turn, have developed their own legislation and regulations to carry out the requirements of CAPTA.

Along with mandated reporting, CAPTA established the National Center on Child Abuse and Neglect to assist states and communities in identification, prevention, and treatment of child abuse and neglect. Since 1988, the National Center on Child Abuse and Neglect Data System (NCANDS) has compiled annual statistics on child maltreatment. For 2002, NCANDS reported referrals of alleged abuse or neglect of more than 3 million children. Of those, 869,000 children were determined by CPS agencies to be victims of abuse or neglect. More than 60% of child victims were neglected by their parents or other caregivers. Close to 20% were physically abused, 10% were sexually abused, and 7% were emotionally abused. Approximately 20% experienced "other" types of maltreatment. (The data included children who experienced more than one type of maltreatment; U.S. Department of Health and Human Services, 2002).

Mandated reporters under CAPTA include physicians, nurses, teachers, psychologists, social workers, guidance counselors, and other professional people who have contact with children. Reports can also be accepted from friends, neighbors, and relatives. In 2002, more than half of the reports to CPS agencies were made by professionals. Federal and state laws protect professionals from criminal and civil liability in all jurisdictions, unless the report is malicious or without probable grounds. Informant anonymity is also guaranteed in some, but not all, states. State laws vary as to what specific situations require reporting (e.g., ongoing abuse or neglect vs. strong potential for abuse or neglect vs. past abuse or neglect without current risk). Laws also vary as to the degree of certainty necessary for reporting and sanctions for not reporting (Sattler, 1998; Wolfe & McEachran, 1997).

School-based practitioners should be familiar with federal and state laws for mandated reporting and with the CPS agencies in their states and local communities. Since the passage of CAPTA, most school districts have established their own procedures to facilitate mandated reports of suspected abuse and neglect. Often groups of school-based practitioners serve on child protection teams within each school or at the district level. Other school-based practitioners who suspect abuse or neglect of a child can bring their concerns to the child protection team. The team supports the practitioner in examining the concerns and filing the mandatory report to the CPS agency. Members of school child protection teams may also assist the child and family during the investigation process and afterward, as appropriate.

Wissow (1995) outlined several physical signs and symptoms that should arouse concern about potential child abuse and neglect. These include unexplained subnormal growth; specific types of head injuries (e.g., torn upper or lower lip, bilateral black eyes, unexplained dental injury, retinal hemorrhage, traumatic hair loss); skin injuries (e.g., bruises or burns in the shape of an object, bite marks); multiple lesions or injuries in various stages of healing; and bone or skull fractures and other traumas inconsistent with a given explanation. Some researchers have reported that sexually abused children exhibit sexually inappropriate behavior—(e.g., imitating sexual acts, self-stimulation and hyperarousal, exposing, and sexually aggressive or victimizing behavior toward others)—more often than nonabused children do (Finkelhor, 1988; Friedrich & Grambsch, 1992; McClellan et al., 1996). Others have found no significant relationship between sexual abuse and sexual behavioral problems (Drach, Wientzen, & Ricci, 2001). While practitioners should be alert to physical or behavioral signs that may suggest abuse, they should also know that abused children can exhibit a vast array of internalizing and externalizing problems similar to clinically referred children who have not been abused. Accordingly, practitioners should use caution in relying only on physical signs or behavioral problems as indicators of abuse. A child's direct report is a better indicator of potential abuse or neglect than are physical signs or behavioral problems alone.

It is beyond the scope of this book to discuss investigations of child abuse and neglect. Instead, readers are referred to Sattler (1998), who presented extensive guidelines on investigative interviewing techniques and background considerations for child abuse and neglect. Wolfe and McEachran (1997) also reviewed developmental perspectives and assessment of physically abused and neglected children, while Wolfe and Birt (1997) reviewed developmental perspectives and assessment of sexually abused children. Other authors have discussed the roles of school-based practitioners in responding to children who have suffered abuse and neglect (e.g., Brassard, Tyler, & Kehle, 1983; Horton & Cruise, 2001; Slater & Gallagher, 1989; Vevier & Tharinger, 1986).

Comprehensive interviews to evaluate child abuse or neglect should be done only by specially trained investigators. Most school-based practitioners and mental health professionals lack such training. More often, professionals who specialize in social service, forensic, and criminal investigations are the ones who assess child maltreatment. Although school-based practitioners usually do not conduct such investigations, they may be among the first to hear disclosures of abuse or neglect from children (or from interviews with parents and teachers). Brassard et al. (1983) outlined guidelines for responding to children who report sexual abuse. Similar guidelines, listed below, are appropriate for responding to all children who report maltreatment:

- Conduct your interview in a private place.
- Maintain an atmosphere of informality and trust.
- Believe the child (or at least take the child's report at face value).
- Reassure the child that he/she has done nothing wrong and will continue to have your support.
- Do not display negative reactions such as horror, shock, or disapproval of the child or parents.
- Be sensitive to the child's nonverbal cues.
- Ask for clarification if what the child says is ambiguous.
- Use language that the child understands.
- Use the child's terms for body parts and sexual behaviors, but also obtain the child's definition of such terms.
- Do not suggest answers to the child and avoid probing and pressing for answers.

- If it becomes clear that you must make a report to a CPS agency, give the child a clear and understandable reason why such reporting is necessary.
- Do not suggest that the child conceal your interview from the parents.
- Record clear notes of your interview and the child's disclosure statements, as well as your subsequent actions regarding reporting.

Based on the 2002 NCANDS report, more than 80% of perpetrators of child abuse and neglect were parents. Other relatives accounted for 7% and unmarried partners of parents for 3% of perpetrators (U.S. Department of Health and Human Services, 2002). As Sattler (1998) pointed out, children who are maltreated by parents or caregivers face a terrible dilemma. If they disclose the abuse or neglect, they may lose the very people that they depend on for love and nurturance. If they do not disclose, they face the likelihood of continued suffering. Children may be reluctant to disclose abuse because they fear retribution or violence from the abuser, breaking up the family, and/or rejection by friends and relatives. Very young victims of sexual abuse may not understand that the sexual activity is wrong. Adolescents who view the sexual abuse as wrong may still fear retribution, abandonment, rejection, and embarrassment or shame if their peers or members of the community find out. Many children and adolescents may also fear that no one will believe their report. It takes courage for a child to disclose abuse and neglect. It is not your job to determine whether the child is lying, exaggerating a situation, or has a faulty memory. Reacting with disbelief when the child is telling the truth can not only be devastating, but can also perpetuate the abuse or neglect and reduce the chance of any further disclosures.

When children report circumstances or incidents that lead you to suspect abuse or neglect, you must inform the child of your legal obligation to report the information to a CPS agency. This requires breaking confidentiality. You can explain that the law requires you to report situations where children are not safe. You can also repeat the limits of confidentiality stated at the beginning of the interview, such as saying, "Remember what I said at the beginning of our talk? I said that I would have to tell someone if you said you were going to hurt yourself, hurt someone else, or someone has hurt you" (see Chapter 2).

Expect that the disclosure and required reporting will be upsetting and perhaps threatening to the child. Take steps to help the child cope with the anxiety reporting may create. Reassure the child that you will still be there to support him/her. Explain what steps you must take next, such as talking with persons on the school child protection team and filing a report to the state or local CPS agency. Remember that it is not your job to establish evidence that the suspected abuse or neglect actually occurred. Your responsibility is to make the report that will initiate the investigative process. Do not make any personal promises to protect the child. If you suspect that the child is in immediate danger, you and other appropriate school staff (e.g., the school child protection team) must take action to protect the child, such as notifying law enforcement or social service agencies, or notifying parents in cases when they are not suspected perpetrators.

Once a report has been filed with a CPS agency, that agency must determine the likelihood that abuse or neglect has occurred, assess the risk for further abuse, and determine what course of action must be taken to protect the child. This often requires further interviews of the child and family by the CPS investigators. According to the NCANDS report, approximately 30% of reports in 2002 included at least one child who was found to be a victim of abuse or neglect. Sixty-one percent of reports were found to be unsubstantiated for various reasons, including intentionally false reports. The remaining reports were closed for other reasons. Although the majority of reports were unsubstantiated, the 30% that were substantiated underscore the necessity for careful monitoring and reporting of suspected maltreatment of children.

ADOLESCENT ISSUES

Alcohol and Drugs

Each year since 1975, the National Institute on Drug Abuse has sponsored a nationwide survey, Monitoring the Future, to measure national trends in the use of alcohol, nicotine, and illicit substances (Johnston, O'Malley, Bachman, & Schulenberg, 2004). The data from this annual survey are especially useful to keep in mind when interviewing adolescents about their substance use. The 2003 sample for the survey included 48,500 students in 8th, 10th, and 12th grades in 392 schools across the nation. (The total survey also included college students and adults through ages 45.) The good news was a decline in the percent of 12th-grade students reporting lifetime use of an illicit drug from a high of 66% in 1981 to 51% in 2003. Use of illicit drugs other than marijuana dropped from a high of 43% in 1981 to 28% in 2003. The bad news was that 51% of students still reported using illicit drugs (including marijuana), which is an alarming figure. In addition, 77% of 12th-grade students reported having consumed alcohol (more than a few sips), and 54% reported having tried cigarettes.

The general trends from the Monitoring the Future survey show that substance use continues to be widespread among U.S. youth. To give a more differentiated picture of current use of different substances, Table 4.3 lists the percentages of 8th-, 10th-, and 12th-grade students reporting use of various substances over the 30 days preceding the 2003 questionnaires. Consistent with the lifetime data, alcohol, cigarettes, and marijuana top the list, with 21–48% of 12th-grade students reporting their use. Three to 7% of 12th-grade students reported use of smokeless tobacco, amphetamines without a doctor's prescription, and tranquilizers without a prescription. Other drugs were used by 1–2% of 12th-grade students, and heroin was used by less than 1%.

The data in Table 4.3 were drawn from self-reports by a large national sample of students without distinguishing between normal "nonreferred" students versus those who were referred for clinical services. To add to this picture, Table 4.4 shows the percent of nonreferred versus referred 11- to 18-year-olds who reported using alcohol, tobacco, or drugs for nonmedical purposes over the past 6 months on the YSR (Achenbach & Rescorla, 2001). Significantly more referred than nonreferred adolescents reported substance use on the YSR. The percents reporting substance use were somewhat lower on the YSR than in the Monitoring the Future survey, probably because of the broader age range and differences in sampling and questionnaire methods.

Adolescence is certainly a time of experimentation. As you can see from the data in Tables 4.3 and 4.4, for many youth, experimentation includes using alcohol and drugs. When considering such data, it is important to distinguish between substance use as experimentation versus substance abuse and dependency. Accordingly, Sattler (1998) delineated five stages of substance use: experimentation arising from curiosity, risk taking, or peer pressure; social use to gain acceptance in a peer group; instrumental use to manipulate emotions and behavior; habitual use that can lead to abuse; and finally, compulsive use or addiction that leads to dependency. These progressive stages are good to keep in mind for evaluating the severity of adolescents' substance use.

According to DSM-IV, a diagnosis of *substance abuse* disorder can be made when use of a substance leads to "clinically significant impairment or distress, but without signs of tolerance or

TABLE 4.3. Percent of Adolescents Reporting Substance Use in the Past 30 Days in 2003

Type of substance	8th grade	10th grade	12th grade
Alcohol	20	35	48
Cigarettes	7	18	31
Marijuana/hashish	8	17	21
Smokeless tobacco	4	5	7
Amphetamine (without prescription)	3	4	5
Tranquilizers (without prescription)	1	2	3
Inhalants	4	2	2
Hallucinogens	1	2	2
Methamphetamine (crystal meth, "ice")	1	1	2
Cocaine	1	1	2
Crack cocaine	1	1	1
LSD	1	1	1
MDMA (Ecstasy)	1	1	1
Steroids	1	1	1
Heroin	< 1	< 1	< 1
Any illicit drug, including marijuana	10	20	24
Any illicit drug, excluding marijuana	5	7	10

Note. Adapted from Johnston, O'Malley, Bachman, and Schulenberg (2004).

TABLE 4.4. Percent of Adolescents Reporting Alcohol or Drug Use on the Youth Self-Report

YSR problem item[a]	Nonreferred girls	Nonreferred boys	Referred girls	Referred boys
I drink alcohol without my parents' approval	14	10	17	17
I smoke, chew, or sniff tobacco	10	6	28	25
I use drugs for nonmedical purposes (do not include alcohol or tobacco)	4	16	16	13

Note. Items are from the Youth Self-Report (YSR; Achenbach, 2001). Copyright 2001 by T.M. Achenbach. Reprinted by permission.
[a]YSR problem items endorsed as "somewhat or sometimes true" or "very true or often true" over the past 6 months by children ages 11–18.

TABLE 4.5. Sample Questions about Alcohol
and Drug Use

Do you smoke or chew tobacco?
(*If yes*) How often?

Have you ever drunk beer, wine, or liquor?
(*If yes*) When and how often?

Have you ever been drunk from alcohol?
(*If yes*) When and how often?
Do you think you have a problem with alcohol?
Have you ever received any help/treatment for alcohol problems?
Do you want help/treatment for alcohol problems now?

Have you used drugs/been high on drugs?
(*If yes*) When and how often?
What kind of drugs?
Do you think you have a problem with drugs?
Have you ever received any help/treatment for drug problems?
Do you want help/treatment for drug problems now?

Note. Reprinted from McConaughy and Achenbach (2001). Copyright 2001
by S. H. McConaughy and T. M. Achenbach. Reprinted by permission.

withdrawal symptoms." *Substance dependence* occurs when use of a substance leads to clinically significant impairment and signs of tolerance or withdrawal symptoms. Tolerance becomes evident when an individual must increase use of a substance to achieve desired effects or when he/she experiences a decrease in desired effects with use of the same amount of the substance. Withdrawal symptoms vary with the type of substance. DSM-IV considers substance dependence to be more severe than substance abuse. Nicotine and polysubstance use can only be diagnosed as "substance dependence" in DSM-IV, whereas many other substances can be diagnosed for "abuse" or "dependence."

The widespread substance use among U.S. youth certainly puts them at risk for developing substance abuse or dependence. For this reason, it is important to screen for alcohol and drug use in clinical interviews. Table 4.5 lists some open-ended questions that cover tobacco and alcohol use, plus general drug use. When adolescents do report use of substances, you should probe further to determine the frequency of use and whether such use has created problems for them. When adolescents report frequent use that suggests possible substance abuse or dependence, you should try to assess their desire for change and readiness for help or treatment. For example, you can ask adolescents if they have ever received help or treatment and whether they want help or treatment now. If you suspect that an adolescent has a severe alcohol or drug problem, then you may want to do more in-depth interviewing regarding his/her substance use. Sattler (1998) provided several interview protocols for such purposes.

Antisocial Behavior and Trouble with the Law

In addition to asking adolescents about substance use, it is important to screen for antisocial behavior that may lead to trouble with the law. Other sections of the clinical interview may naturally present opportunities to ask about such problems, for example, when discussing activities

TABLE 4.6. Sample Questions about Trouble with the Law

Have you ever been in trouble with the law or police?
(*If yes*) What kind of trouble?
What happened when you got in trouble with the law/police?

Have you ever been in any traffic accidents/had any traffic tickets?
(*If yes*) What kind of accidents?

Do you belong to a gang?
(*If yes*) Tell me about the gang.
Has your gang ever gotten into trouble with the law or police?

Note. Reprinted from McConaughy and Achenbach (2001). Copyright 2001 by S. H. McConaughy and T. M. Achenbach. Reprinted by permission.

with friends or family. You can then follow up such discussions with probes about activities that may have led to trouble with the law. If you do not have opportunities to ask such questions earlier in the interview, you can ask directly about trouble with the law and gang activities, as shown in Table 4.6.

Researchers on conduct disorders have described two different developmental paths for antisocial behavior. One pattern involves early onset (e.g., age 6 or younger) of aggressive and antisocial behavior that seems to be strongly associated with children's temperaments and poor parent–child relationships. Another pattern involves later onset of antisocial behavior among adolescents who associate with troubled or delinquent peers (Moffit, 1993; McMahon & Estes, 1997). Children who show early onset of aggressive, antisocial behavior tend to have severe problems that continue into adulthood. Very early interventions are crucial for changing such patterns of behavior. However, adolescents who begin antisocial behavior later in life may or may not continue such patterns into adulthood. A lot depends on what consequences adolescents experience in response to their antisocial behavior. If they are arrested and put into the criminal justice system, their expected outcomes are bleak. If, instead, they enter into treatment programs or court diversion programs, they may change their course of behavior. For example, problem-solving training and multisystemic treatment programs have shown promising results with antisocial adolescents (Henggeler & Lee, 2003; Kazdin, 2003).

To provide some background on the prevalence of adolescents' antisocial behaviors, Table 4.7 shows the percent of 11- to 18-year-olds who reported antisocial behavior on the YSR (Achenbach & Rescorla, 2001). You can see that rates of all such problems were higher in clinically referred than nonreferred children. Still, over one-third of nonreferred children reported that they break rules and hang around with kids who get into trouble. These data underscore the importance of asking adolescents about such behaviors in clinical interviews. When adolescents do report such problems, you can explore options for changing antisocial behaviors before they lead to serious social or legal consequences.

Dating and Romances

According to a 1997 national survey by the U.S. Centers for Disease Control and Prevention, 38% of 9th-grade students and 61% of 12th-grade students reported having had sexual intercourse (Institute for Youth Development, 1999). Although these data represent a slight decrease from

TABLE 4.7. Percent of Adolescents Reporting Antisocial Behavior on the Youth Self-Report

YSR problem item[a]	Nonreferred girls	Nonreferred boys	Referred girls	Referred boys
I break rules at home, school, or elsewhere	34	43	77	81
I hang around with kids who get into trouble	35	44	49	55
I cut classes or skip school	12	10	26	26
I run away from home	3	4	22	18
I set fires	2	6	7	14
I steal at home	3	4	10	18
I steal from places other than home	3	4	15	20

Note. Items are from the Youth Self-Report (YSR; Achenbach, 2001). Copyright 2001 by T.M. Achenbach. Reprinted by permission.
[a]YSR problem items endorsed as "somewhat or sometimes true" or "very true or often true" over the past 6 months by children ages 11–18.

1991 figures, they still indicate high percentages of high school students who are sexually active. More alarming are 1997 data showing that 7% of students reported initiating sexual intercourse before age 13. Other research has shown that young people who had sexual intercourse at an early age are significantly more likely to have multiple lifetime partners. Fifty-seven percent of girls and 74% of boys who had sexual intercourse before age 14 reported 6 or more lifetime sexual partners.

Increased sexual feelings can certainly add a vital and exciting dimension to the lives of adolescents. Being attracted to someone and developing intimate relationships are opportunities for growth. However, early onset of sexual activity and high frequency of sexual partners put adolescents at significant risk for HIV infection, other sexually transmitted diseases (STDs), and teenage pregnancy. Early onset of sexual activity may also increase girls' risks for coercive sex and exploitation: 22% of girls who had sex before age 13 reported that it was nonvoluntary, and 49% reported it was unwanted. Moreover, teenage pregnancy and single motherhood raise risks of dropping out of high school, receiving fewer employment opportunities, and ending up welfare dependent.

Asking about sexual activity in clinical interviews may produce discomfort for many adolescents. Discussion of sexual practices with adolescents may also be a sensitive, or even taboo, topic for some parents and school staff. For example, some fundamentalist parents in my clinical practice explicitly asked whether my child clinical interview would include questions about sex. Some school districts may also have policies about discussing sexual practices with students. When adolescents, or adults, do have concerns, it is important to explain your purpose for discussing such topics. For example, you can explain that you may want to ask about dating and romantic relationships to learn more about an adolescent's social interactions and whether he/she is at risk for unsafe sex practices.

Table 4.8 lists sample questions interviewers can ask about dating, romances, and sexual activity. These are only intended as screening questions. Use your own judgment about their appropriateness for each interviewee. In some cases, you should also consider the gender of the

TABLE 4.8. Sample Questions about Dating and Romances

How do you think your parents feel about your friends?

Do you date/go to dances/parties?
How do you feel about dating/parties?

Do you have a boyfriend/girlfriend?
Have you had sex with your girlfriend/boyfriend?
What do you know about safe sex?

Note. Reprinted from McConaughy and Achenbach (2001). Copyright 2001 by S. H. McConaughy and T. M. Achenbach. Reprinted by permission.

interviewer and interviewee. For example, it may not be appropriate for a male interviewer to ask girls questions about their sexual activity, especially when there is reason to suspect that they have experienced sexual abuse. When you do ask such sensitive questions, do so in a neutral, professional manner, and be prepared to handle any embarrassment that may arise. Ask only enough questions to evaluate risk without violating an adolescent's sense of privacy. Also be cautious that your questions are not misinterpreted as showing personal interest. If an adolescent's reports lead you to suspect ongoing abuse or imminent risk for abuse, you must break confidentiality and follow legal reporting requirements as discussed in an earlier section. Inform the adolescent of these requirements and remind him/her of the limits of confidentiality that you stated at the beginning of the interview.

Confidentiality Issues with Adolescents

Adolescents who use alcohol or drugs or have committed illegal acts may be reluctant to report such problems for fear of getting into trouble. Others may not want to discuss their sexual activity out of embarrassment or fear that someone else will find out about them. In such cases, confidentiality is likely to be a major issue. You should carefully consider your ethical and professional responsibilities for dealing with confidentiality before beginning your clinical interviews on these topics. And you should clearly state the limits on confidentiality at the beginning of the interview. As indicated earlier in this chapter and Chapter 2, ethical and legal standards require you to break confidentiality when there is reason to suspect harm or danger to self, harm or danger to others, or child abuse. However, APA and NASP ethical standards do not explicitly require breaking confidentiality to report illegal substance use or criminal behavior that does not present a danger to others. (See Jacob & Hartshorne, 2003, for more detailed discussion of legal and ethical issues regarding confidentiality.)

One approach is to inform adolescents ahead of time that you will report concerns about substance use or illegal activities to their parents or guardians. You may also want to report unsafe sexual practices that increase health risks or risks for exploitation or abuse. Such reports are necessary when these issues are the main reasons for referral or are the focus of assessment for specific treatment programs. For example, some clinics and treatment programs require adolescents to sign a release allowing clinicians to share information about substance abuse or illegal activities with parents. When you take this route, you run the risk that adolescents will deny such problems. It is, therefore, important to establish rapport early on and to explain clearly the purpose of your interview and assessment.

In other cases, you may choose to keep reports of substance use or illegal activities confidential in order to help an adolescent move toward acknowledging the severity of the problems and accepting appropriate treatment. The federal Public Health Services Act (1987) includes comprehensive privacy rules that protect the confidentiality of patient records for persons, including minor adolescents, who enter into substance abuse treatment programs (Confidentiality of Alcohol and Drug Abuse Patient Records, 1987). In addition, at least 20 states give minors the right to seek drug treatment without their parents' consent (Gudeman, 2003). In any case, you should have a clear strategy for dealing with the limits of confidentiality prior to interviewing adolescents about their substance use or illegal activities, as well as their sexual activity.

Case Example: Kelsey Watson

Fourteen-year-old Kelsey Watson's case illustrates the special issues that can arise with adolescents. Kelsey grew up in a semirural community, where she had experienced a great deal of instability in her home life. Her biological father was an alcoholic who had left the family when Kelsey was a young child. Her mother suffered from Bipolar Disorder and had been hospitalized several times for psychiatric treatment. When her mother was sick, Kelsey was cared for by various relatives. At age 12 Kelsey moved to a large city to live with a maternal aunt for a year. There she attended an alternative school for children with learning and behavioral problems. She ran away from her aunt's home several times and became involved with a street gang. At age 13 Kelsey was hospitalized in a psychiatric unit because of suicide attempts. She was diagnosed with Major Depression and placed on antidepressant medication (Prozac). After her release from the hospital, Kelsey returned to live with her mother for 6 months. At age 14 Kelsey was placed in the custody of the state social service agency because of unmanageable behavior and runaway episodes. She then moved into a residential group home but continued to have home visits with her mother.

After Kelsey entered the group home, she began attending eighth grade in the local school district. There she was referred for a psychological evaluation of her behavioral and emotional functioning. The psychologist's clinical interview with Kelsey was a critical component of the evaluation. The psychologist took special care to establish rapport with her, while at the same time explaining the purpose of the interview. Kelsey arrived dressed in a tank top and short skirt. She had short, spiked colored hair and wore rings in her nose, left eyebrow, and both ears. She had a tattoo on her right arm. The psychologist greeted her without commenting on her appearance. She explained that the interview was part of Kelsey's evaluation and that she would be writing a report summarizing what she learned. She told Kelsey that they could talk about what would go into the report at the end of the interview. Because Kelsey had a history of suicide attempts, the psychologist made sure that Kelsey understood the limits of confidentiality. She clearly explained the legal requirements for reporting any concerns that Kelsey might hurt herself or hurt others or that she might be in danger of being hurt by someone else. Kelsey said she understood these limits and agreed to participate in the interview.

Although Kelsey was nervous and tense at first, she was cooperative and seemed eager to discuss her feelings and personal issues. In fact, she seemed to thrive on the individual attention. The interview covered most of the topic areas discussed in this chapter and Chapter 3 (see Table

3.1), along with adolescent issues regarding alcohol and drugs (Table 4.5), trouble with the law (Table 4.6), and dating and romances (Table 4.8).

Kelsey's interview raised particular concerns about several key adolescent issues. First and foremost was Kelsey's accounts of past suicide attempts and self-mutilation. Kelsey said, "I cut my wrists with glass and razor blades and tried to OD on caffeine pills. That's how I ended up in the mental hospital." She said that slashing her wrists made her feel "good, sort of like a high." When questioned further, Kelsey said she was no longer cutting herself and currently did not have any thoughts of killing herself. She thought that if she died, "she would probably go somewhere— heaven or hell—probably to hell." Sometimes, she said, she still felt like she wanted to die—"it was confusing"—but she reported no current plans to commit suicide. Kelsey noted that she was currently seeing a "shrink" at the group home, but that she and her therapist had not developed any contract stating that she would not commit suicide.

A second concern was Kelsey's prior association with deviant or fringe peer groups in the city. Kelsey reported that at least one of her wrist-slashing episodes was part of a "cult thing" that she did with her city friends. Kelsey described herself as a "Satanist." She said that she and her friend Jillian had slashed their wrists together and then had tried to drink their blood "to give themselves more power." Kelsey's reports of cult activities were certainly worrisome, but she did not mention any antisocial activities that had led to trouble with police. Kelsey said that she continued to write letters to Jillian, but had no other contact with her or other city friends since she had returned home.

A third concern was Kelsey's reported use of alcohol and drugs. She freely admitted to getting drunk on beer and wine several times in the past, as well as using marijuana, LSD, pills (Valium), and heroin. She said she liked the "nice" feeling she had the two times she had shot up with heroin. She had not tried cocaine. Most of her substance use occurred during the year she spent in the city. In the clinical interview, Kelsey said she continued to use marijuana about once a month when she could get it, and she smoked "about a pack of cigarettes a day, when I can afford them." She had not drunk any alcohol in the past month, and really didn't like it as much as marijuana. Although drugs were harder to come by now, Kelsey said she still had urges to get high.

Kelsey's active sexual behavior was a fourth concern. She reported that she started having sex at age 12 with a 14-year-old boy, José, whom she had met in the city. She "was crazy about José" and "slept with him" about six times. When the psychologist asked what she meant by "sleeping with José," Kelsey looked embarrassed but then clearly described having had intercourse. Sometimes, she said, José used a condom, but not always. Kelsey wanted to "get a shot for birth control," but had never seen a gynecologist and had never visited Planned Parenthood. However, she said she would like to learn more about safe sex. Kelsey also stated that she had never been sexually or physically abused by any of her cult members in the city. After she returned home, Kelsey found a new boyfriend, Eric. She reported that they engaged in oral sex and anal sex and sometimes intercourse. She said that she "would do anything for Eric" and thought about him all the time. Kelsey also reported having had several gay friends in the city. She once tried oral sex with a girl, but thought it was embarrassing.

The summary of Kelsey's history and her clinical interview revealed serious emotional and behavioral problems at the time of the school-based evaluation. Although she was in state custody and under treatment for depression, Kelsey remained at risk for suicide, substance abuse, and sexually related problems, including teenage pregnancy, HIV and other STDs, and sexual exploitation. Kelsey's pattern of problems called for intense interventions on several fronts, involving both school and community agencies. We will return to Kelsey's case in Chapter 7 to learn more about other people's perspectives on her functioning and potential intervention strategies.

SUMMARY

This chapter discussed interviewing children about their home situation and family relations, self-awareness and feelings, and special issues appropriate for adolescents—alcohol and drugs; antisocial behavior and trouble with the law; and dating and romances. Research findings were included for each topic to provide a framework for talking about these issues and interpreting children's interview reports. Segments of clinical interviews with Bruce Garcia, Karl Bryant, and Catherine Holcomb illustrated interview strategies and different issues that can arise in clinical interviews. Kelsey Watson's case illustrated specific concerns that can arise with adolescents. The Kinetic Family Drawing and incomplete sentences were discussed as examples of interviewing techniques that can provide breaks from more direct questioning.

APPENDIX 4.1

What I Think and Feel

Directions: Here are some sentences I'd like you to finish for me. It will help me to get to know you and learn how you think and feel about things. You can say whatever you think, and I will write what you say right here [point to the blank in the sentence]. There aren't any right or wrong answers—it is just what you think and feel. Here is the first one [read sentence].

What I like best is _____.

What I like least is _____.

Most grown people are _____.

My mother thinks I am _____.

My father thinks I am _____.

My teacher thinks I am _____.

Other kids in my class think I am _____.

My friends think I am _____.

My mother makes me feel _____.

My father makes me feel _____.

My sister/brother makes me feel _____.

I am _____.

When my mother gives me jobs, I _____.

When there is no one to help me, I _____.

When my teacher tells me to do something, I _____.

When my teacher corrects me, I _____.

When I don't know what the book says, I _____.

When I have hard homework, I _____.

About My Feelings

Directions: Complete each of these sentences about feelings in your own words, using examples of how you feel.

I felt afraid when _____

_____.

I am really good at _____

_____.

I get excited when _____

_____.

Most of the time I feel _____

_____.

I am happy when _____

_____.

I feel upset when _____

_____.

I am sad when _____

_____.

I am calm when _____

_____.

I was really mad when _____

_____.

I am thankful for _____

_____.

I am lonely when _____

_____.

5

Interviews with Parents

Communication with parents is an essential component of assessment and intervention planning for children. As Barkley (2006) states so well, "No other adult is more likely than the parents to have the wealth of knowledge about, history of interactions with, or sheer time spent with a child." This unique relationship affords parents special expertise about their children that cannot be duplicated by any other informants. Interviews with parents are especially useful for the following purposes:

- To establish rapport and mutual respect between the interviewer and parent.
- To learn the parent's current concerns about the child.
- To identify and prioritize the child's specific problems that would be appropriate targets for interventions.
- To identify the child's strengths and competencies that can be marshaled to bolster interventions.
- To learn more about key areas of the child's history and current circumstances that are relevant for understanding identified problems.
- To learn which interventions, if any, have already been attempted.
- To assess the prima facie effectiveness of previous interventions.
- To assess the acceptability and feasibility of future interventions.

Despite their value, parent interviews can sometimes be challenging for school-based practitioners due to time constraints, scheduling difficulties, or other factors. Some parents may also be reluctant to be interviewed about personal and family issues in school settings. These challenges make it all the more important that you use your interview time efficiently to gather key information, while still eliciting parents' concerns and unique perspectives on their children.

As indicated in Chapter 1, clinical interviews are best viewed as one of several assessment methods for gaining knowledge about a child's functioning and need for help. If practitioners routinely use other assessment methods along with interviews, they can tailor their interviews to achieve goals to which interviews are best suited. For example, if parents are asked routinely to complete a background questionnaire prior to being interviewed, you can use interview time to ask for details about key areas of developmental, medical, educational, and family history that affect the child's current functioning. Likewise, if parents complete standardized behavioral rating scales prior to the interview, you do not have to waste precious interview time asking about all possible problem areas. Instead, you can focus on parents' main concerns about their child and the specific problems revealed on the rating scales.

This chapter discusses parent interviews with a special emphasis on semistructured formats. The first two sections cover issues regarding confidentiality and questioning strategies for parent interviews. To guide the interview process with parents, a reproducible format for the Semi-structured Parent Interview (McConaughy, 2004a), which is the main focus of this chapter, is provided in Appendix 5.1. Other assessment methods that can dovetail with parent interviews are also discussed. A concluding section covers structured diagnostic interviews with parents to assess specific symptoms of psychiatric disorders.

DISCUSSING CONFIDENTIALITY AND PURPOSE WITH PARENTS

With the exception of certain emergency situations (e.g., abuse, suicide risk), assessment of children younger than 18 requires informed consent from parents or other legal guardians. The IDEA outlines requirements for informed consent for comprehensive evaluations of students with suspected disabilities. Each state also has its own regulations for interpreting and carrying out the mandates of the IDEA. These state regulations usually include specific formats for obtaining informed consent from parents. The Family Education Rights and Privacy Act (FERPA; 1974, Public Law 93-830) and its modifications also define confidentiality and parental rights regarding release of information from school records. Briefly, FERPA grants parents rights to access their children's official educational records and requires parental consent for release of records to other agencies, except in limited circumstances, such as school transfer, subpoenas, or requests by state educational agencies or accrediting agencies. Respect for client privacy is also a mandate in the ethical codes of most mental health professional organizations, including the ACA, APA, NASP, and NASW.

School-based practitioners should be familiar with federal and state laws, as well as their own professional ethical codes, regarding privacy and release of information about children and families. They should also be familiar with their school district's policies and procedures. Armed with this knowledge, discussion of purposes and limits of confidentiality can become the entrée for the parent interview. If a parent interview is part of a comprehensive special education evaluation, then, by law, written informed consent must be obtained prior to any assessment of the child, including the parent interview. Parents' written consent should also be obtained prior to any other formal assessment of the child.

As Jacob (2002) pointed out, informed consent involves three key elements: It is knowing, competent, and voluntary. This means that parents must have a clear understanding of what they are consenting to; they must be legally competent to give such consent; and the consent must be given without coercion or undue enticement. If a parent has already signed a written consent form prior to the interview appointment, you should still review the consent form to make sure that the parent understands what he/she has agreed to. If a parent has not signed a written consent form, then you should obtain a signature prior to asking questions about the child. In either case, you need to review the legal limits of confidentiality in a clear and concise way and explain how information from the interview will be released to any other parties. You should also explain that you will be including information from the parent in your written evaluation reports.

As discussed in Chapter 3, exceptions to confidentiality occur when there is a clear and imminent danger to another individual or to the child directly. Under state statutory law and case law, school personnel also have a legal obligation to take steps to ensure the safety of students under school supervision. Jacob and Hartshorne (2003) and Sattler (1998) are excellent sources for detailed discussions of legal and ethical issues regarding confidentiality and disclosure. As they recommend, any written consent form should contain some statement that outlines the limits of confidentiality. An example is the following:

> I understand that there may be circumstances under which the law requires school personnel or clinician(s) to disclose confidential information. These circumstances include: (a) abuse or neglect of minors and (b) situations which may pose a danger to my child or others.

The Semistructured Parent Interview (McConaughy, 2004a; see Appendix 5.1) begins with a standard introduction about confidentiality and the purpose of the interview. The phrasing of the introduction assumes that parents have already received and signed a written consent form, and that parents have completed a background questionnaire and standardized rating scales prior to their interview appointment. (The questionnaire and rating scales are discussed in a later section of this chapter.) You can adapt this introduction to fit the particular circumstances of your interview:

> "Thank you for taking your time to meet with me today and for completing the various questionnaires that you received before our meeting. I have reviewed the information that you provided on these forms. In this interview, I would like to hear more about your concerns about [child's name]. Your perspective as a parent is very important for understanding him [her].
>
> "To begin, let's talk about confidentiality issues. You have already voluntarily consented to have [child's name] receive an evaluation. This interview is part of my evaluation of [child's name]. The information you provide will be summarized in a written evaluation report. My usual practice is not to include direct quotations of parents' comments in written reports. I will try to respect your privacy by not reporting information that is not relevant for understanding [child's name]'s functioning and planning appropriate interventions/treatment. We can discuss what information will and will not be included in a written evaluation report at the end of this interview, if you wish.
>
> "There are circumstances under which the law requires clinicians to disclose confidential information. These circumstances include when there is reason to suspect child abuse or when the child poses a danger to self or a danger to other persons. Do you understand these limits to confidentiality?"

STRATEGIES FOR INTERVIEWING PARENTS

The ideal interview climate is one of open and responsive collaboration between the interviewer and parent, with each party showing respect for the other. However, as pointed out in Chapter 1, clinical interviews are not like ordinary conversations. Because their purpose is essentially information gathering, clinical interviews can arouse considerable anxiety in many parents. Some parents may be reluctant to discuss personal matters because they are afraid of what the information might reveal about themselves, their children, or their family, or what may happen next. Some parents may actually fear you as an interviewer, because they feel socially inferior or ignorant or think that you blame them for their children's difficulties. Other parents may view you as some kind of "miracle worker" who has all the answers for dealing with their children's problems. Parents from different ethnic or cultural backgrounds may feel that you are not capable of understanding their views and attitudes about their children, or may feel, for some reason, that you are insensitive to their ethnic or cultural views. In addition, some parents themselves may have had unpleasant experiences in school, which have made them leery of dealing with any school-based practitioners.

Any one or more of the above parental perspectives can raise a barrier to good clinical interviewing. Being sensitive to these potential perspectives is the first step toward ameliorating their impact. It is important to take time to establish rapport with parents, while also using interview time efficiently. Addressing parents as experts on their children is a good way to show respect. You can start by stating that they, the parents, probably know their child better than anyone else. Then assure parents that their perspective is important for understanding the child. Be careful to phrase questions in ways that do not assign blame to parents (or teachers) for the child's problems. Also avoid starting the interview with reports of teachers' concerns or a litany of people's negative comments about the child. Instead, explain that you want to hear the parents' views on their child's functioning and what they think might help to address their concerns about their child.

Many of the interviewing strategies discussed in Chapter 2 for semistructured clinical interviews with children also apply to parent interviews. As a general strategy, semistructured interviews with parents can be built around a series of open-ended questions to introduce a topic, followed by more focused questions about specific problems or areas of concern. As the interview progresses, you can use several strategies to facilitate effective communication. Busse and Beaver (2000) used the acronym PACERS for the following strategies: paraphrasing, attending, clarifying, eliciting, reflecting, and summarizing.

Paraphrasing is restating or summarizing the content of what has been said by the interviewee. To paraphrase what the parent has said without restating every word exactly, use key words or phrases. This shows that you heard what was said and gives the parent the opportunity to agree or correct misconceptions.

Attending involves comments that show the interviewee that you are paying attention. These include "minimal encouragers" (e.g., "uh-huh") and repeating one or two key words (e.g., "You're feeling discouraged . . . ") to encourage the parent to say more about something.

Clarifying involves paraphrasing or restating comments or asking questions to ensure that you, the interviewer, have understood what the interviewee said. You can also ask more specific questions to elicit specific examples of a problem (or competency) that the parent reported about the child. Section II of the Semistructured Parent Interview gives examples of clarifying probes about specific problems: "When [child's name] has this problem(s), what exactly does he [she] do? What does he [she] say? Give me some examples of this problem." These kinds of questions help to define the problem in concrete, observable terms.

Eliciting involves asking questions or stating direct requests to gather more information or to obtain specific details. Polite direct requests in the form of a "soft command" (e.g., "Tell me more about _____") make it clear that you want more information. However, you should use these requests sparingly so as not to make the interview seem like an interrogation, especially when interviewing anxious or angry parents. You can also ask specific questions to gather details about antecedents, consequences, and circumstances surrounding specific problems of concern, as outlined in Section II of the Semistructured Parent Interview. One caveat is not to disguise judgmental statements in the form of clarifying questions (e.g., "Don't you think that Andy would do better if you supervised his homework?")

Reflecting involves rephrasing affect or the emotional aspects of the interviewee's statements. This is different from paraphrasing because instead of focusing on the content of what was reported, it validates or clarifies the parent's reactions to the problem (e.g., "Sounds like it is pretty frustrating for you to always have to remind Andy to do his homework"). Reflecting can help maintain rapport by showing empathy for, and concern about, the difficulties faced by the parent. It is also important to pay attention to nonverbal cues, such as facial expressions, gestures, and tone of voice, to ascertain the emotional aspects of what parents report. Another caveat, however, is to avoid letting reflective statements turn the interview into a rant or diatribe of negative feelings or complaints about the child or other people. Too much negativity can undermine constructive problem solving later on. You also run the risk of sounding patronizing if you seem too sympathetic.

Summarizing is stating the key issues and themes that have been covered on a topic. This is different from paraphrasing because it covers more information and a longer time span of the interview. Summarizing is a good way to end one topic and move to another. It is also a good strategy for moving the interview along when a parent is getting off track or is going into excessive detail about some topic. At the end of the entire interview, you should summarize the key themes and concerns that were discussed in order to provide closure. Concluding the interview with a summary is also a good way to move into discussing what information you want to highlight in your written evaluation reports and/or follow-up meetings with other people.

Many of the "dos and don'ts" listed in Table 2.2 for child clinical interviews also apply to parent interviews, with appropriate modifications for speaking to adults. Among these, several "don'ts" are especially good to keep in mind. Avoid asking too many factual questions that make the interview seem like an interrogation or fact-finding mission. Avoid questions with obvious right answers or desirable responses. Avoid "why" questions that elicit motives or may seem accusatory to parents. Avoid using psychological or educational jargon, especially if it may not be understood, may seem demeaning, or make you seem superior to the parent.

Interviewing Culturally or Linguistically Diverse Parents

Interviewing parents with different ethnic or cultural backgrounds from the interviewer presents additional challenges. Several other authors have provided guidelines for assessing children and families from diverse cultural and linguistic backgrounds. Rhodes et al. (2005) devoted an entire book to this topic. Sattler (1998) provided a good summary of demographics and special issues to consider when interviewing African Americans, Hispanic Americans, Asian Americans, Native Americans, and refugees. Castillo, Quintana, and Zamarripa (2000) and Nuttall et al. (2003) also provided guidelines for assessing children from different cultural and ethnic groups, as discussed in Chapter 2. Drawing from these authors and my own experiences, the following key recommendations can be applied to parent interviews:

• Choose a neutral place that is private and comfortable for the parent interview. Avoid using offices of authority figures (e.g., the principal's office) or the child's classroom. Provide chairs appropriately sized for adults. Avoid sitting behind a desk because this can seem intimidating.

• Determine the parent's preferred language before beginning the interview. If the parent speaks English, do not assume that this is the preferred language or that the parent necessarily will understand the nuances of interview questions in English.

• If necessary, use a well-trained interpreter or another adult family member or trusted person as an interpreter. Avoid using children or siblings of the referred child as interpreters. Be sure to explain the purpose of the interview to the interpreter. Ask the interpreter to translate the parent's responses verbatim rather than paraphrasing or making his/her own interpretations of what the parent meant.

• As indicated earlier, provide a clear, concise explanation of privacy and confidentiality. Tell the parent that you plan to take notes to remember the interview, and that you will keep your notes in a confidential, secure place. If you want to tape-record the interview, ask the parent's permission ahead of time. (Tape recording may be very intimidating to some parents.)

• Speak clearly and avoid idioms, slang expressions, and statements with double meanings. At the same time, do not talk down to parents in a way that suggests they have low intelligence.

• Try to be sensitive and respectful of parents' cultural perspectives and value systems, even if they are different from your own. Try to see the strengths of different cultural coping mechanisms that can be marshaled for interventions.

• Try to avoid making judgments about children and families based on stereotypes or preconceived notions regarding ethnic and cultural backgrounds, socioeconomic status, or child-rearing practices.

TOPIC AREAS FOR SEMISTRUCTURED PARENT INTERVIEWS

The Semistructured Parent Interview (McConaughy, 2004a) in Appendix 5.1 is organized in a modular fashion for the six topic areas listed in Table 5.1. Interviewers can pick and choose topic areas and questions, depending on the referral concerns about a particular child. Interviewers can also skip certain topics or questions because of time constraints, parental sensitivities, or school policies regarding subject matter for interviews. The interview protocol lists sample questions for each topic area in the left-hand column. You should feel free to adapt these questions to fit your own style or the flow of the interview. The right-hand column provides space to record notes of parents' responses.

Concerns about the Child

After explaining confidentiality and purpose, it is usually good to begin the interview by asking parents for their current concerns about the child (Section I). This gives parents the message that you are there to hear what they have to say first. It also validates their unique expertise on their child. After hearing the major concerns, you can ask more specific questions about when they first became concerned about each problem area and how long the problem(s) has existed.

If parents' concerns are primarily about academic problems, you can move to questions in Section IV about school functioning, and later ask questions from other sections of the protocol, as

TABLE 5.1. Topic Areas for Semistructured Parent Interviews

  I. Concerns about the child

  II. Behavioral or emotional problems
      Specific nature of the problems
      Priorities for interventions
      Antecedents and consequences of priority problem(s)
      Other possible problem areas

  III. Social functioning
      Friends
      Social problems
      Fights/aggression
      Anxiety/depression
      Regarding adolescents
          Dating/romances
          Trouble with the law
          Alcohol/drugs

  IV. School functioning
      Subjects/grades/activities
      Special help/school services
      Teachers
      Homework
      Learning problems
      Retention
      School behavior problems
      Other school concerns

  V. Medical and developmental history
      Medical history
      Developmental history and temperament

  VI. Family relations and home situation
      Family composition
      Home environment
      Family relations
      Rules/punishments
      Chores/rewards
      Home environment

appropriate. If the parents' concerns are mostly about behavioral or emotional problems, you can move directly to questions in Section II.

Behavioral or Emotional Problems

The questions in Section II follow the general format for *behavioral interviewing* that has been discussed by many other authors (e.g., Busse & Beaver, 2000; Hughes & Baker, 1990; Merrell, 2003; Kratochwill & Shapiro, 2000; Shapiro & Kratochwill, 2000; Sheridan et al., 1996; Zins &

Erchul, 2002). Behavioral interviewing was developed in the context of behavioral consultation models (e.g., Bergan & Kratochwill, 1990; Sheridan et al. 1996) that involve four general stages of assessment and intervention planning: (1) identifying a problem; (2) analyzing the problem; (3) developing an intervention plan; and (4) evaluating the intervention plan. Interviewers can use the questions from Section II of the Semistructured Parent Interview, shown in Table 5.2, to accomplish the first two stages of this process.

The first step in identifying a problem is to obtain descriptions of the specific nature of the problem and the conditions under which the problem occurs. To do this, ask the parent to describe specific behaviors that can be observed and recognized by other people (e.g., "What exactly does the child do? What does he/she say?"). Then ask about the duration and frequency of each identified problem and the circumstances under which it occurs (e.g., "How long has he/she

TABLE 5.2. Sample Questions about Behavioral or Emotional Problems

Specific nature of the problems

When [child's name] has this problem, what exactly does he/she do? What does he/she say? Give me some examples of this problem.
Ask the parent to give specific descriptions of the problem. If there is more than one problem, ask about each one.

How long has he/she been having this problem?

How often does this problem occur?

Under what circumstances does this problem occur? Where and when does this problem usually occur?
Ask for specific descriptions of where and when each problem occurs at home and/or school.

Priorities for interventions

Which of the problems we have discussed are you most concerned about now? Which do you think is the most important to address now?

How would you rank the other problems in terms of your concerns and their importance for interventions?

Antecedents and consequences of priority problem(s)

Let's talk about the problem(s) you think are of most concern. What usually happens before this problem occurs? What seems to set it off?
If more than one area of concern, ask about the top two or three problems.

What usually happens after this problem occurs?
What do you do? What do other people do?

How do you usually deal with this problem at home?
How do you feel/react when this problem occurs?
What usually happens at school if this problem occurs?
How does [child's name] feel/react when this happens?

Replacement behaviors

What would be acceptable or alternative behavior related to this problem? What would you like to see [child's name] do instead?

What does [child's name] do well? What do you see as his/her strengths that might help address this problem(s)?

been having this problem? How often does this problem occur? Where and when does this problem usually occur?"). If the parent identifies more than one problem, ask for a description of each problem, and then ask the parent to prioritize the problems for planning interventions. Prioritizing may be hard for some parents who want to fix everything immediately. However, you can explain that it works better to select only a few problems to focus on at any one time, because this will allow you to collaborate better on appropriate interventions.

Functional Behavioral Assessment

After selecting two or three key problems, you can move to identifying antecedents and consequences of each specific problem, using questions such as those listed in Table 5.2. Identifying antecedents and consequences is important for obtaining a *functional behavioral assessment* (FBA) of each problem. Through FBA, you can develop hypotheses about why the problem is occurring and identify circumstances in the environment that are maintaining the problem. An underlying assumption of FBA is that problem behaviors serve some function or purpose for a child. Though there may be various reasons for problem behaviors, an FBA distills these down to three basic functions: (1) to increase social attention; (2) to escape or avoid aversive (unpleasant) tasks or situations; or (3) to serve as self-reinforcement (pleasure). You can then move from hypotheses about the function of problem behaviors to develop a *behavioral intervention plan* (BIP). The 1997 amendments to the IDEA and its 1999 regulations require an FBA and BIP for children with disabilities under certain circumstances, such as changes in educational placement or school exclusion. Although these uses tend to be reactive applications, FBA and BIPs can be used as proactive strategies to develop positive behavioral support systems for many children in special education and general education settings (Crone, Horner, & Hawkin, 2004). Other authors have given detailed accounts of the steps for conducting an FBA and developing BIPs (e.g., see Fisher, 2003; McComas, Hoch, & Mace, 2000; Nelson, Roberts, & Smith, 1998). The U.S. Office of Special Education website also provides documents to assist practitioners in conducting FBAs and developing BIPs (Sugai et al., 1999; www.pbis.org/english/Center_Products.htm).

A key strategy for developing a good intervention plan is to identify acceptable alternative behaviors that might "replace" a child's problem behaviors. You should also look for strengths and competencies that can be marshaled in interventions. Table 5.2 lists additional questions that interviewers can ask about replacement behaviors and strengths (e.g., "What would be acceptable or alternative behavior related to this problem? What would you like to see [child's name] do instead? What does [child's name] do well?"). These questions turn the focus toward positive characteristics of the child, which can become important building blocks for a BIP. Focusing on the positive can strengthen rapport with parents of children who have behavioral or emotional problems, who often hear nothing but negative reports about their children.

Standardized Parent Rating Scales

The last part of Section II includes space for recording problem areas that have been reported by parents on standardized parent rating scales. This section is built on the assumption that the parent has completed a standardized parent rating scale prior to the interview. When this is done, interviewers can examine the scoring profiles to identify areas in which the child exhibits severe problems compared to normative samples. Table 5.3 summarizes characteristics of several standardized parent rating scales that can easily be incorporated into multimethod assessment procedures. The table lists the number of items and scales for each instrument, characteristics of the normative samples, and contact information for the publisher of each instrument.

Each of the instruments listed in Table 5.3 provides a scoring profile of scales that assess different patterns of problems and/or competencies. Standard scores for each scale help you identify areas in which a parent reported unusual problems or strengths for the child compared to normative samples of boys or girls of the same age range. For example, the ASEBA CBCL/6–18 (Achenbach & Rescorla, 2001) includes scales measuring empirically derived patterns of problems (Withdrawn/Depressed, Somatic Complaints, Anxious/Depressed, Social Problems, Thought Problems, Attention Problems, Rule-Breaking Behavior, Aggressive Behavior), plus problems consistent with DSM-IV diagnoses, as well as children's competencies (Activities, Social, School). The Adolescent Symptom Inventory–4 Parent Checklist (ASI-4; Gadow & Sprafkin, 1998) and Child Symptom Inventory–4 Parent Checklist (CSI-4; Gadow & Sprafkin, 2002) assess problems consistent with DSM-IV disorders. The BASC-2 Parent Rating Scales (Reynolds & Kamphaus, 2004) includes a variety of problem scales (Hyperactivity, Aggression, Conduct Problems, Anxiety, Depression, Somatization, Attention Problems, Atypicality, Withdrawal) and adaptive scales (Adaptability, Social Skills, Leadership, Activities of Daily Living, Functional Communication). The Behavioral and Emotional Rating Scale—Second Edition (BERS-2; Epstein, 2004) assesses patterns of behavioral and emotional strengths (Interpersonal Strengths, School Functioning, Intrapersonal Strengths, Family Strengths, Affective Strengths, and Career Strengths). Other rating scales listed in Table 5.3 assess problems and/or social behaviors and social skills.

After examining the scoring profile of a standardized rating scale, you can list problem scales with deviant scores in the spaces provided in Section II of the Semistructured Parent Interview protocol. This list can prompt you to ask parents about problem areas that have not already been discussed. If parents acknowledge concerns about these problem areas, you can ask further questions about circumstances surrounding the problems and whether anything has been done to address the problems. You can also ask about situations outside the home that might affect the child's behavior. It is usually good to avoid going into much detail in this part of the interview so as not to overwhelm the parent or prolong the interview. However, questions about other possible problems can broaden the focus for formulating a comprehensive picture of the child.

Social Functioning

Section III of the Semistructured Parent Interview contains questions about children's social functioning, as shown in Table 5.4. Section III questions are modeled on similar questions for child clinical interviews, as discussed in Chapters 3 and 4. The similarity between parent and child interview questions makes it easier to compare the two perspectives on the child's social functioning.

Section III begins with open-ended questions about the child's friendships (e.g., "How many close friends does [child's name] have?"), and social activities (e.g., "Do other kids come to your house to play/do things with [child's name]? Does he/she belong to any clubs or social groups?"). Additional questions ask about social problems, fights, aggressive behavior, anxiety, and depression. Each of the latter three topic areas begins with a structured question, asking whether the child has exhibited that type of problem. Interviewers can check boxes on the form to indicate the

TABLE 5.3. Examples of Published Standardized Parent Rating Scales

Instrument and scales	Items and scales	Normative samples	Publisher
ASEBA[a] Child Behavior Checklist for Ages 1½–5 (CBCL/1½–5; Achenbach & Rescorla, 2000)	100 items *Problem Scales* Total Problems, Internalizing, Externalizing, Emotionally Reactive, Anxious/Depressed, Somatic Complaints, Withdrawn, Sleep Problems, Attention Problems, Aggressive Behavior, Affective Problems, Anxiety Problems, Pervasive Developmental Problems, Attention/Deficit Hyperactivity Problems, Oppositional Defiant Problems	Combined norms for boys and girls, ages 1½–5	Research Center for Children, Youth, and Families, Inc. One South Prospect Street Burlington, VT 05401-3456 802-264-6432 www.ASEBA.org
ASEBA[a] Child Behavior Checklist For Ages 6–18 (CBCL/6–18; Achenbach & Rescorla, 2001)	20 competence and 120 problem items *Problem Scales* Total Problems, Internalizing, Externalizing, Withdrawn/Depressed, Somatic Complaints, Anxious/Depressed, Social Problems, Thought Problems, Attention Problems, Rule-Breaking Behavior, Aggressive Behavior, Affective Problems, Anxiety Problems, Attention/Deficit Hyperactivity Problems, Oppositional Defiant Problems, Conduct Problems *Competence/Adaptive Scales* Total Competence, Activities, Social, School	Separate norms for boys and girls, ages 6–11 and 12–18	Research Center for Children, Youth, and Families, Inc. One South Prospect Street Burlington, VT 05401-3456 802-264-6432 www.ASEBA.org
Adolescent Symptom Inventory–4 Parent Checklist (ASI-4; Gadow & Sprafkin, 1998)	120 items *Problem Scales* 15 DSM-IV Disorders	Separate norms for boys and girls, ages 12–18 (secondary school)	Checkmate Plus P.O. Box 696 Stony Brook, NY 11790-0696 800-779-4292 www.checkmateplus.com
Behavior Assessment System for Children–2 Parent Rating Scales (BASC-2 PRS; Reynolds & Kamphaus, 2004)	134–160 items *Problem Scales* Behavioral Symptoms Index, Externalizing, Internalizing, Hyperactivity, Aggression, Conduct Problems (ages 6–18), Anxiety, Depression,	Separate norms for boys and girls, ages 2–5, 6–11, 12–18	American Guidance Service 4201 Woodland Road Circle Pines, MN 55014-1796 800-328-2560 www.agsnet.com

Measure	Content	Norms	Publisher/Contact
(continued from previous page)	Somatization, Attention Problems, Atypicality, Withdrawal *Competence/Adaptive Scales* Adaptive Skills Composite, Adaptability, Social Skills, Leadership (ages 6–18), Activities of Daily Living, Functional Communication		
Behavioral and Emotional Rating Scale (2nd edition) Parent Rating Scale (BERS-2; Epstein, 2004)	57 items *Competence/Adaptive Scales* Total Strengths Score, Interpersonal Strengths, School Functioning, Intrapersonal Strengths, Family Strengths, Affective Strengths, Career Strengths	Separate norms for boys and girls, ages 5–18	PRO-ED 8700 Shoal Creek Boulevard Austin, TX 78757-6897 800-879-3202 www.proedinc.com
Child Symptom Inventory–4 Parent Checklist (CSI-4; Gadow & Sprafkin, 2002)	97 items *Problem Scales* 13 DSM-IV Disorders	Separate norms for boys and girls, ages 5–12 (elementary school)	Checkmate Plus P.O. Box 696 Stony Brook, NY 11790-0696 800-779-4292 www.checkmateplus.com
Conners Rating Scales—Revised Parent Form (CRS-R-P; Conners, 1997)	27 items (short form) *Problem Scales* ADHD Index, Oppositional, Hyperactivity, Cognitive Problems/Inattention	Separate norms for boys and girls, ages 3–5, 6–8, 9–11, 12–14, 15–17	MHS P.O. Box 950 North Tonawanda, NY 14120-0950 800-456-3003 www.mhs.com
Devereux Behavior Rating Scale School Form (DBRS; Naglieri, LeBuff, & Pfeiffer, 1993)	40 items *Problem Scales* Total Problems, Interpersonal Problems, Inappropriate Behaviors/Feelings, Depression, Physical Symptoms/Fears	Separate norms for boys and girls, ages 5–12 and 13–18	Harcourt Assessment, Inc. 19500 Academic Court San Antonio, TX 78204-2498 800-211-8378 www.psychcorpcenter.com
Early Childhood Inventory–4 Parent Checklist (ECI-4; Gadow & Sprafkin, 2000)	120 items *Problem Scales* 14 DSM-IV Disorders Developmental Deficits Index Peer Conflict Scale	Separate norms for boys and girls, ages 3–6 (pre-elementary school)	Checkmate Plus P.O. Box 696 Stony Brook, NY 11790-0696 800-779-4292 www.checkmateplus.com

(continued)

TABLE 5.3. (continued)

Instrument and scales	Items and scales	Normative samples	Publisher
Home and Community Social Behavior Scales (HCSBS; Merrell & Caldarella, 2001)	64 items *Problem Scales* Antisocial Behavior Total, Defiant/Disruptive, Antisocial/Aggressive *Competence/Adaptive Scales* Social Competence Total, Peer Relations, Self-Management/Compliance	Combined norms for boys and girls, ages 5–11 and 12–18	Assessment–Intervention Resources 2285 Elysium Avenue Eugene, OR 97401 541-338-8736 www.assessment-intervention.com
Preschool and Kindergarten Behavioral Scales—Second Edition Parent Form (PKBS-2-P; Merrell, 2002a)	76 items *Problem Scales* Total Problem Behavior, Internalizing, Externalizing *Competence/Adaptive Scales* Total Social Skills, Social Cooperation, Social Interaction, Social Independence	Combined norms for boys and girls, ages 3–6	PRO-ED 8700 Shoal Creek Boulevard Austin, TX 78757-6869 800-879-3202 www.proedinc.com
Social Skills Rating System—Parent Form (SSRS-P; Gresham & Elliott, 1990)	49–55 items *Problem Scales* Total Problems, Internalizing, Externalizing, Hyperactive (ages 6–11) *Competence/Adaptive Scales* Total Social Skills, Cooperation, Assertion, Responsibility, Self-Control	Separate norms for boys and girls, ages 3–5, grades K–6 and 7–12	American Guidance Service 4201 Woodland Road Circle Pines, MN 55014-1796 800-328-2560 www.agsnet.com

[a]ASEBA, Achenbach System of Empirically Based Assessment.

TABLE 5.4. Sample Questions about Social Functioning

Friends

How many close friends does [child's name] have? Do you think that is enough friends?
How do you feel about his/her choice of friends?

Do other kids come to your house to play/do things with [child's name]?
Does he/she go to other kids' houses?

Does he/she belong to any clubs or social groups (e.g., Scouts, YMCA, teams)?
Does he/she go to church/belong to any church or spiritual groups?

Social problems

Does [child's name] have any problems getting along with other kids (e.g., not liked, teased/picked on, feel left out)?
☐ Yes   ☐ No   ☐ Don't know

(If yes) Tell me more about his/her social problems.
Has anything been done to try to help him/her with social problems (e.g., see a counselor, social skills group, friendship group)?

Fights/aggression

Does [child's name] ever get into physical fights with other kids?
☐ Yes   ☐ No   ☐ Don't know

(If yes) How often?
What usually starts the fights?
How do they usually end?
Has anything been done to try to help him/her avoid fighting?

Do you think he/she has trouble controlling his/her temper?
Has he/she ever used a weapon or object (e.g., stick, stone) to hurt other kids?
Does he/she belong to a gang?

Anxiety/depression

Does [child's name] seem unusually anxious or worried about things?
☐ Yes   ☐ No   ☐ Don't know

(If yes) Tell me more about that.
What does he/she worry about?
Has [child's name] ever seemed very sad or depressed for a long period of time?
☐ Yes   ☐ No   ☐ Don't know

(If yes) Tell me more about that.
Has he/she ever made comments about wanting to harm or kill himself/herself?
Has he/she ever attempted to harm or kill himself/herself?
If yes, probe more regarding plans, attempts, access to methods, etc. Review confidentiality and legal reporting requirements. Discuss need for intervention.

Note. Reprinted from McConaughy (2004a). Copyright 2004 by S. H. McConaughy. Reprinted by permission.

parent's responses to each lead-in question ("yes," "no," "don't know"). If a parent answers "yes," then the interviewer can ask more specific questions to learn about the nature of the problem.

When parents report depression, it is important to follow up with questions about suicidal thoughts or attempts (e.g., "Has he/she ever made comments about wanting to harm or kill himself/herself? Has he/she ever attempted to harm or kill himself/herself?"). In cases where parents report suicidal thoughts or attempts, you should ask more specific questions regarding plans, how many attempts, access to methods (e.g., guns in the house, lethal pills), and deterrents to suicide. When there is sufficient cause to indicate risk for suicide, then you will need to discuss limits to confidentiality and legal reporting requirements, as well as need for intervention. Chapter 8 provides more detailed guidelines for assessing suicide risk.

Section III provides a format for querying parents about potential problems that is different from the behavioral interviewing format in Section II. If you do not want to conduct an FBA in the parent interview, you can skip Section II and use Section III to ask parents about behavioral and emotional problems. You can also select questions from Section III to cover potential problems that were not discussed in Section II. If a parent has not completed a standardized rating scale prior to the interview, Section III provides a structure for asking about potential problems of both an internalizing and externalizing nature.

The last part of Section III (see Appendix 5.1) includes questions for parents of adolescents that are modeled on similar questions for the child clinical interview. These cover dating and romances, trouble with the law, and alcohol and drug use. Interviewers can check boxes on the form to indicate the parent's responses to lead-in questions about trouble with the law and alcohol or drug problems. When parents report that an adolescent does have problems in these areas, the interviewer can ask questions about the nature of the problems, whether there have been any interventions or treatment for the problems, and whether the parent thinks the adolescent needs treatment.

School Functioning

Section IV of the Semistructured Parent Interview provides questions about children's school functioning, as shown in Table 5.5. Some of the questions about school subjects, teachers, and homework parallel similar questions in the child clinical interview. However, parents are asked about these areas in more detail. The initial questions are useful for all parents, to obtain their views on their child's school performance and relationships with school staff.

Section IV also includes questions about learning problems, special help or school services, retention, school behavior problems, and other school concerns. A structured lead-in question asks whether the child has exhibited problems in each of these areas. Because these questions focus more specifically on school problems, they may not be necessary or appropriate for parents of children who function well in school.

To facilitate efficiency in parent interviews, lead-in questions about learning problems, special help or school services, retention, and school behavior problems are tied to similar questions listed on the Child and Family Information Form (McConaughy & Achenbach, 2004a) in Appendix 5.2. This background questionnaire covers demographic information, the child's school history, medical and developmental history, family history, and current living situation. As a routine practice, parents can be asked to complete the Child and Family Information Form prior to appointments for the parent interview and assessment of their child. You can then review the

TABLE 5.5. Sample Questions about School Functioning

Subjects/grades/activities

What are [child's name]'s best subject areas in school? What does he/she like best?
What are [child's name]'s worst subject areas, if any? What does he/she like the least in school?

What kind of grades does he/she get? *Ask about each subject area.*
Have his/her grades changed remarkably in any area?

What are his/her extracurricular activities (e.g., sports, clubs, school play, band, choir)?
Does [child's name] have any problems with school attendance/skipping classes?

Teachers

How many teachers does [child's name] have?
How does he/she get along with each teacher?
How does he/she get along with the principal and other school staff?
Is there anyone at school who is especially important to him/her?

Homework

How much homework does [child's name] typically have? How do you feel about the amount of homework he/she has?

Does he/she have any trouble with homework?
(*If yes*) Tell me more about that.
When and where does he/she usually do homework?
How long does homework usually take?
How much time do you think he/she should spend on homework?
Does he/she get any help with homework?
(*If yes*) How does that work out?

Learning problems

Does [child's name] have learning problems?
☐ Yes   ☐ No   ☐ Don't know
[*See Child and Family Information Form*]

(*If yes*) What kind of learning problems?
Why do you think [child's name] is having learning problems right now?
How long has he/she had these problems?
What has been done to address these problems?

Special help/school services

Does [child's name] receive any special help/special services in school?
☐ Yes   ☐ No   ☐ Don't know
[*See Child and Family Information Form*]

(*If yes*) What kind of help?
Probe for special education, IEP, remedial instruction/Title I services, Section 504 plan, peer tutoring, individual aide, behavior plan, guidance services, school psychologist.

How long has he/she had this special help?
How often does he/she get this help?
What kinds of help has he/she had in the past?

Do you think this is enough help/the right kind of help?
What else would you like to have happen for [child's name] at school?

(continued)

TABLE 5.5. *(continued)*

Retention

Has [child's name] ever been retained/held back a grade?

☐ Yes   ☐ No   ☐ Don't know
[*See Child and Family Information Form*]

(*If yes*) When? For what reason?
How did [child's name] feel about being retained/held back?
How did you feel about his/her being retained/held back?

School behavior problems

Does [child's name] have behavior problems at school?

☐ Yes   ☐ No   ☐ Don't know
[*See Child and Family Information Form*]

(*If yes*) What kind of problems?
What usually happens at school when he/she has these problems?
What has been done to address these problems?

Other school concerns

Do you have other school concerns?

☐ Yes   ☐ No   ☐ Don't know
[*See Child and Family Information Form*]

(*If yes*) What kind of concerns?
What has been done to address these concerns?
If you could change something about school, what would it be?
What would you especially like to see happen for [child's name] at school?

Note. Reprinted from McConaughy (2004a). Copyright 2004 by S. H. McConaughy. Reprinted by permission.

questionnaire prior to your parent interview to learn about particular areas of concern. You can check boxes ("yes," "no," "don't know") in Section IV of the Semistructured Parent Interview protocol to indicate how parents responded to each question on the Child and Family Information Form. During your interview, you can then ask parents to elaborate on areas reported as problems. If parents have not completed the Child and Family Information Form ahead of time, you can ask about each school problem area, as appropriate.

When parents report that their child has learning problems in school, it is important to elicit their perspectives on these problems and learn what they think about any special help to address the problems. When asking about school services, it is important to probe for several possibilities (e.g., special education, IEP, remedial instruction/Title I services, Section 504 plan, peer tutoring, individual aide, behavior plan, guidance services, school psychologist), because parents may not think some of these constitute "special help." Teachers may or may not report similar problems and may have more detailed information on school interventions (see Chapter 6). In my experience, lack of sufficient or appropriate services has often been a key parental complaint and source of tension between parents and school staff.

It is also good to ask whether the child has repeated a grade, because grade retention can be a marker for past, current, and future learning or behavioral problems. It is estimated that as many as 15% of U.S. students are held back each year, even though research has indicated that retention is not an effective strategy for improving educational success (National Association of

School Psychologists, 2003a). Retention is often a key worry for elementary school children and may have negative effects on their self-confidence. Section IV also includes questions about school behavior problems. However, if these have already been covered in earlier parts of the parent interview (e.g., Section I), it is not necessary to ask parents about such problems again.

In interviews with parents, school-based practitioners should make a special effort to maintain a neutral stance regarding children's school problems and special help or services so as to encourage parents to express their views openly. Appearing too closely aligned with school staff can undermine rapport and become a barrier to obtaining parental cooperation in intervention efforts.

Medical and Developmental History

Section V covers aspects of medical and developmental history. Learning about the child's history is important for understanding the nature of current problems. Interviewers of parents in mental health and medical settings often devote considerable time to taking medical and developmental histories (e.g., Barkley, 2006; Barkley & Murphy, 2006). However, asking detailed questions about the child's history can become very tedious and unnecessarily prolong parent interviews for school-based assessments. To reduce time requirements, the questions in Section V are tied to similar questions on the Child and Family Information Form (Appendix 5.2). If parents have completed this background questionnaire prior to the interview, you can take the same approach as the one noted for questions about school problems. That is, review the Child and Family Information Form ahead of time and ask for elaboration only on medical and developmental problems reported present by parents. If parents have not completed the Child and Family Information Form, you can briefly review each area listed in Section V of the parent interview.

Family Relations and Home Situation

Section VI of the Semistructured Parent Interview asks about the child's family and the home environment. This section was placed last in the protocol because it can be a very sensitive area of discussion for many parents. As indicated earlier, some parents may be reluctant to discuss what transpires at home because they consider these private matters. Parents may also worry that school-based practitioners blame them and the home situation for their child's problems. If you begin your interview with such sensitive topics, parents may be unwilling to continue or may be less forthcoming when discussing other issues.

Some of the questions in Section VI are tied to the Child and Family Information Form. With this in mind, you can use that background questionnaire as an entrée to asking about family composition and the home environment. If the parents are divorced or separated, it is important to learn who has legal custody and what visiting arrangements have been made for the child. In cases without joint custody arrangements, you should ask what information, if any, may be shared with the noncustodial parent. The Child and Family Information Form contains specific questions about family history of medical, mental health, and learning problems as well as the child's current living situation. After reviewing this information, you can ask about specific problems that parents reported on the questionnaire. If parents have not completed the Child and Family Information Form, you can ask more general questions about the family and home environment (e.g., "Is there anything about your home or living situation that is a problem for you or the family?

TABLE 5.6. Sample Questions about Family Relations and Home Situation

<u>Family relations</u>

How does [child's name] get along with members of the family/people in your home?
Ask about the child's relationship with each member of the family, as appropriate: father, mother, stepparents, other adults in home, other caregivers, siblings, stepsiblings.

Who does [child's name] get along with best?
Who does [child's name] get along with least?

Do members of the family have trouble getting along?

Do you have any problems getting along with members of the family (e.g., spouse/partner, your children, relatives, other adults or children in the home)?

<u>Rules/punishments</u>

What are the rules/expectations about behavior in your home? Who makes the rules?
How do you think [child's name] feels about the rules?
What kinds of punishments/discipline procedures are used in your home?
Do children ever get spanked/physically punished for bad behavior?

Who usually gives the punishments/disciplines children in the family?
Do you and your spouse/partner agree on punishments/discipline?
How do you think [child's name] feels about the punishments/discipline?

Have you ever talked with someone else about punishment/discipline (e.g., counselor, teacher, friend, relative)?
Would you like help in discipline or behavior management?

<u>Chores/rewards</u>

What happens when a child does something good or special?
Do you give out any special rewards or treats for good behavior/accomplishments?
Does this ever happen for [child's name]?

Does [child's name] have any special chores/jobs at home?
Does he/she get an allowance? (*If yes*) What does he/she have to do for it?
Does he/she have a paying job outside the home?

Note. Reprinted from McConaughy (2004a). Copyright 2004 by S. H. McConaughy. Reprinted by permission.

Have there been any recent changes or stresses in your living situation or family? Do any family members have medical or mental health problems that might affect [child's name]?").

Other questions in Section VI parallel questions in the child clinical interview (see Chapters 3 and 4). These concern family relations, rules and punishments, and chores and rewards for the child, as shown in Table 5.6. Answers to these types of questions can be very helpful for planning interventions for children with behavioral and emotional problems. For example, some parents may resort to harsh or excessive punishments (e.g., frequent spanking; no TV for the rest of the year; "grounding" for long periods of time) that are ineffective for changing children's behavior. Other parents may report few or no rules or punishments in the home and poor supervision of their children's whereabouts. Research has shown strong associations between children's externalizing problems and poor parental supervision and/or harsh discipline strategies (McMahon & Estes, 1997; McMahon & Forehand, 2003). Asking about reward systems in the home can also identify positive incentives for the child that might be incorporated into school-based interventions. Asking about chores can give some indication whether the child has age-appropriate responsibilities and opportunities to earn monetary rewards, such as an allowance.

Some parents may report no use of rewards in the home, which could exacerbate problems arising from ineffective discipline and harsh punishments.

As indicated earlier, interviewers should frame questions about family issues in ways that do not imply that parents have caused their children's problems. Instead, the challenge is to recruit parents' cooperation in identifying problems and developing appropriate interventions. Helping parents feel respected and treated as equal partners with school staff in problem-solving efforts can go a long way toward building effective home–school collaboration on behalf of children with learning and behavior problems (Kay, Fitzgerald, & McConaughy, 2001; McConaughy, Kay, & Fitzgerald, 2000).

STRUCTURED DIAGNOSTIC INTERVIEWS WITH PARENTS

For certain purposes, school-based practitioners may want to determine whether a child meets criteria for a DSM-IV psychiatric diagnosis. Countless research studies have focused on children with psychiatric diagnoses. Among these are epidemiological studies that have examined the prevalence of psychiatric disorders in general population samples. Doll (1996) reviewed 12 epidemiological studies published after 1986. Based on prevalence rates from these studies, she estimated that a hypothetical school of 1,000 students could be expected to have between 180 to 220 students with diagnosable psychiatric disorders. Such high prevalence estimates suggest that large percentages of school-age children (18–22%) exhibit behavioral and emotional problems that warrant mental health services. From her review, Doll (1996) concluded that "the numbers alone are overwhelming," especially when you consider that the National Association of School Psychologists (1992) recommended a ratio of one school psychologist per 1,000 students.

Utility of Psychiatric Diagnoses

Given the unmet needs identified in research studies, new efforts are being made to forge links between community mental health clinics and schools to provide services to children with mental health problems (Nastasi, 1998; National Association of School Psychologists, 2003b). Psychiatric diagnoses are especially useful for referrals for mental health services in or outside of school. For such cases, psychiatric diagnoses may facilitate communication between school-based practitioners and professionals in mental health and hospital settings (e.g., psychiatrists, clinical psychologists, social workers). In addition, psychiatric diagnoses are often required for reimbursements by third-party payers, including Medicaid, private insurance companies, and health maintenance organizations (HMOs).

Although some experts have questioned the utility of psychiatric diagnoses for planning school-based interventions (Gresham & Gansle, 1992), they can be useful for identifying children who are eligible for certain types of services. For example, children with disabilities may be eligible for a Section 504 plan under the Rehabilitation Act of 1973 (Rehabilitation Act, 1973) and its revisions in the Americans with Disabilities Act of 1990 (Americans with Disabilities Act, 1990). A psychiatric diagnosis is one form of "disability" covered in these federal civil rights statutes. Section 504 plans outline accommodations in the general education setting, which can serve as alternatives to special education services. Use of section 504 plans is often the route taken for children with ADHD. Children with diagnoses of mood disorders (depression or anxiety) and some children with CD or ODD may also qualify for Section 504 plans. The key determinant is whether the child's disability has a negative impact on "learning" or "alertness" and interferes with life functioning.

Psychiatric diagnoses are not required for eligibility for special education services under the IDEA. Instead, the IDEA has its own definitions of disabilities, including mental retardation (MR), specific learning disabilities (LD), emotional disturbance (ED), and seven other categories. However, a psychiatric diagnosis may provide additional assessment information that is helpful in deciding whether a child meets the IDEA criteria for a disability. For example, children with diagnoses of mood disorders may qualify as having ED. Some children with diagnoses of disruptive disorders (ADHD, CD, ODD) may also qualify as having ED, though this usage has generated controversy among school-based practitioners and administrators (Skiba & Grizzle, 1991, 1992). Children with ADHD (but no ED or LD) may be eligible for special education under the IDEA disability category of "other health impairment," which also covers other chronic health conditions (e.g., seizure disorders, cerebral palsy).

DSM-IV lists specific features, or symptoms, for over 40 numerically coded disorders of childhood and adolescence. Several adult disorders may also be used for children and adolescents. Table 5.7 lists examples of DSM-IV diagnoses that are commonly applied to children and adolescents. For each disorder, practitioners must decide whether the child exhibits a specified list of symptoms over a particular period of time (e.g., the past 6 or 12 months). They must then determine whether each symptom reported as "present" produces "clinically significant impairment" in social, academic, or occupational functioning, or impairment in different settings (e.g., home, school, or work). Some diagnoses require that at least some of the symptoms have occurred before a certain age (e.g., prior to age 7 for ADHD). Practitioners must also rule out other diagnoses that might account for the symptoms. An individual qualifies for the diagnosis if he/she exhibits the required number of symptoms, shows impairment, and meets other specified criteria (e.g., age of onset).

Structured Parent Interviews

Interviews with parents are key assessment procedures for making DSM-IV diagnoses. The American Academy of Pediatrics (2000) has also stressed the importance of parent interviews in its guidelines for assessment of ADHD. Since the 1970s, much effort has been devoted to developing highly structured protocols for interviewing parents about diagnostic criteria. Many of the

---

TABLE 5.7. Common DSM-IV Diagnoses Applied to Children and Adolescents

Attention-Deficit/Hyperactivity Disorder	Bipolar I Disorder: Manic Episode (296.xx)[a]
Combined Type (314.01)	Bipolar Disorder: Mixed Episode (296.xx) [a]
Predominantly Inattentive Type (314.00)	Dysthymic Disorder (300.4)
Predominantly Hyperactive–Impulsive Type, 314.01)	Generalized Anxiety Disorder (300.02)
Conduct Disorder (312.8)	Obsessive–Compulsive Disorder (300.3)
Oppositional Defiant Disorder (313.81)	Major Depressive Disorder (296.xx) [a]
Separation Anxiety Disorder (309.21)	Specific Phobia (300.29)
	Social Phobia (300.23)

[a]DSM-IV has specific criteria for the fourth and fifth digit codes indicated by the "xx" for these diagnoses.

parent interviews have parallel forms for children. However, research has shown much higher reliability and validity of structured diagnostic interviews with parents than with children (for reviews, see McConaughy, 2000b; Saigh, 1992).

The Diagnostic Interview for Children and Adolescents–IV (DICA-IV; Reich, 2000; Reich, Welner, Herjanic, et al., 1999) and the NIMH Diagnostic Interview Schedule for Children—Version IV (NIMH DISC-IV; Shaffer et al., 2000) are two examples of highly structured diagnostic interviews. A computerized version of DICA-IV is distributed by Multi-Health Systems (www.mhs.com). A computerized version of the NIMH DISC-IV is distributed by the Columbia University Department of Psychiatry (www.c-disc.com/disc.htm). The DICA-IV covers 28 DSM-IV diagnoses applicable to children. The NIMH DISC-IV covers approximately 30 diagnoses. Both of these interviews employ a standard set of questions and probes with specific response criteria. Questions are organized into a branching hierarchy with skip functions. A modular format allows interviewers to focus on subsets of specific diagnoses. The Child and Adolescent Psychiatric Assessment (CAPA; Angold & Costello, 2000) and Schedule for Affective Disorders and Schizophrenia for School-Age Children (K-SADS; Ambrosini, 2000) are other examples of diagnostic interviews. The CAPA and K-SADS are somewhat less structured than the DICA-IV and NIMH DISC-IV, but they still follow a standard set of questions and probes.

The structured diagnostic interviews were developed primarily for mental health assessment and research. Though it is good to be aware of these interview protocols, their length and detail render them impractical for most school-based assessments. For example, the full DICA-IV has approximately 1,600 questions, and the full NIMH DISC-IV has as many 3,000 questions. Administration time can vary from about 1 hour to 2 or 3 hours, depending on the number of diagnoses selected by the interviewer and symptoms endorsed by parents. All of the published diagnostic interviews require special training to administer.

Appendix 5.3 offers the Structured Diagnostic Interview for Parents as an alternative to the lengthier published interviews to screen for DSM-IV diagnoses. This parent interview is adapted from a structured diagnostic interview for assessing children with ADHD (Barkley, 2006; Barkley & Murphy, 2006). Practitioners can copy the interview protocol for their own use. It covers symptoms and other diagnostic criteria for all the DSM-IV disorders listed in Table 5.7, except Obsessive–Compulsive Disorder (OCD). Screening questions at the end of the interview cover OCD, plus Tic Disorders, Tourette's Disorder, and Psychotic Disorders. You can select disorders for your interview to match referral complaints about the child. However, for screening purposes, it is usually good to cover several of the more common disorders, such as ADHD, ODD, CD, Separation Anxiety Disorder, Dysthymic Disorder, or Major Depression, and perhaps Generalized Anxiety Disorder.

Practitioners who use the Structured Diagnostic Interview for Parents should have had appropriate training in theory and practice for making DSM-IV diagnoses. They should also have access to the DSM-IV manual (American Psychiatric Association, 2000) as a reference source for details regarding specific diagnoses. The interview should take about an hour or less, depending on how many symptoms a parent endorses as "present." More than an hour is likely to become very tedious for you and the parent. The interview may take longer if parents want to elaborate on certain symptoms. In these cases, you can limit the time requirements by explaining that they can tell you more about the child's symptoms after you have gone through all the questions. The protocol provides the following standard introduction for the interview:

"Now I need to ask you a number of very specific questions about a variety of behavioral, social, or emotional problems that children sometimes have difficulties with. As I ask you about these things, keep in mind that some of these things are not bad or abnormal and may be seen sometimes in healthy, normal children. I want you to tell me if your child does any of these things to a degree that you consider to be inappropriate for someone of his/her age and sex."

For some cases, you may want to use the Structured Diagnostic Interview for Parents (Appendix 5.3) instead of the Semistructured Parent Interview (Appendix 5.1) discussed in previous sections. Or you may decide to use both interview protocols, though this will, of course, require more time. For school-based assessments that do not require psychiatric diagnoses, the Semistructured Parent Interview is probably the better option, because of its flexibility and more conversational format. It also provides a more comprehensive assessment of a child's functioning and is more directly tied to issues that are important for school-based interventions. Regardless of which format you choose for the parent interview, data are needed from other sources for formulating conclusions about the child and making DSM-IV diagnoses.

CONCLUDING THE PARENT INTERVIEW

To conclude the parent interview, thank parents for sharing their perspectives and feelings about their child. Then briefly summarize what you learned about the child's current functioning: major problem areas, environmental and family circumstances surrounding the problems, and the child's competencies and strengths. Make sure that the "release of information to other parties" clause is clearly indicated on the parental consent form. You should also review the limits of confidentiality discussed at the beginning of the interview. Then discuss what family information you plan to report to other parties. Be open to excluding information that parents may not want to share with others. For school-based evaluations, in particular, it may not be necessary to include sensitive family history or circumstances in the home that are not directly relevant for placement decisions or intervention planning. If you plan to write a report, summarize the type of information that will be included and inform parents who will receive copies of your written reports. You should also tell parents about any follow-up meetings you will have with other parties, such as teachers. Whenever possible, arrange a subsequent meeting with parents to discuss the results of your complete evaluation, plans for any additional data collection, and potential interventions for the child.

SUMMARY

This chapter discussed the use of clinical interviews to obtain parents' perspectives on their children's functioning and offered guidelines for questioning strategies with parents, including suggestions for interviewing culturally and linguistically diverse parents. The Semistructured Parent Interview (Appendix 5.1) provides a framework with which to discuss a variety of issues that may be relevant to school-based interventions. The interview protocol first addresses parents' concerns about their children and then moves to more specific behavioral and emotional problems.

Practitioners can use this part of the interview to obtain a functional behavioral assessment of specific problems of concern. Interview questions about social functioning, school functioning, family relations, and home environment mirror similar inquiries in child clinical interviews. This parallel format facilitates comparisons between parents' and children's perspectives on these topics. More structured questions review medical and developmental history that may impinge upon a child's current functioning. The format of the Semistructured Parent Interview is built upon the assumption that practitioners will also use other procedures for obtaining parent reports, including standardized parent rating scales and background questionnaires. The Child and Family Information Form (Appendix 5.2) is a background questionnaire directly tied to the Semistructured Parent Interview.

Some practitioners may also want to obtain psychiatric diagnoses for certain purposes. The Structured Diagnostic Interview for Parents (Appendix 5.3) offers a format for interviewing parents about symptoms and criteria for common DSM-IV disorders applicable to children. The modular formats of the Structured Diagnostic Interview for Parents and the Semistructured Parent Interview allow practitioners to select topics and questions to fit their assessment purposes.

Semistructured Parent Interview

Child's name _____ Age _____ Gender _____
                First   Middle   Last

                                                              Relationship
Parent's name _____ to child _____
                First   Middle   Last

Interviewer's name _____ Date ____ / ____ / ____
                    First   Middle   Last   Month   Day   Year

CONFIDENTIALITY AND PURPOSE OF THE INTERVIEW

Thank you for taking your time to meet with me today and for completing the various questionnaires that you received before our meeting. I have reviewed the information that you provided on these forms. In this interview, I would like to hear more about your concerns about [child's name]. Your perspective as a parent is very important for understanding him/her.

To begin, let's talk about confidentiality issues. You have already voluntarily consented to have [child's name] receive an evaluation. This interview is part of my evaluation of [child's name]. The information you provide will be summarized in a written evaluation report. My usual practice is not to include direct quotations of parents' comments in written reports. I will try to respect your privacy by not reporting information that is not relevant for understanding [child's name]'s functioning and planning appropriate interventions/treatment. We can discuss what information will and will not be included in a written evaluation report at the end of this interview, if you wish.

There are circumstances under which the law require clinicians to disclose confidential information. These circumstances include when there is reason to suspect child abuse or when the child poses a danger to self or a danger to other persons. Do you understand these limits to confidentiality?

I. CONCERNS ABOUT THE CHILD	RESPONSES/COMMENTS
What concerns you most about [child's name]? *If the parent has more than one concern, list each area of concern.*	
When did you first become concerned about this? *If the parent has more than one concern, note when first concerned for each.*	
How long has this been a problem? *If the parent has more than one concern, note duration for each area of concern.* *If the parent's main concerns are about academic problems, ask questions in Section IV first and then return to Sections II and III. If the main concerns are about behavioral or emotional problems, continue with Section II.*	

(continued)

II. BEHAVIORAL OR EMOTIONAL PROBLEMS

Does [child's name] currently have behavioral or emotional problems?

☐ Yes   ☐ No   ☐ Don't know

(If yes) What kinds of problems?

Specific Nature of the Problems

When [child's name] has this problem, what exactly does he/she do? What does he/she say? Give me some examples of this problem. *Ask the parent to give specific descriptions of the problem. If there is more than one problem, ask about each one.*

How long has he/she been having this problem?

How often does this problem occur?

Under what circumstances does this problem occur? Where and when does this problem usually occur? *Ask for specific descriptions of where and when each problem occurs at home and/or school.*

Priorities for Interventions

Which of the problems we have discussed are you most concerned about now? Which do you think is the most important to address now?

How would you rank the other problems in terms of your concerns and their importance for interventions?

Antecedents and Consequences of Priority Problem(s)

Let's talk about the problem(s) you think are of most concern. What usually happens before this problem occurs? What seems to set it off? *If more than one area of concern, ask about the top two or three problems.*

What usually happens after this problem occurs? What do you do? What do other people do?

How do you usually deal with this problem at home?
How do you feel/react when this problem occurs?
What usually happens at school if this problem occurs?
How does [child's name] feel/react when this happens?

RESPONSES/COMMENTS

(continued)

113

	RESPONSES/COMMENTS

Replacement Behaviors

What would be acceptable or alternative behavior related to this problem? What would you like to see [child's name] do instead?

What does [child's name] do well? What do you see as his/her strengths that might help address this problem(s)?

Other Possible Problem Areas

If behavior rating scales (e.g., ASEBA Child Behavior Checklist or BASC-2 Parent Rating Scale) have been completed and scored prior to the interview, list all problem scales with scores in the borderline or clinical ranges (compared to the relevant normative sample). Summarize the results for the parent. Ask about problem areas that were not discussed as major concerns.

Before our meeting, you completed a questionnaire about [child's name]'s behavior. The questionnaire listed behaviors that can be scored on scales describing different problem areas. Your ratings produced scores indicating severe problems in:

_____

_____

_____

_____

_____

_____

_____

_____

We have already discussed some of these problem areas. What about the problem areas we have not discussed. How much are you concerned about these problems?

Under what circumstances do these problems occur?

What is currently being done to address these problems?

Are there any other areas where you think [child's name] has behavioral or emotional problems?

Do you have concerns about situations outside of your home that might affect [child's name]'s behavior or emotional functioning?

(continued)

	RESPONSES/COMMENTS
III. SOCIAL FUNCTIONING Now, let's talk about [child's name]'s social relationships and social behavior.	

Friends

How many close friends does [child's name] have? Do you think that is enough friends? How do you feel about his/her choice of friends?

Do other kids come to your house to play/do things with [child's name]?
Does he/she go to other kids' houses?

Does he/she belong to any clubs or social groups (e.g., Scouts, YMCA, teams)?
Does he/she go to church/belong to any church or spiritual groups?

Social Problems

Does [child's name] have any problems getting along with other kids (e.g., not liked, teased/picked on, feel left out)?
☐ Yes   ☐ No   ☐ Don't know

(*If yes*) Tell me more about his/her social problems.
Has anything been done to try to help him/her with social problems (e.g., see a counselor, social skills group, friendship group)?

Fights/Aggression

Does [child's name] ever get into physical fights with other kids?
☐ Yes   ☐ No   ☐ Don't know

(*If yes*) How often?
What usually starts the fights?
How do they usually end?
Has anything been done to try to help him/her avoid fighting?

Do you think he/she has trouble controlling his/her temper?
Has he/she ever used a weapon or object (e.g., stick, stone) to hurt other kids?
Does he/she belong to a gang?

Anxiety/Depression

Does [child's name] seem unusually anxious or worried about things?
☐ Yes   ☐ No   ☐ Don't know

(*If yes*) Tell me more about that.
What does he/she worry about?

(continued)

Anxiety/Depression *(cont.)*
Has [child's name] ever seemed very sad or depressed for a long period of time?
☐ Yes   ☐ No   ☐ Don't know

(If yes) Tell me more about that.
Has he/she ever made comments about wanting to harm or kill himself/herself?
Has he/she ever attempted to harm or kill himself/herself?
If yes, probe more regarding plans, attempts, access to methods, etc. Review confidentiality and legal reporting requirements. Discuss need for intervention.

REGARDING ADOLESCENTS:

Dating/Romances
Does he/she date? Have a boyfriend/girlfriend? Do you think he/she is sexually active? Does he/she know about safe sex practices?

Trouble with the Law
Has [child's name] ever been in trouble with the law or police?
☐ Yes   ☐ No   ☐ Don't know

(If yes) For what?
What happened when [child's name] got in trouble with the law/police?

Has [child's name] ever been in any traffic accidents? Had any traffic tickets?
☐ Yes   ☐ No   ☐ Don't know

Alcohol/Drugs
Does [child's name] smoke or chew tobacco?
☐ Yes   ☐ No   ☐ Don't know

Has [child's name] ever drunk beer, wine, or liquor?
☐ Yes   ☐ No   ☐ Don't know

Has [child's name] ever been drunk from alcohol?
☐ Yes   ☐ No   ☐ Don't know

(If yes) When and how often?
Do you think he/she has a problem with alcohol?

Has he/she ever received any help/treatment for alcohol problems?
Do you think he/she needs help/treatment for alcohol problems now?

RESPONSES/COMMENTS

(continued)

116

	RESPONSES/COMMENTS

Alcohol/Drugs *(cont.)*
Has [child's name] used drugs/been high on drugs?
☐ Yes ☐ No ☐ Don't know

(If yes) When and how often?
What kind of drugs?
Do you think he/she has a problem with drugs?

Has he/she ever received any help/treatment for drug problems?
Do you think he/she needs help/treatment for drug problems now?

IV. SCHOOL FUNCTIONING
Now let's discuss how [child's name] is doing in school.

Subjects/Grades/Activities
What are [child's name]'s best subject areas in school? What does he/she like best?
What are [child's name]'s worst subject areas, if any? What does he/she like the least in school?

What kind of grades does he/she get?
Ask about each subject area.
Have his/her grades changed remarkably in any area?

What are his/her extracurricular activities (e.g., sports, clubs, school play, band, choir)

Does [child's name] have any problems with school attendance/skipping classes?

Teachers
How many teachers does [child's name] have?
How does he/she get along with each teacher?
How does he/she get along with the principal and other school staff?
Is there anyone at school who is especially important to him/her?

Homework
How much homework does [child's name] typically have? How do you feel about the amount of homework he/she has?

(continued)

	RESPONSES/COMMENTS

Homework *(cont.)*

Does he/she have any trouble with homework?
(*If yes*) Tell me more about that.
When and where does he/she usually do homework?
How long does homework usually take?
How much time do you think he/she should spend on homework?
Does he/she get any help with homework?
(*If yes*) How does that work out?

Learning Problems

Does [child's name] have learning problems?
☐ Yes ☐ No ☐ Don't know
[*See Child and Family Information Form*]

(*If yes*) What kind of learning problems?
Why do you think [child's name] is having learning problems right now?
How long has he/she had these problems?
What has been done to address these problems?

Special Help/School Services

Examine the parent's responses on the Child and Family Information Form prior to your parent interview. Check "yes," "no," or "don't know" for the parent's reports about problems in each area listed below. Ask for more detail about problems marked "yes," as appropriate. If the parent has not completed the Child and Family Information Form, then ask about each problem area.

Does [child's name] receive any special help/special services in school?
☐ Yes ☐ No ☐ Don't know
[*See Child and Family Information Form*]

(*If yes*) What kind of help?
Probe for special education, IEP, remedial instruction/Title I services, Section 504 plan, peer tutoring, individual aide, behavior plan, guidance services, school psychologist.

How long has he/she had this special help?
How often does he/she get this help?
What kinds of help has he/she had in the past?

Do you think this is enough help/the right kind of help?
What else would you like to have happen for [child's name] at school?

(continued)

118

	RESPONSES/COMMENTS

Retention

Has [child's name] ever been retained/held back a grade?

☐ Yes ☐ No ☐ Don't know
[*See Child and Family Information Form*]

(*If yes*) When? For what reason?
How did [child's name] feel about being retained/held back?
How did you feel about his/her being retained/held back?

School Behavior Problems

Does [child's name] have behavior problems at school?

☐ Yes ☐ No ☐ Don't know
[*See Child and Family Information Form*]

(*If yes*) What kind of problems?
What usually happens at school when he/she has these problems?
What has been done to address these problems?

Other School Concerns

Do you have other school concerns?

☐ Yes ☐ No ☐ Don't know
[*See Child and Family Information Form*]

(*If yes*) What kind of concerns?
What has been done to address these concerns?

If you could change something about school, what would it be?

What would you especially like to see happen for [child's name] at school?

V. MEDICAL AND DEVELOPMENTAL HISTORY

Examine the parent's responses on the Child and Family Information Form prior to your parent interview. Check "yes," "no," or "don't know" for the parent's reports about problems in each area listed below. Ask for more detail about problems marked "yes," as appropriate. If the parent has not completed the Child and Family Information Form, then ask about each problem area.

Now, I would like to talk about [child's name]'s medical and developmental history. I have reviewed the information that you reported on the *Child and Family Information Form.* I would like to hear a little more about the problems you marked "yes."

(continued)

	RESPONSES/COMMENTS

Medical History

Current medications for behavior problems
☐ Yes ☐ No ☐ Don't know
[*See Child and Family Information Form*]

Current medications for other purposes
☐ Yes ☐ No ☐ Don't know
[*See Child and Family Information Form*]

Illnesses, accidents, operations, medical problems
☐ Yes ☐ No ☐ Don't know
[*See Child and Family Information Form*]

Allergies
☐ Yes ☐ No ☐ Don't know
[*See Child and Family Information Form*]

Problems with pregnancy and newborn period
☐ Yes ☐ No ☐ Don't know
[*See Child and Family Information Form*]

Developmental History and Temperament

Developmental delays
☐ Yes ☐ No ☐ Don't know
[*See Child and Family Information Form*]

Problems in temperament
☐ Yes ☐ No ☐ Don't know
[*See Child and Family Information Form*]

Problems in early behavior
☐ Yes ☐ No ☐ Don't know
[*See Child and Family Information Form*]

VI. FAMILY RELATIONS AND HOME SITUATION

Now I would like to talk about [child's name]'s family relations and home situation. I have reviewed the information you provided on the Child and Family Information Form. I want to hear your perspective on the family and home situation.

Family Composition

Who does [child's name] live with most of the time?
If the parents are divorced or separated, ask about visiting arrangements with each family.

Does he/she go to day care/have a day care provider other than the family? How well does that work out?

(continued)

120

Home Environment

Is there anything about your home or living situation that is a problem for you or the family (e.g., other persons living in the home, work situation, financial problems, neighborhood violence)?

Do any family members have medical or mental health problems that might affect [child's name]?

Have there been any recent major changes or stresses in your living situation or family?

Has anything happened to [child's name] that was very upsetting for him/her?
Probe further in cases of possible abuse or neglect: what happened, when, was it reported to authorities? Review confidentiality and legal reporting requirements in cases of suspected abuse.

Family Relations

How does [child's name] get along with members of the family/people in your home?
Ask about the child's relationship with each member of the family, as appropriate: father, mother, stepparents, other adults in home, other caregivers, siblings, stepsiblings.

Who does [child's name] get along with best? Who does [child's name] get along with least?

Do members of the family have trouble getting along?
Do you have any problems getting along with members of the family (e.g., spouse/partner, your children, relatives, other adults or children in the home)?

Rules/Punishments

What are the rules/expectations about behavior in your home? Who makes the rules?
How do you think [child's name] feels about the rules?
What kinds of punishments/discipline procedures are used in your home?
Do children ever get spanked/physically punished for bad behavior?

RESPONSES/COMMENTS

(continued)

121

Rules/Punishments *(cont.)*	RESPONSES/COMMENTS
Who usually gives the punishments/disciplines children in the family? Do you and your spouse/partner agree on punishments/discipline? How do you think [child's name] feels about the punishments/discipline? Have you ever talked with someone else about punishment/discipline (e.g., counselor, teacher, friend, relative)? Would you like help in discipline or behavior management? **Chores/Rewards** What happens when a child does something good or special? Do you give out any special rewards or treats for good behavior/accomplishments? Does this ever happen for [child's name]? Does [child's name] have any special chores/jobs at home? Does he/she get an allowance? (*If yes*) What does he/she have to do for it? Does he/she have a paying job outside the home?	

ASSESSING PSYCHIATRIC DIAGNOSES

This interview protocol is not intended for making psychiatric diagnoses, as defined in the American Psychiatric Association's (2000) *Diagnostic Manual for Mental Disorders—Fourth Edition, Text Revision* (DSM-IV). Interviewers should use other protocols to gather parent reports about symptoms and criteria for childhood DSM-IV disorders. The Structured Diagnostic Interview for Parents (Appendix 5.3) is an example of a brief structured diagnostic interview that can be used for this purpose. Other examples are the National Institutes of Mental Health's Diagnostic Interview Schedule for Children—Version IV (Shaffer et al., 2000) and the Diagnostic Interview for Children and Adolescents–IV (Reich et al., 1999).

CONCLUSION OF THE PARENT INTERVIEW

Conclude the interview by thanking the parent for sharing his/her perspective and feelings about the child. Briefly summarize the interview information about the child's current functioning: major problem areas, circumstances surrounding the problems, and the child's competencies and strengths. Tell the parent what family information will be included in a written evaluation report.

Review the limits of confidentiality. Discuss any concerns the parent may have about reporting information from the interview and/or parent questionnaires. Tell the parent who will receive copies of any written evaluation reports, as agreed upon in prior informed consents. Inform the parent of any follow-up meetings with school staff or other parties to discuss the evaluation results. If possible, arrange a follow-up meeting with the parent to discuss results of the evaluation and appropriate interventions or treatments, if needed.

APPENDIX 5.2

Child and Family Information Form

Today's date ___ / ___ / ___   Filled out by _____   Relationship to child _____

Mo. Day Year

Child's name _____

First   Middle   Last

Child's birthdate ___ / ___ / ___ Age ___ ☐ Boy ☐ Girl   Child's ethnic group/race _____

Mo. Day Year

Child's address _____

Street   City   State   Zip code

Health insurance for child: ☐ None ☐ Medicaid ☐ Private company (specify): _____

PERSONS WITH LEGAL CUSTODY OF CHILD

1. Name _____ Relationship to child _____

First   Middle   Last

Address _____

Street   City   State   Zip code

Home phone _____ Work phone _____ Cell phone _____

Birthdate ___ / ___ / ___ Highest education completed _____ Ethnic group/race _____

Mo. Day Year

Type of work _____ Place of work _____

Work day/hours _____ OK to contact at work? ☐ No ☐ Yes—when? _____

2. Name _____ Relationship to child _____

First   Middle   Last

Address _____

Street   City   State   Zip code

Home phone _____ Work phone _____ Cell phone _____

Birthdate ___ / ___ / ___ Highest education completed _____ Ethnic group/race _____

Mo. Day Year

Type of work _____ Place of work _____

Work day/hours _____ OK to contact at work? ☐ No ☐ Yes—when? _____

Whom does the child live with

Is the child adopted? ☐ No ☐ Yes   on a regular basis? _____

OTHER ADULTS AND CHILDREN LIVING IN THE CHILD'S HOME

Please list all other adults and children living with the child, if not listed above. Include stepsiblings, foster children, and related and unrelated adults.

Name	Age	Gender	Relationship to child
_____	_____	_____	_____
_____	_____	_____	_____
_____	_____	_____	_____

(continued)

Child and Family Information Form *(page 2 of 7)*

CHILD'S FULL OR HALF SIBLINGS NOT LIVING IN THE CHILD'S HOME

Name   Age   Gender   Relationship to child

_____ _____ _____ _____

_____ _____ _____ _____

_____ _____ _____ _____

BEST PERSON TO CONTACT FOR APPOINTMENTS FOR CHILD (if different from persons with legal custody)

Name _____ Relationship to child _____
           First   Middle   Last

Address _____
                   Street   City   State   Zip code

Home phone _____ Work phone _____ Cell phone _____

CHILD'S BIRTH PARENTS IF NOT PERSONS WITH LEGAL CUSTODY

1. Father's name _____ Birthdate ___/___/___
                 First   Middle   Last   Mo. Day Year

Address _____
                   Street   City   State   Zip code

Type of work _____ Highest education completed _____

Living? ☐ Yes ☐ No—year of death _____ Cause of death _____

Reason not living with child? _____ How often does he see the child? _____

2. Mother's name _____ Birthdate ___/___/___
                 First   Middle   Last   Mo. Day Year

Address _____
                   Street   City   State   Zip code

Type of work _____ Highest education completed _____

Living? ☐ Yes ☐ No—year of death _____ Cause of death _____

Reason not living with child? _____ How often does she see the child? _____

Because we occasionally do follow-up evaluations of our services or need to contact families for other reasons, we would appreciate having the names of two people who would know where to contact you if we are unable to reach you.

1. Name _____ Phone _____
           First   Middle   Last

Address _____
                   Street   City   State   Zip code

2. Name _____ Phone _____
           First   Middle   Last

Address _____
                   Street   City   State   Zip code

(continued)

Child and Family Information Form *(page 3 of 7)*

CONCERNS ABOUT CHILD

What are your concerns about the child? _____
_____
_____

What are the child's strengths? _____
_____
_____

What would you like to see happen for the child? _____
_____
_____

CHILD'S SCHOOL HISTORY

Child's school _____ Grade _____ Teacher _____

OK to contact school staff about the child? ☐ No   ☐ Yes—best person to contact _____

School address _____ Phone _____
           Street   City   State   Zip code

                                    If yes, please describe:

1. Has the child had learning problems?   ☐ No ☐ Yes _____
2. Has the child had behavior problems in school? ☐ No ☐ Yes _____
3. Has the child had social problems in school? ☐ No ☐ Yes _____
4. Is the child receiving any special help in school? ☐ No ☐ Yes _____
   (e.g., tutoring, special education, Section 504
   plan, guidance counselor?
5. Has the child ever been held back a grade? ☐ No ☐ Yes _____
6. Other school problems?   ☐ No ☐ Yes _____

CHILD'S MEDICAL HISTORY

Child's physician/pediatrician _____ Phone _____

Physician's address _____
                           Street   City   State   Zip code

Date of last complete check-up ___ / ___ / ___ Outcome _____
                                Mo. Day Year

1. Does the child take any medication for behavioral or emotional problems?   ☐ No ☐ Yes—
   please describe below:

Name of medication:	Dose	Purpose	Effect	Doctor
_____	_____	_____	_____	_____
_____	_____	_____	_____	_____
_____	_____	_____	_____	_____

(continued)

125

2. Does the child take any medication now for any other purpose? ☐ No ☐ Yes—please describe below:

Name of medication:	Dose	Purpose	Effect	Doctor
_____	____	_____	_____	_____
_____	____	_____	_____	_____
_____	____	_____	_____	_____

3. Has the child experienced any severe illnesses, accidents, operations, disabilities or handicaps, or repeated medical problems? ☐ No ☐ Yes—please describe below:

Type of problem	Age	Treatment	Doctor
_____	____	_____	_____
_____	____	_____	_____
_____	____	_____	_____

4. Does the child have allergies (e.g., dust, pollen, pets, certain foods)? ☐ No ☐ Yes—please describe below:

_____

_____

5. Are you concerned about any aspect of the child's health? ☐ No ☐ Yes—please describe below:

_____

_____

_____

_____

PREGNANCY AND NEWBORN PERIOD

Birthweight: ___ / ___
   Pounds Ounces

Please indicate if any of the following occurred during the pregnancy or the newborn period for your child:

If yes, please describe:

1. Medical problems during mother's pregnancy with this child (e.g., bleeding, infections, high blood pressure, diabetes, convulsions, large weight gain, injuries, operations)? ☐ No ☐ Yes _____

2. Did the mother take medications during the pregnancy? ☐ No ☐ Yes _____

3. Did the mother smoke during the pregnancy? ☐ No ☐ Yes _____

4. Did the mother drink alcohol during the pregnancy? ☐ No ☐ Yes _____

5. Did the mother use drugs during the pregnancy? ☐ No ☐ Yes _____

(continued)

If yes, please describe:

6. Did the mother experience unusual stress during the pregnancy (e.g., marital problems, job, financial, problems with living situation, problems with other people)? □ No □ Yes _____

7. Were there any problems with labor or the delivery (e.g., prolonged labor, bleeding, breech birth, forceps used, Cesarean section)? □ No □ Yes _____

8. Was the child born prematurely? □ No □ Yes _____

9. Did the child have any problems during the newborn period (e.g., born blue, birth defects, yellow jaundice, seizures, infections, injuries, feeding or sleep problems)? □ No □ Yes _____

10. Was the child difficult to care for as a baby? □ No □ Yes _____

DEVELOPMENTAL DELAYS

If yes, please describe:

1. Have you noticed any problems in the child's development? □ No □ Yes _____

2. Were any of the following difficult or slow to develop for the child? □ No □ Yes _____

   a. Walking alone □ No □ Yes _____

   b. Speaking □ No □ Yes _____

   c. Bowel training □ No □ Yes _____

   d. Bladder training □ No □ Yes _____

   e. Staying dry at night □ No □ Yes _____

   f. Tying shoes □ No □ Yes _____

   g. Riding bike □ No □ Yes _____

   h. Reading □ No □ Yes _____

   i. Writing □ No □ Yes _____

CHILD'S TEMPERAMENT

If yes, please describe:

1. Is the child overactive? □ No □ Yes _____

2. Does the child have trouble paying attention? □ No □ Yes _____

3. Does have trouble staying with one activity? □ No □ Yes _____

4. Does the child go from happy to sad quickly, without any little apparent cause? □ No □ Yes _____

5. Does the child get frustrated easily? □ No □ Yes _____

6. Does the child get upset by abrupt changes? □ No □ Yes _____

(continued)

If yes, please describe:

7. Are the child's emotional responses unpredictable? ☐ No ☐ Yes _____

8. Does it take the child a long time to warm up to new situations or new people? ☐ No ☐ Yes _____

9. Does the child react strongly to physical pain? ☐ No ☐ Yes _____

10. Does the child react strongly to other things? ☐ No ☐ Yes _____

CHILD'S EARLY BEHAVIOR

If yes, please describe:

1. Has the child had any problems in the following areas: If yes, please describe: ☐ No ☐ Yes _____
   a. Discipline ☐ No ☐ Yes _____
   b. Temper ☐ No ☐ Yes _____
   c. Fighting ☐ No ☐ Yes _____
   d. Moods ☐ No ☐ Yes _____
   e. Relationships with others ☐ No ☐ Yes _____
   f. Other behaviors ☐ No ☐ Yes _____

FAMILY HISTORY

Has any relative of the child had any of the following problems?

If yes, please describe:

1. Neurological disease (e.g., seizures, fits or spells, weaknesses) ☐ No ☐ Yes _____

2. Chronic disease (e.g., diabetes, thyroid, heart disease, stroke) ☐ No ☐ Yes _____

3. Mental illness (e.g., schizophrenia, bipolar or manic–depressive disorder, depression, anxiety, nervous breakdown) ☐ No ☐ Yes _____

4. Mental retardation ☐ No ☐ Yes _____

5. Learning problems ☐ No ☐ Yes _____

6. Behavior problems ☐ No ☐ Yes _____

7. Excessive use of alcohol ☐ No ☐ Yes _____

8. Drug problems, drug addiction ☐ No ☐ Yes _____

9. Trouble with the law ☐ No ☐ Yes _____

10. Trouble holding a job ☐ No ☐ Yes _____

11. Suicidal behavior ☐ No ☐ Yes _____

12. Violent behavior ☐ No ☐ Yes _____

13. Other problems ☐ No ☐ Yes _____

14. Has anyone in the child's family seen a psychologist, psychiatrist, or other mental health worker? ☐ No ☐ Yes _____

(continued)

CURRENT LIVING SITUATION

Do any of the following problems apply to the child's
current living situation?   If yes, please describe:

1. Marital or relationship problems   ☐ No   ☐ Yes _____
   between the child's major caregivers
2. Problems with siblings or other   ☐ No   ☐ Yes _____
   persons living in the home
3. Problems with work situation   ☐ No   ☐ Yes _____
4. Problems with present living situation ☐ No ☐ Yes _____
   or neighborhood
5. Recent major changes or stresses in ☐ No   ☐ Yes _____
   the child's living situation or family
6. Violence in the home or neighborhood ☐ No   ☐ Yes _____
7. Alcohol or drug problems in the home ☐ No   ☐ Yes _____
   or neighborhood
8. Other problems   ☐ No   ☐ Yes _____

PLEASE WRITE DOWN ANYTHING ELSE YOU THINK WE SHOULD KNOW

_____
_____
_____
_____
_____
_____
_____
_____
_____
_____
_____
_____
_____
_____
_____
_____
_____

Structured Diagnostic Interview for Parents

Informant's name: _____   Relationship to child _____
First   Middle   Last

Child's name: _____   Child's birthdate: ____ / ____ / ____
First   Middle   Last   Mo. Day Year

Now I need to ask you a number of very specific questions about a variety of behavioral, social, or emotional problems that children sometimes have difficulties with. As I ask you about these things, keep in mind that some of these things are not bad or abnormal and may be seen sometimes in healthy, normal children. I want you to tell me if your child does any of these things to a degree that you consider to be inappropriate for someone of his/her age and sex.

Oppositional Defiant Disorder (ODD 313.81)

Diagnosis requires four or more symptoms. Symptoms must be inappropriate for child's age; must have lasted at least the past 6 months; and must produce clear evidence of clinically significant impairment in social, academic, or occupational functioning.

I am going to ask you some specific questions about your child's behavior during the past 6 months. For each of the behaviors I ask you about, please tell me if your child shows that behavior to a degree that is inappropriate, compared to other children of your child's age.

A. Oppositional Defiant Symptoms
During the past 6 months, did your child show any of the following:

☐ Yes ☐ No ☐ Don't know   1. Often loses temper
☐ Yes ☐ No ☐ Don't know   2. Often argues with adults
☐ Yes ☐ No ☐ Don't know   3. Often actively defies or refuses to comply with adults' requests or rules
☐ Yes ☐ No ☐ Don't know   4. Often deliberately annoys people
☐ Yes ☐ No ☐ Don't know   5. Often blames others for his/her own mistakes or misbehavior
☐ Yes ☐ No ☐ Don't know   6. Is often touchy or easily annoyed by others
☐ Yes ☐ No ☐ Don't know   7. Is often angry or resentful
☐ Yes ☐ No ☐ Don't know   8. Is often spiteful or vindictive

B. Have these behaviors existed for at least the last 6 months?
☐ Yes ☐ No ☐ Don't know

C. At what age did these behaviors first cause problems for your child? ____ (years)

D. Have these behaviors created problems or impairment for your child in either of the following areas?
☐ Yes ☐ No ☐ Don't know   Social relations with others
☐ Yes ☐ No ☐ Don't know   Academic performance

E. Exclusion Criteria: Symptoms occur only during a Psychotic Disorder or Mood Disorder, or if criteria are met for Conduct Disorder.

Check here if all requirements are met.
☐ ODD (313.81)

(continued)

Conduct Disorder (312.8)

Diagnosis requires three or more symptoms during previous 12 months and at least once during the past 6 months; the symptoms must presently be causing impairment in social or academic functioning:

Now I want to ask you about some other things your child may have done. For these behaviors, I want you to think about the past 12 months and tell me whether any of these have occurred during that time.

A. Conduct Disorder Symptoms

During the past 12 months, did your child do any of the following:

☐ Yes ☐ No ☐ Don't know   1. Often bullies, threatens, or intimidates others

☐ Yes ☐ No ☐ Don't know   2. Often initiates physical fights

☐ Yes ☐ No ☐ Don't know   3. Has used a weapon that can cause serious physical harm to others (e.g., a bat, brick, broken bottle, knife, gun)

☐ Yes ☐ No ☐ Don't know   4. Has been physically cruel to people

☐ Yes ☐ No ☐ Don't know   5. Has been physically cruel to animals

☐ Yes ☐ No ☐ Don't know   6. Has stolen while confronting a victim (e.g., mugging, purse snatching, extortion, armed robbery)

☐ Yes ☐ No ☐ Don't know   7. Has forced someone into sexual activity

☐ Yes ☐ No ☐ Don't know   8. Has deliberately engaged in fire setting with the intention of causing serious damage

☐ Yes ☐ No ☐ Don't know   9. Has deliberately destroyed others' property (other than by fire setting)

☐ Yes ☐ No ☐ Don't know   10. Has broken into someone else's house, building, or car

☐ Yes ☐ No ☐ Don't know   11. Often lies to obtain goods or favors or to avoid obligations (i.e., "cons" others)

☐ Yes ☐ No ☐ Don't know   12. Has stolen items of nontrivial value without confronting a victim (e.g., shoplifting, but without breaking and entering; forgery)

☐ Yes ☐ No ☐ Don't know   13. Often stays out at night despite parental prohibitions
Must begin before age 13 years to be counted as a symptom

☐ Yes ☐ No ☐ Don't know   14. Has run away from home overnight at least twice while living in parent's home, foster care, or group home
Count as a symptom if it occurred once without child returning for a lengthy period

☐ Yes ☐ No ☐ Don't know   15. Is often truant from school
If so, at what age did he/she begin doing this? _____ (years)
Must begin before age 13 years to be counted as a symptom

B. Have three of these behaviors occurred during the last 12 months?
☐ Yes ☐ No ☐ Don't know

C. Has at least one of these behaviors occurred during the past 6 months?
☐ Yes ☐ No ☐ Don't know

D. Did any of these behaviors occur prior to age 10 years?
☐ Yes ☐ No ☐ Don't know

E. Have these behaviors created problems or impairment for your child in either of the following areas?
☐ Yes ☐ No ☐ Don't know   Social relations with others
☐ Yes ☐ No ☐ Don't know   Academic performance

(continued)

F. Exclusion Criteria: For ages 18 or older, criteria are met for Antisocial Disorder and Personality Disorder.

Check one subtype if all requirements are met.

☐ CD, Childhood-Onset Type (312.81) [*onset of at least one symptom prior to age 10 years*]

☐ CD, Adolescent-Onset Type (312.82) [*absence of any symptoms prior to age 10 years*]

Severity

☐ Mild [*few, if any, conduct problems in excess of those required to make the diagnosis and conduct problems cause only minor harm to others*]

☐ Moderate [*number of conduct problems and effect on others is intermediate between "mild" and "severe"*]

☐ Severe [*many conduct problems have occurred in excess of those required to make the diagnosis, or conduct problems cause considerable harm to others*]

Disruptive Behavior Disorder NOS

This category is for disruptive disorders characterized by conduct problems or oppositional defiant behaviors that do not meet criteria for CD or ODD, but that produce clinically significant impairment

☐ Disruptive Behavior Disorder NOS (312.9)

Attention-Deficit/Hyeractivity Disorder (ADHD 314.01 or 314.00)

Diagnosis requires six inattention symptoms and/or six hyperactive–impulsive symptoms. Symptoms must also be inappropriate for child's age, have lasted at least the past 6 months, and have caused some impairment prior to age 7 years; presently must be causing impairment in two situations (home, school, or work functioning); and must be producing clear evidence of clinically significant impairment in social or academic functioning.

Let me ask you about some other behaviors that your child may have shown during the past 6 months. Again, for each of the behaviors I ask you about, please tell me if your child shows that behavior to a degree that is inappropriate compared to other children of your child's age.

A. Inattention Symptoms
During the past 6 months, did your child show any of the following:

☐ Yes ☐ No ☐ Don't know   1. Often fails to give close attention to details or makes careless mistakes in schoolwork, work, or other activities

☐ Yes ☐ No ☐ Don't know   2. Often has difficulty sustaining attention in tasks or play activities

☐ Yes ☐ No ☐ Don't know   3. Often does not seem to listen when spoken to directly

☐ Yes ☐ No ☐ Don't know   4. Often does not follow through on instructions and fails to finish schoolwork, chores, or duties at work.
Inquire to be sure this is not due solely to oppositional behavior or failure to understand instructions.

☐ Yes ☐ No ☐ Don't know   5. Often has difficulty organizing tasks and activities

☐ Yes ☐ No ☐ Don't know   6. Often avoids, dislikes, or is reluctant to engage in tasks that require sustained mental effort (such as schoolwork or homework)

☐ Yes ☐ No ☐ Don't know   7. Often loses things necessary for tasks or activities (e.g., toys, school assignments, pencils, books, or tools)

(continued)

☐ Yes ☐ No ☐ Don't know   8. Is often easily distracted by extraneous stimuli

☐ Yes ☐ No ☐ Don't know   9. Is often forgetful in daily activities

B. Hyperactive–Impulsive Symptoms
    During the past 6 months, did your child show any of the following:

☐ Yes ☐ No ☐ Don't know   1. Often fidgets with hands or feet of squirms in his/her seat.

☐ Yes ☐ No ☐ Don't know   2. Often leaves his/her seat in the classroom or in other situations in which remaining seated is expected

☐ Yes ☐ No ☐ Don't know   3. Often runs about or climbs excessively in situations in which it is inappropriate to do so
    For adolescents, this may be limited to subjective feelings of restlessness.

☐ Yes ☐ No ☐ Don't know   4. Often has difficulty playing or engaging in leisure activities quietly

☐ Yes ☐ No ☐ Don't know   5. Is often "on the go" or often acts as if "driven by a motor"

☐ Yes ☐ No ☐ Don't know   6. Often talks excessively

☐ Yes ☐ No ☐ Don't know   7. Often blurts out answers before questions have been completed

☐ Yes ☐ No ☐ Don't know   8. Often has difficulty awaiting his/her turn

☐ Yes ☐ No ☐ Don't know   9. Often interrupts or intrudes on others (e.g., butts into conversations or games)

C. Have these behaviors existed for at least the past 6 months?
☐ Yes ☐ No ☐ Don't know

D. At what age did these behaviors first cause problems for your child? ____ (years)
    [*Onset by age 7*]

E. During the past 6 months, have these behaviors caused problems for this child in any of these situations?
☐ Yes ☐ No ☐ Don't know   At home
☐ Yes ☐ No ☐ Don't know   In school
☐ Yes ☐ No ☐ Don't know   At day care or with babysitters

F. Have these behaviors created problems or impairment for your child in any of the following areas?
☐ Yes ☐ No ☐ Don't know   Social relations with others
☐ Yes ☐ No ☐ Don't know   Academic performance

G. Exclusion Criteria: Symptoms occur only during a Pervasive Developmental Disorder or Psychotic Disorder or are better accounted for by another mental disorder, such as a Mood, Anxiety, Dissociative, or Personality Disorder.

Check one subtype if all requirements are met.
☐ ADHD, Combined Type (314.01) [*meets criteria for both inattention and hyperactive–impulsive symptoms*]
☐ ADHD, Predominantly Inattentive Type (314.00) [*meets criteria only for inattention symptoms*]
☐ ADHD, Predominately Hyperactive–Impulsive Type (314.01) [*meets criteria only for hyperactive–impulsive symptoms*]
☐ ADHD NOS (Not Otherwise Specified) (314.9) [*for disorders with prominent symptoms that do not meet full criteria for any subtype of ADHD*]
    For individuals (especially adolescents and adults) who currently have symptoms that no longer meet full criteria, specify "In Partial Remission."

(continued)

133

ANXIETY AND MOOD DISORDERS

Now I would like to ask you some questions about your child's emotions in general and his/her emotional reactions to some specific situations. I'll begin by asking you about any specific fears that your child may have. Then I will ask you about his/her general mood or emotional condition throughout much of the day. Let's start with some specific fears that your child may have.

Specific Phobia (300.29)

Diagnosis requires that all criteria, A–F, be met.

☐ Yes ☐ No ☐ Don't know   A. Does your child show a marked and persistent fear that is excessive or unreasonable in response to the presence of or the anticipation of a specific objects or situation? For instance, in response to or anticipation of certain animals, heights, being in the dark, thunderstorms or lightning, flying, receiving an injection, seeing blood, or any other things or situations?

If A is present, answer the following question then proceed to B–G below; otherwise, skip to the next disorder. If any of the criterion B–F is not met, skip to the next disorder.

What specifically is your child fearful of? _____

☐ Yes ☐ No ☐ Don't know   B. Does your child have this anxious or fearful reaction almost invariably when exposed to the specific thing or situation?

This may include a panic attack in the presence of the feared object or situation; or anxiety expressed by crying, tantrums, freezing, or clinging. Also, children do not need to recognize that their fear is excessive or unreasonable to qualify for this diagnosis.

☐ Yes ☐ No ☐ Don't know   C. Does your child attempt to avoid this thing or situation, or, if he/she must be exposed to it, does he/she endure it with intense anxiety or distress?

D. Does your child's avoidance of, anticipation of, or anxious reaction to this thing or situation interfere significantly with any of the following?
   Only one of these conditions needs to be endorsed for this criterion to be met.
☐ Yes ☐ No ☐ Don't know   His/her normal routine
☐ Yes ☐ No ☐ Don't know   Academic functioning
☐ Yes ☐ No ☐ Don't know   Social activities
☐ Yes ☐ No ☐ Don't know   Social relationships

E. Does having this fear cause him/her marked distress?
☐ Yes ☐ No ☐ Don't know

F. Has your child had this fearful or anxious reaction to this thing, situation, or event over a period of at least the past 6 months?
☐ Yes ☐ No ☐ Don't know

G. Exclusion Criteria: Phobia or anxiety is better accounted for by another mental disorder, such as Obsessive–Compulsive Disorder, Posttraumatic Stress Disorder, Separation Anxiety Disorder, Social Phobia, or Panic Disorder.
☐ Yes ☐ No ☐ Don't know

Check here if all requirements are met.

☐ Specific Phobia (300.29)

(continued)

Social Phobia (300.23)

Diagnosis requires that all criteria, A–F, be met; in addition, the child must have developed the capacity for age-appropriate social relationships with familiar people, and the anxiety must occur in peer settings (not just in interactions with adults).

A. What about social situations?

☐ Yes ☐ No ☐ Don't know   1. Does your child show a marked and persistent fear that is excessive or unreasonable in response to the presence of, or the anticipation of, a social or performance situation in which he/she is exposed to unfamiliar people or to possible scrutiny by others?

☐ Yes ☐ No ☐ Don't know   2. Does your child fear that he/she will act in a way that will be embarrassing or humiliating, or that he/she will be so anxious that it will be humiliating or embarrassing for him/her?

If parts 1 and 2 of A are present, answer the next question and then proceed with remaining criteria that follow; otherwise, skip to the next disorder. If any of the remaining criteria below are not met, skip to the next disorder.

3. What specific social situation is your child fearful of? _____

_____

B. Does your child have this anxious or fearful reaction almost invariably when exposed to this situation? *This may include a panic attack or anxiety expressed by crying, tantrums, freezing, clinging, or shrinking from this social situation with unfamiliar people. Also, children do not need to recognize that their fear is excessive or unreasonable to qualify for this diagnosis.*

☐ Yes ☐ No ☐ Don't know

C. Does your child attempt to avoid this situation, or if he/she must be exposed to it, does he/she endure it with intense anxiety of distress?

☐ Yes ☐ No ☐ Don't know

D. Does your child's avoidance of, anticipation of, or anxious reaction to this situation interfere significantly with any of the following?

☐ Yes ☐ No ☐ Don't know   His/her normal routine

☐ Yes ☐ No ☐ Don't know   Academic functioning

☐ Yes ☐ No ☐ Don't know   Social activities

☐ Yes ☐ No ☐ Don't know   Social relationships

E. Does having this fear cause him/her marked distress?

☐ Yes ☐ No ☐ Don't know

F. Has your child had this fearful or anxious reaction to this situation for at least the past 6 months?

☐ Yes ☐ No ☐ Don't know

G. Exclusion Criteria: Phobia or anxiety is due to the direct physiological effects of a substance or a general medical condition, or is better accounted for by another mental disorder, such as Panic Disorder, Separation Anxiety Disorder, Body Dysmorphic Disorder, a Pervasive Developmental Disorder, or Schizoid Personality Disorder.

Check here if all requirements are met.

☐ Social Phobia (300.23)   *(continued)*

Separation Anxiety Disorder (309.21)

Diagnosis requires that at least three symptoms be present (see A below) for at least 4 weeks. The symptoms must have developed before age 18 years and must produce clinically significant distress or impairment in social, academic, or other important areas of functioning, and other disorders must be excluded, as indicated below.

A. Separation Anxiety Disorder Symptoms

Now let's talk about how your child reacts emotionally when he/she must be away from you or when he/she must leave home for activities in the community. Does your child show any of the following?

☐ Yes ☐ No ☐ Don't know   1. Recurrent, excessive distress when separation from home, or from a parent or major attachment figure, occurs or is anticipated

☐ Yes ☐ No ☐ Don't know   2. Persistent and excessive worry about losing a parent or major attachment figure or about possible harm occurring to such a figure

☐ Yes ☐ No ☐ Don't know   3. Persistent and excessive worry that an unexpected or untoward event will lead him/her to become separated from a parent or major attachment figure (e.g., getting lost or being kidnapped)

☐ Yes ☐ No ☐ Don't know   4. Persistent reluctance or refusal to go to school or elsewhere because of fear of separation

☐ Yes ☐ No ☐ Don't know   5. Persistent and excessive fear or reluctance to be alone, or without a parent or major attachment figure at home, or without such a parent or caregiver when in other settings

☐ Yes ☐ No ☐ Don't know   6. Persistent reluctance or refusal to go to sleep without being near a major attachment figure or to sleep away from home

☐ Yes ☐ No ☐ Don't know   7. Repeated nightmares involving the theme or topic of separation from a parent or other caregiver

☐ Yes ☐ No ☐ Don't know   8. Repeated complaints of physical symptoms, such as headaches, stomachaches, nausea, or vomiting, when separation from a parent or major attachment figure occurs or is anticipated

If three or more symptoms were endorsed, proceed with remaining criteria; otherwise, skip to next disorder. If any of the remaining criteria below are not met, skip to the next disorder.

B. Have these fears existed for at least 4 weeks?
☐ Yes ☐ No ☐ Don't know

C. At what age did these behaviors first cause problems for your child? ____ (years)
Symptoms must have developed before age 18 years.

D. Have these worries created distress for your child or impairment in any of the following areas?
☐ Yes ☐ No ☐ Don't know   Social relations with others
☐ Yes ☐ No ☐ Don't know   Academic performance
☐ Yes ☐ No ☐ Don't know   Any other areas of functioning

(continued)

E. Exclusion Criteria: Symptoms occur only during Pervasive Developmental Disorder, Schizophrenia, or other Psychotic Disorder, or are not better accounted for by Panic Disorder.

Check here if all requirements are met.

☐ Separation Anxiety (309.21)

☐ Early Onset (before age 6 years): ____ (years)

Generalized Anxiety Disorder (300.02)

Diagnosis requires that criteria A and B be met; at least one symptom in criterion C be present for at least 6 months on more days than not; that symptoms produce clinically significant distress or impairment in social, academic, or other important areas of functioning; and that other disorders be excluded, as indicated below:

Now let's talk about whether your child tends to be generally anxious or to worry a lot, compared to other children of his/her age group.

A. Does your child show excessive anxiety and worry about a number of events or activities, such as work activities, school performance, or other situations?
☐ Yes ☐ No ☐ Don't know

B. Has this anxiety or worry occurred on more days than not for at least the last 6 months?
☐ Yes ☐ No ☐ Don't know

C. Does your child find it difficult to control his/her worry?
☐ Yes ☐ No ☐ Don't know

D. Generalized Anxiety Disorder Symptoms
Has your child's anxiety or worry been associated with any of the following behaviors for more days than not over the past 6 months?
Only one condition needs to be present for this criterion to be met.
☐ Yes ☐ No ☐ Don't know   1. Restlessness or feeling keyed up or on edge
☐ Yes ☐ No ☐ Don't know   2. Being easily fatigued or tired
☐ Yes ☐ No ☐ Don't know   3. Difficulty concentrating or mind going blank
☐ Yes ☐ No ☐ Don't know   4. Irritability
☐ Yes ☐ No ☐ Don't know   5. Muscle tension
☐ Yes ☐ No ☐ Don't know   6. Sleep disturbance or difficulties falling asleep, staying asleep, or restless and unsatisfying sleep

E. Have these worries created distress for your child or impairment in any of the following areas?
☐ Yes ☐ No ☐ Don't know   Social relations with others
☐ Yes ☐ No ☐ Don't know   Academic performance
☐ Yes ☐ No ☐ Don't know   Any other areas of functioning

F. Exclusion Criteria: Anxiety or worry are confined to features of another mental disorder, such as being worried about having a panic attack (Panic Disorder), being embarrassed in public (Social Phobia), being contaminated (Obsessive–Compulsive Disorder), having multiple physical complaints (Somatization Disorder), or having a serious illness (Hypochondriasis); or if the anxiety is associated with Posttraumatic Stress Disorder, the disturbance is due to the direct physiological effects of a substance (e.g., drug abuse, medication) or a general medical condition (e.g., hyperthyroidism) or occurs exclusively during a Mood Disorder, a Psychotic Disorder, or a Pervasive Developmental Disorder.

(continued)

Check here if all requirements are met.

☐ Generalized Anxiety Disorder (300.02)

Dysthymic Disorder (300.4)

Diagnosis requires that depressed mood exist for most of the day, for more days than not, for at least 1 year, that at least two symptoms from B exist; that the child has never been without the symptoms in A and B below for 2 consecutive months during the first year of the disturbance; that all exclusionary criteria are met; and that the symptoms cause clinically significant distress or impairment in social, academic, or other important areas of functioning.
    I would like to speak with you now about your child's mood for most of the time.

A. Does your child show depressed mood or irritability for most of the day, by either his/her own report or your own observations of your child?
☐ Yes ☐ No ☐ Don't know

Has this depressed mood occurred more days than not for at least the past 12 months?
☐ Yes ☐ No ☐ Don't know

If the two questions in A were endorsed, proceed with remaining criteria for this disorder; otherwise, skip to next disorder. If any of the remaining criteria are not met, skip to the next disorder.

B. Does your child show any of the following difficulties while he/she is depressed?
☐ Yes ☐ No ☐ Don't know   1. Poor appetite or overeating
☐ Yes ☐ No ☐ Don't know   2. Insomnia (trouble falling asleep) or hypersomnia (excessive sleeping)
☐ Yes ☐ No ☐ Don't know   3. Low energy or fatigue
☐ Yes ☐ No ☐ Don't know   4. Low self-esteem
☐ Yes ☐ No ☐ Don't know   5. Poor concentration or difficulty making decisions
☐ Yes ☐ No ☐ Don't know   6. Feelings of hopelessness

If two or more of symptoms in 1–6 were endorsed, proceed. If not, skip to the next disorder.

C. During the 12 months or more that your child has shown this depressed mood, has he/she ever been without this depressed mood or the other difficulties. *If he/she has not had any remission of symptoms for at least 2 months, check yes.*
☐ Yes ☐ No ☐ Don't know

D. Has this depressed mood created distress for your child or impairment in any of the following areas?
☐ Yes ☐ No ☐ Don't know   Social relations with others
☐ Yes ☐ No ☐ Don't know   Academic performance
☐ Yes ☐ No ☐ Don't know   Any other areas of functioning

E. Exclusion Criteria: Meets criteria for Major Depressive Episode during the first year of his/her mood disorder, or if the disorder is better accounted for by Major Depressive Disorder; Manic Episode, Mixed (Manic–Depressive) Episode, or the disorder described above occurs exclusively during the course of a chronic Psychotic Disorder, such as Schizophrenia or Delusional Disorder, or is the result of the direct physiological effects of a substance or a general medical condition.

(continued)

138

Check here if all requirements are met.

☐ Dysthymic Disorder (300.4)

Major Depressive Disorder (296.xx)

Diagnosis requires that at least five or more of the symptoms listed in A below have been present for a 2-week period; that this represents a change from previous functioning; that at least one of the symptoms is depressed mood or loss of interest of pleasure; that the symptoms create clinically significant distress or impairment in school, academic, or other important areas of functioning; and that all exclusion criteria are met.

A. Major Depressive Episode Symptoms

Let's continue to talk about your child's mood or emotional adjustment. Has your child developed any of the following for at least a 2-week period of time?

☐ Yes ☐ No ☐ Don't know   1. Depressed or irritable mood most of the day nearly every day for at least 2 weeks
This can be determined by the child's own report or by the parents' or others' observations.

☐ Yes ☐ No ☐ Don't know   2. Marked diminished interest in pleasure in all or almost all activities most of the day, nearly every day for at least 2 weeks
This can be by the child's own report or by the parents' or others' observations.

If either 1 or 2 was endorsed, proceed with remaining criteria; otherwise, skip to the next disorder.

☐ Yes ☐ No ☐ Don't know   3. Significant weight loss, when not dieting

☐ Yes ☐ No ☐ Don't know   Significant weight gain

☐ Yes ☐ No ☐ Don't know   Decrease or increase in appetite nearly every day

☐ Yes ☐ No ☐ Don't know   Failed to meet expected weight gains

☐ Yes ☐ No ☐ Don't know   4. Insomnia (trouble falling asleep) or hypersomnia (excessive sleep) nearly every day

☐ Yes ☐ No ☐ Don't know   5. Agitated or excessive movement nearly every day
Must be supported by parents' or others' observations.

☐ Yes ☐ No ☐ Don't know   Or lethargic, sluggish, slow moving, or significantly reduced movement or activity nearly every day
Must be supported by the parents' or others' observations.

☐ Yes ☐ No ☐ Don't know   6. Fatigue or loss of energy nearly every day

☐ Yes ☐ No ☐ Don't know   7. Feelings of worthlessness or excessive or inappropriate guilt nearly every day
This should not be self-reproach or guilt about being sick.

☐ Yes ☐ No ☐ Don't know   8. Diminished ability to think or concentrate, or indecisiveness, nearly every day
Can be determined by child's selfreport or parents' or others' observations.

☐ Yes ☐ No ☐ Don't know   9. Recurrent thoughts of death

☐ Yes ☐ No ☐ Don't know   Or recurrent thoughts of suicide

☐ Yes ☐ No ☐ Don't know   Or suicide attempt or a specific plan for committing suicide

If five or more of symptoms in 1–9 were endorsed, proceed. If not, skip to the next disorder.

(continued)

B. Have any of these symptoms of depression created distress for your child or impairment in any of the following areas?

☐ Yes ☐ No ☐ Don't know   Social relations with others

☐ Yes ☐ No ☐ Don't know   Academic performance

☐ Yes ☐ No ☐ Don't know   Any other areas of functioning

C. Exclusive Criteria: If the symptoms are due to direct physiological effects of a substance or a general medical condition; if the symptoms are better accounted for by clinical Bereavement after the loss of a loved one or by Schizoaffective Disorder; if the symptoms are superimposed on Schizophrenia, Schizophreniform Disorder, Delusional Disorder, Psychotic Disorder NOS, or there has been a Manic Episode, a Mixed Episode, or a Hypomanic Episode.

Check here if all requirements are met.

☐ Major Depressive Disorder (296.xx)

Code for single episode is 296.2x, recurrent episode is 296.3x; see pp. 375–376 of DSM-IV-TR (American Psychiatric Association, 2000) for additional specifications about the disorder.

Depressive Disorder NOS

Code this only when there is clinically significant depression with impairment, but when full criteria for Major Depressive Disorder, Dysthymic Disorder, Adjustment Disorder with Depressed Mood, or Adjustment Disorder with Mixed Anxiety and Depressed Mood are not met.

☐ Depressive Disorder NOS (311)

Bipolar I Disorder: Manic Episode (296.xx)

Diagnosis requires that the child has had a distinct period of at least 1 week of abnormally and persistently elevated, expansive, or irritable mood, or any period of such mood that resulted in hospitalization; and has had at least three of the symptoms listed in B below (or four if mood was primarily irritable) to a significant degree. Also, the symptoms must create clinically significant impairment in social, academic, or other important areas of functioning, and exclusion criteria must be met.

I have some questions to ask you about your child's moods or emotional adjustment.

A. Has your child ever experienced a period of time that lasted at least 1 week:

☐ Yes ☐ No ☐ Don't know   1. In which his/her mood was unusually and persistently elevated; that is, he/she felt abnormally happy, giddy, joyous, or ecstatic, well beyond normal feelings of happiness?

☐ Yes ☐ No ☐ Don't know   2. Or in which his/her mood was abnormally and persistently expansive; that is, your child felt able to accomplish everything he/she decided to do, felt nearly superhuman in his/her ability to do anything he/she wished to do, or felt as if his/her abilities were without limits?

☐ Yes ☐ No ☐ Don't know   3. Or in which his/her mood was abnormally and persistently irritable; that is, he/she was unusually touchy, too easily prone to anger or temper outbursts, too easily annoyed by events or by others, or abnormally cranky?

If any of the above were endorsed, proceed with B; otherwise skip to next disorder.

(continued)

B. During the week or more that your child showed this abnormal and persistent mood, did you notice any of the following to be persistent and/or occurring to an abnormal or significant degree?

☐ Yes ☐ No ☐ Don't know   1. Showed inflated self-esteem or felt grandiose about self well beyond what would be characteristic for his/her level of abilities

☐ Yes ☐ No ☐ Don't know   2. Showed a decreased need for sleep; for instance, he/she stated that he/she felt rested after only 3 hours of sleep

☐ Yes ☐ No ☐ Don't know   3. Was more talkative than usual or seemed to feel reassured to keep talking

☐ Yes ☐ No ☐ Don't know   4. Skipped from one idea to another in speech, as if his/her ideas were flying by rapidly

☐ Yes ☐ No ☐ Don't know   Or stated that he/she felt that his/her thoughts were racing or flying by at an abnormal rate of speed

☐ Yes ☐ No ☐ Don't know   5. Was distractible; that is, his/her attention was too easily drawn to unimportant or irrelevant events or things around him/her

☐ Yes ☐ No ☐ Don't know   6. Showed an increase in goal-directed activity; that is; he/she became unusually and persistently productive or directed more activity than normal toward the tasks he/she wanted to accomplish

☐ Yes ☐ No ☐ Don't know   Or seemed very agitated, overly active, or abnormally restless

☐ Yes ☐ No ☐ Don't know   7. Showed an excessive involvement in pleasurable activities that have a high likelihood of negative, harmful, or painful consequences

If three or more symptoms above were endorsed, proceed with remaining criteria; otherwise, skip to next disorder.

C. Remaining Criteria

☐ Yes ☐ No ☐ Don't know   1. Was this disturbance in your child's mood enough to cause severe impairment, disruption, or difficulties with social relationships, academic performance, or other important activities?

☐ Yes ☐ No ☐ Don't know   2. Or did your child's abnormal mood cause him/her to be hospitalized to prevent harm to himself/herself or others?

☐ Yes ☐ No ☐ Don't know   3. Or did your child have hallucinations [explain] or bizarre ideas [psychotic thinking], or feel or act paranoid [as if others were intentionally out to harm him/her]?

If one or more of the criteria 1–3 were endorsed, proceed.

D. Exclusion Criteria: Symptoms meet criteria for a Mixed Episode or Schizoaffective Disorder, are the direct physiological effects of a substance or a general medical condition, or are superimposed on Schizophrenia, Schizophreniform Disorder, Delusional Disorder, or Psychotic Disorder NOS. Also, if the child meets criteria for ADHD, give diagnosis of Manic Episode only if the child meets the criteria after excluding distractibility (5, above) and psychomotor agitation (second part of 6, above).

Check here if all requirements are met.

☐ Bipolar I Disorder: Manic Episode (296.xx)

Code 296.0x if single Manic Episode; 206.4x if multiple episodes and most recent was Manic Episode.

(continued)

141

Bipolar I Disorder: Mixed Episode

Code this disorder if criteria are met both for a Manic Episode and for a Major Depressive Episode nearly every day for at least 1 week; disturbance causes clinically significant impairment; and symptoms are not the result of a substance or a general medical condition.

☐ Bipolar I Disorder: Mixed Episode (296.6x)

Bipolar I Disorder: Other Types of Episodes

☐ Bipolar I Disorder: Most Recent Episode Hypomanic (296.40)
Code this disorder if criteria are met for a Hypomanic Episode (a milder form of Manic Episode; see p. 368 of DSM-IV-TR), and there has previously been at least one Manic or Mixed Episode.

☐ Bipolar I Disorder: Most Recent Episode Depressed (296.5x)
Code this disorder if criteria are met for a Major Depressive Episode as described earlier, and there has previously been at least one Manic or Mixed Episode.

☐ Bipolar I Disorder: Most Recent Episode Unspecified (296.7)
Code this disorder if criteria, except for duration, are met for a Manic, Hypomanic, Mixed, or Major Depressive Episode; there has previously been at least one Manic or Mixed Episode; disturbance causes clinically significant impairment; and symptoms are not the result of a substance or a general medical condition.

Other Mental and Developmental Disorders

☐ Yes ☐ No ☐ Don't know
1. Does this child have any things about which he/she seems obsessed, or is he/she unable to get his/her mind off a particular topic?
If present, review diagnostic criteria for Obsessive–Compulsive Disorder in the DSM-IV-TR (American Psychiatric Association, 2000).

☐ Yes ☐ No ☐ Don't know
2. Does this child have any unusual behaviors he/she must perform, such as dressing, bathing, mealtime, or counting rituals?
If present, review diagnostic criteria for Obsessive–Compulsive Disorder in the DSM-IV-TR (American Psychiatric Association, 2000).

☐ Yes ☐ No ☐ Don't know
3. Does this child demonstrate any nervous tics or other repetitive, abrupt nervous movements or vocal noises?
If present, review diagnostic criteria for Tourette's Disorder or other Tic Disorders in the DSM-IV-TR (American Psychiatric Association, 2000).

☐ Yes ☐ No ☐ Don't know
4. Has this child made comments or acted in such a way that he/she seemed to see things, hear things, or feel things on his/her skin that really did not exist (hallucinations)?
If present, review diagnostic criteria for Psychotic Disorders in the DSM-IV-TR (American Psychiatric Association, 2000).

☐ Yes ☐ No ☐ Don't know
5. Has this child ever reported bizarre or very strange or peculiar ideas that seemed very unusual compared to other children (delusions)?
If present, review diagnostic criteria for Psychotic Disorders in the DSM-IV-TR (American Psychiatric Association, 2000).

6

Interviews with Teachers

No school-based assessment would be complete without teachers' reports about a child's functioning in school. Teachers are often the ones who initiate referrals for school-based assessments and interventions. Over the course of the school year, teachers have many opportunities to observe children's academic performance, behavior, and social interactions. As teachers become more experienced, they accumulate knowledge about patterns of behavior and academic progress that they come to regard as "typical" for children of different ages. From this knowledge base, teachers become attuned to individual children who seem to be "atypical" compared to other children. Teachers are also likely to know about school-based services available to children in their community. For these reasons, it is important to obtain information from teachers about children's school performance, competencies, and problems. Interviews with teachers are especially useful for the following purposes:

- To learn the teacher's current concerns about the child.
- To identify and prioritize the child's specific problems that would be appropriate targets for school-based interventions.
- To identify the child's strengths and competencies that can be marshaled to bolster interventions.
- To learn about aspects of the child's educational history that are relevant for understanding identified problems.
- To learn what interventions, if any, have already been attempted.
- To assess the prima facie effectiveness of previous interventions.
- To assess the acceptability and feasibility of future interventions.

Specific interview formats have been developed for interviewing teachers about academic problems and wider aspects of the school environment. An example is Shapiro's (2004) Teacher Interview Form for Academic Problems, which focuses on reading, mathematics, and writing. Another is The Instructional Environment System–II (TIES-II; Yesseldyke & Christenson, 1993), which focuses on teachers' instructional goals, teaching strategies, and the classroom environment. The Academic Intervention Monitoring System (AIMS; Elliott, DiPerna, & Shapiro, 2001) includes teacher interviews and teacher rating scales for developing, monitoring, and evaluating classroom-based interventions for academic difficulties. Readers are referred to these sources for in-depth discussions of teacher interviews for consultation about specific academic interventions.

Many authors have also written about interviews with teachers in the context of school behavioral consultation models (e.g., Bergan & Kratochwill, 1990; Knoff, 2002; Kratochwill et al., 2002; Zins & Erchul, 2002). Other authors have expanded these approaches into "conjoint behavioral consultation" which involves interviewing teachers and parents together to create positive working partnerships (Busse & Beaver, 2000; Sheridan et al., 1996). As discussed in Chapter 5, behavioral interviewing seeks to identify specific problem behaviors that can be targeted for interventions. The goal is to obtain a functional behavioral assessment (FBA) that posits hypotheses about the functions of specific problem behaviors (e.g., to gain attention, to avoid something, or to obtain self-reinforcement). The FBA is then used to develop a behavioral intervention plan (BIP). Interviewing teachers is usually the first step for problem identification and problem solving. After interventions are implemented, teacher interviews can also aid in monitoring progress and evaluating the effectiveness of interventions.

This chapter discusses generic teacher interviews that can fit into the multimethod assessment model discussed in Chapter 1. It also mirrors the discussion of parent interviews in the previous chapter. The first two sections cover confidentiality issues and questioning strategies for teachers. The next section describes the Semistructured Teacher Interview (McConaughy, 2004b; see Appendix 6.1), which is the main focus of this chapter. Standardized teacher rating scales are also summarized as other assessment methods that can dovetail with teacher interviews.

DISCUSSING CONFIDENTIALITY WITH TEACHERS

School-based practitioners should be fully aware of federal and state laws regarding parental consent, confidentiality, and release of information about students, as indicated in the previous chapter on parent interviews. They should also be familiar with school district policies regarding confidentiality and release of information. As a general rule, school-based practitioners should obtain informed parental consent before interviewing teachers as part of a formal assessment of a child. If the teacher interview is part of a special education evaluation, then the IDEA and state regulations govern the timing and format for obtaining parental consent. Practitioners should also obtain parental consent before interviewing teachers as part of other formal assessment procedures, such as psychological evaluations, behavioral consultation, and referrals of children and families for mental health services or services from other agencies outside of school.

Sometimes practitioners may want to talk with teachers for screening purposes or as part of team-based support services in school. For example, school-based practitioners may want to discuss student needs and classroom accommodations in "prereferral" teams that support general education teachers. For these broader purposes, prior informed parental consent is usually not necessary. However, practitioners should be thoroughly familiar with their school district's policies regarding such procedures. As best practice, it behooves school administrators to inform parents of all children about the support services available in their school. This way, parents will not be surprised or upset when they learn that a school-based practitioner (e.g., guidance counselor or school psychologist) has discussed concerns about their child with the teacher. When screening or prereferral discussions lead to requests for formal evaluation, then practitioners must obtain the required parental consent before gathering more teacher reports through interviewing and other assessment procedures.

Even when parents have given prior consent for practitioners to obtain information from teachers, you should explain clearly to teachers what information will be reported to others. For example, teacher reports are especially important to include in written evaluation reports. Practitioners may also want to share teachers' perspectives with parents or other parties in follow-up discussions of a child. Teachers' perspectives are essential for subsequent school-based consultations about a child.

To protect confidentiality of teacher reports, practitioners should refrain from naming individual teachers in written reports and avoid quoting teachers' exact words. Exceptions are circumstances that require reports of suspected child abuse or neglect, suicide risk (see Chapter 8), or when a child poses a threat to other persons (see Chapter 9). In other cases teachers may view naming or quoting their specific comments as a violation of trust, which can lead to reluctance to share their observations and true opinions in future interviews. Some parents may also react negatively when they learn exactly what a teacher said about their child. Bad feelings from either party can undermine future problem solving and collaboration between parents and teachers.

As a general practice, you can inform teachers that you will summarize or paraphrase their comments in reports to other parties. If a child has only one teacher, then of course it will be obvious which teacher provided the information. Still, omitting the teacher's name in a written report will make the information seem less personally tied to that teacher. If a child has more than one teacher, you can cite each teacher's position (e.g., language arts teacher, math teacher, special educator), summarize the general consensus among the teachers, and then indicate certain classes or subject areas in which the child has problems or does particularly well. These reporting practices are especially important for written evaluation reports, because such reports often become part of the student record and may be read again long after particular teachers have had contact with the child.

The Semistructured Teacher Interview (McConaughy, 2004b) in Appendix 6.1 begins with the following standard introduction:

"Thank you for taking your time to meet with me today and for completing the various questionnaires that you received before our meeting. I have reviewed the information that you provided on these forms. In this interview, I would like to hear more about your concerns about [child's name]. Your perspective(s) is important for evaluating [child's name]'s functioning.

"The information you provide will be summarized in a written evaluation report. My usual practice is not to include direct quotations of teachers' comments in written reports. However, I may have to report information to appropriate legal authorities or others (such as parents) if there is reason to suspect child abuse or when the child poses a danger to self or a danger to other persons. In such cases, I may have to quote what you said directly, but I will try to confer with you about that ahead of time."

Readers should see Jacob (2002) and Jacob and Hartshorne (2003) for more detailed discussions of ethics and legal requirements regarding confidentiality and disclosure of information.

INTERVIEWING STRATEGIES WITH TEACHERS

As a general rule, teacher interviews are best conducted with the teachers who know a child best or who spend the most time with the child. For children in preschool or elementary grades, there is usually one lead teacher who will be the best informant on behavioral and academic functioning. If the child has other teachers for "special" classes (e.g., art, music, gym, special education), interviewing at least one of them as well can provide additional perspectives. Children in middle, junior, or high school settings usually have multiple teachers. For these children, it is usually good to obtain information from more than one teacher. One approach is to interview one (or more) teachers who know the child well, and then to gather additional information from other teachers using other procedures, such as teacher rating scales. Due to time constraints, it may not be practical to conduct individual interviews with multiple teachers.

An alternative approach is to interview several teachers simultaneously. To do this, you can ask each teacher to give his/her perspective on the child in a round-robin fashion. However, this method also takes more time and runs the risk of missing information if certain teachers fail to express their views in a group. Interviewing several teachers at once also runs the risk of reinforcing negative views of the child if the interview degenerates into a mutual complaint session. In such cases interviewers should try to move the interview toward a more positive problem-solving process that involves open exchange of information without pejorative judgments of the child or teachers involved.

Many of the questioning strategies for parent interviews and child clinical interviews also apply to semistructured teacher interviews. Such interviews with teachers can include open-ended questions and follow-up probes for different topic areas. PACERS (Busse & Beaver, 2000), described in Chapter 5, can facilitate effective communication between interviewers and teachers: paraphrasing, attending, clarifying, eliciting, reflecting, and summarizing.

Interviewers should strive to convey respect toward teachers for their special expertise about children and curricula. By virtue of their work with many children, teachers can provide unique perspectives on a particular child's learning and behavior compared to other children. Teachers also have special knowledge about academic requirements for their different subjects and grade levels. Teachers may or may not agree on their perspectives about a child. However, each teacher's viewpoint can add important information for understanding the child's functioning and his/her relationship with that teacher. Some parents may blame teachers for their child's problems. Some teachers, in turn, may blame parents. As an interviewer, you should strive to maintain a neutral stance to avoid aligning yourself with either parents or teachers. Instead, you can acknowledge each teacher's point of view and seek additional information as needed.

Given the demands and routines of the typical school day, teachers are likely to have limited time for participating in interviews. It is important to respect their time constraints in order to obtain their cooperation. Whenever possible, let the teacher choose the time for the interview. Choose a place that affords privacy for teachers and the child concerned. Many school buildings have private conference rooms for such purposes. A staff member's office may be another choice.

If you conduct the teacher interview in a classroom, choose a time when no children are present (e.g., a free period or before or after school).

TOPIC AREAS FOR SEMISTRUCTURED TEACHER INTERVIEWS

The Semistructured Teacher Interview (McConaughy, 2004b; Appendix 6.1) is organized in a modular fashion for six topic areas, as listed in Table 6.1. Practitioners can select topic areas and questions to fit concerns about a particular child, as well as skip certain topics or questions to save time or to abide by school policies regarding subject matter for interviews. The Semistructured Teacher Interview is modeled on the format used for the Semistructured Parent Interview discussed in Chapter 5 (Appendix 5.1). The interview protocol lists sample questions for each topic area in the left-hand column and provides space for notes in the right-hand column. Interviewers can adapt questions to fit their own style and the flow of conversation.

Concerns about the Child

Section I begins by asking teachers to describe their current concerns about the child. If several teachers participate in the interview, ask each teacher to articulate his/her concerns. You can list each area of concern in the space in the right-hand column. Then ask the teachers when they first became concerned about each problem and how long the problem has been going on. If the teachers' main concerns are about academic problems, you can move to questions in Section III. If their main concerns are about school behavioral and emotional problems, then move directly to

TABLE 6.1. Topic Areas for Semistructured
Teacher Interviews

  I.   Concerns about the child

 II.   School behavior problems
       Specific nature of the problems
       Priorities for interventions
       Antecedents and consequences of priority problem(s)
       Other possible problem areas

III.   Academic performance
       Subjects/grades/activities
       Teachers
       Homework

 IV.   Teaching strategies
       Strategies
       Retention

  V.   School interventions for behavior problems

 VI.   Special help/services

Section II. Many teachers may be concerned about both academic and school behavior problems, given that research has show strong links between poor academic performance and behavioral and emotional problems. In these cases, you can decide which area to address first.

School Behavior Problems

Section II of the teacher interview follows a format similar to the section on behavioral and emotional problems in the parent interview. This section follows the general approach of behavioral interviewing. The first step is to ask teachers to describe each problem in specific, observable terms and to give examples of it. Then ask teachers about the duration and frequency of each problem and the circumstances surrounding it.

When teachers have concerns about several problems, it is important to prioritize them so that you can target specific problems for interventions and additional data collection. As is the case with many parents, some teachers may want to address all of their concerns at once. When this happens, you can explain that behavioral interventions work best when you focus only on a few key problems at any one time. After selecting two or three problem behaviors that concern teachers most, ask them to identify antecedents and consequences surrounding the behaviors. Answers to these questions help to develop hypotheses for FBA, as discussed in Chapter 5. You can also ask teachers how they usually deal with the identified problems in their classrooms and what would be acceptable replacement behaviors. Gathering this information will help you learn which strategies have already been tried and what behaviors teachers expect from children in their classrooms. It is also important to ask teachers about children's strengths and competencies, which can form positive aspects of your school intervention plans.

Standardized Teacher Rating Scales

The last part of Section II includes spaces for recording problem areas reported by teachers on standardized teacher rating scales. As in the parent interview, this part of the interview assumes that teachers have been asked to complete such rating scales prior to the interview. When this has been done, you can examine the scoring profiles to identify areas in which teachers have reported severe problems, compared to normative samples. Table 6.2 lists examples of standardized teacher rating scales that can easily be incorporated into multimethod assessment. The table summarizes the number of items and scales for each instrument, characteristics of the normative samples, and contact information for the publisher.

The instruments listed in Table 6.2 provide standard scores that compare a child's scores to normative samples of boys or girls of the same age range. The scoring profiles consist of scales for different patterns of teacher-reported problems and/or competencies. For example, the Academic Competence Evaluation Scales (ACES; DiPerna & Elliott, 2000) has scales for teachers' reports of children's academic skills plus behaviors that "enable" good academic performance (interpersonal skills, engagement, motivation, study skills). The ASEBA TRF (Achenbach & Rescorla, 2001) includes problem scales corresponding to those on the ASEBA CBCL/6–18 for parents, plus scales for adaptive functioning and academic performance. The ASI-4 Teacher Checklist (Gadow & Sprafkin, 1998) and CSI-4 Teacher Checklist (Gadow & Sprafkin, 2002) assess DSM-IV disorders, similar to the parent versions. The BASC-2 Teacher Rating Scale (Reynolds & Kamphaus, 2004) has problem and adaptive scales similar to the BASC-2 Parent Rating Scale, plus an addi-

TABLE 6.2. Examples of Published Standardized Teacher Rating Scales

Instrument	Items and scales	Normative samples	Publisher
Academic Competence Evaluation Scales/Teacher Form (ACES; DiPerna & Elliott, 2000)	73 items *Competence/Adaptive Scales* Academic Enablers Total Score, Interpersonal Skills, Engagement, Motivation, Study Skills, Academic Skills Total Score, Reading/Language Arts, Mathematics, Critical Thinking	Combined norms for boys and girls, grades K–2, 3–5, 6–8 and 9–12	Harcourt Assessment, Inc. 19500 Academic Court San Antonio, TX 78204-2498 800-211-8378 www.psychcorpcenter.com
ASEBA[a] Caregiver–Teacher's Report Form for Ages 1½–5 (C-TRF; Achenbach & Rescorla, 2000)	100 items *Problem Scales* Total Problems, Internalizing, Externalizing, Emotionally Reactive, Anxious/Depressed, Somatic Complaints, Withdrawn, Attention Problems, Aggressive Behavior, Affective Problems, Anxiety Problems, Pervasive Developmental Problems, Attention/Deficit Hyperactivity Problems, Oppositional Defiant Problems	Combined norms for boys and girls, ages 1½–5	Research Center for Children, Youth, and Families, Inc. One South Prospect Street Burlington, VT 05401-3456 802-264-6432 www.ASEBA.org
ASEBA[a] Teacher's Report Form (TRF; Achenbach & Rescorla, 2001)	6 adaptive items and 120 problem items *Problem Scales* Total Problems, Internalizing, Externalizing, Withdrawn/Depressed, Somatic Complaints, Anxious/Depressed, Social Problems, Thought Problems, Attention Problems, Rule-Breaking Behavior, Aggressive Behavior, Affective Problems, Anxiety Problems, Attention/Deficit Hyperactivity Problems, Oppositional Defiant Problems, Conduct Problems, Inattention and Hyperactivity–Impulsivity subscales *Competence/Adaptive Scales* Total Adaptive Functioning, Working Hard, Behaving Appropriately, Learning, Happy, Academic Performance	Separate norms for boys and girls, ages 6–11 and 12–18	Research Center for Children, Youth, and Families, Inc. One South Prospect Street Burlington, VT 05401-3456 802-264-6432 www.ASEBA.org
Adolescent Symptom Inventory–4 Teacher Checklist (ASI-4; Gadow & Sprafkin, 1998)	79 items *Problem Scales* 11 DSM-IV Disorders Academic Performance	Separate norms for boys and girls, ages 12–18 (secondary school)	Checkmate Plus P.O. Box 696 Stony Brook, NY 11790-0696 800-779-4292 www.checkmateplus.com

(continued)

149

TABLE 6.2. (continued)

Instrument	Items and scales	Normative samples	Publisher
Behavior Assessment System for Children–2 Teacher Rating Scales (BASC-2 TRS; Reynolds & Kamphaus, 2004)	134–160 items *Problem Scales* Behavioral Symptoms Index, Externalizing, Internalizing, Hyperactivity, Aggression, Conduct Problems (ages 6–18), Anxiety, Depression, Somatization, Attention Problems, Learning Problems, Atypicality, Withdrawal *Competence/Adaptive Scales* Adaptive Skills Composite, Adaptability, Social Skills, Leadership (ages 6–18), Study Skills (ages 6–18), Functional Communication	Separate norms for boys and girls, ages 2–5, 6–11, and 12–18	American Guidance Service 4201 Woodland Road Circle Pines, MN 55014-1796 800-328-2560 www.agsnet.com
Behavioral and Emotional Rating Scale (2nd edition) Teacher Rating Scale (BERS-2; Epstein, 2004)	52 items *Competence/Adaptive Scales* Total Strengths Score, Interpersonal Strengths, School Functioning, Intrapersonal Strengths, Family Strengths, Affective Strengths	Separate norms for boys and girls, ages 5–18	PRO-ED 8700 Shoal Creek Boulevard Austin, TX 78757-6897 800-879-3202 www.proedinc.com
Child Symptom Inventory–4 Teacher Checklist (CSI-4; Gadow & Sprafkin, 2002)	77 items *Problem Scales* 12 DSM-IV Disorders Academic Performance	Separate norms for boys and girls, ages 5–12 (elementary school)	Checkmate Plus P.O. Box 696 Stony Brook, NY 11790-0696 800-779-4292 www.checkmateplus.com
Conners Rating Scales—Revised—Teacher Form (CRS-R-T; Conners,1997)	28 items (short form) *Problem Scales* ADHD Index, Oppositional, Hyperactivity, Cognitive Problems/Inattention	Separate norms for boys and girls, ages 3–5, 6–8, 9–11, 12–14, 15–17	MHS P.O. Box 950 North Tonawanda, NY 14120-0950 800-456-3003 www.mhs.com

Instrument	Items and scales	Norms	Publisher
Devereux Behavior Rating Scale–School Form (DBRS; Naglieri, LeBuff, & Pfeiffer, 1993)	40 items *Problem Scales* Total Problems, Interpersonal Problems, Inappropriate Behaviors/Feelings, Depression, Physical Symptoms/Fears	Separate norms for boys and girls, ages 5–12 and 13–18	Harcourt Assessment, Inc. 19500 Academic Court San Antonio, TX 78204-2498 800-211-8378 www.psychcorpcenter.com
Early Childhood Inventory–4 Teacher Checklist (ECI-4; Gadow & Sprafkin, 2000)	87 items *Problem Scales* 11 DSM-IV Disorders Developmental Deficits Index Peer Conflict Scale	Separate norms for boys and girls, ages 3–6 (pre-elementary school)	Checkmate Plus P.O. Box 696 Stony Brook, NY 11790-0696 800-779-4292 www.checkmateplus.com
Preschool and Kindergarten Behavioral Scales—Second Edition Teacher version (PKBS-2-T; Merrell, 2002a)	76 items *Problem Scales* Total Problem Behavior, Internalizing, Externalizing *Competence/Adaptive Scales* Total Social Skills, Social Cooperation, Social Interaction, Social Independence	Combined norms for boys and girls, ages 3–6	PRO-ED 8700 Shoal Creek Boulevard Austin, TX 78757-6869 800-879-3202 www.proedinc.com
School Social Behavior Scales—Second Edition (SSBS-2; Merrell, 2002b)	64 items *Problem Scales* Antisocial Behavior Total, Hostile/Irritable, Antisocial/Aggressive, Defiant/Disruptive *Competence/Adaptive Scales* Social Competence Total, Peer Relations, Self-Management/Compliance, Academic Behavior	Combined norms for boys and girls, grades K–6 and 7–12	Assessment–Intervention Resources 2285 Elysium Avenue Eugene, OR 97401 541-338-8736 www.assessment-intervention.com
Social Skills Rating System—Teacher Form (SSRS-T; Gresham & Elliott, 1990)	40–57 items *Problem Scales* Total Problems, Internalizing, Externalizing, Hyperactive (ages 6–11) *Competence/Adaptive Scales* Total Social Skills, Cooperation, Assertion, Responsibility	Separate norms for boys and girls, ages 3–5; grades K–6 and 7–12	American Guidance Service 4201 Woodland Road Circle Pines, MN 55014-1796 800-328-2560 www.agsnet.com

151

*ASEBA, Achenbach System of Empirically Based Assessment.

tional adaptive scale for study skills. The BERS-2 Teacher Rating Scale (Epstein, 2004) assesses patterns of behavioral and emotional strengths similar to the BERS-2 Parent Rating Scale. Other rating scales focus on teachers' reports of social behaviors and social skills, paralleling similar forms for parents.

In the spaces provided in Section II of the Semistructured Teacher Interview, you can record problem areas in which a child has obtained deviant scores on one or more standardized teacher rating scales. This list can serve as a prompt to ask teachers about problems that have not already been discussed in the interview. You can then ask further questions about circumstances surrounding any of these additional problems and whether anything has been done to address them. You can also ask about situations in and outside of school that might affect the child's behavior. It is usually good to avoid going into much detail about other problems, so as not to unnecessarily prolong the interview. However, questions about other possible problems can broaden the focus for formulating conclusions and planning interventions.

Academic Performance

Section III of the Semistructured Teacher Interview provides questions about children's academic performance, as shown in Table 6.3. These questions are similar to questions about school

---

TABLE 6.3. Sample Questions about Academic Performance

Subjects/grades/activities

What are [child's name]'s best subject areas in school? What does he/she like best?
What are [child's name]'s worst subject areas, if any? What does he/she like the least in school?
What grades has [child's name] received in the most recent marking period?
Ask about each subject area.

Have [child's name]'s grades changed remarkably in any area?
What are his/her extracurricular activities (e.g., sports, clubs, school play, band, choir)?
Does [child's name] have any problems with school attendance/skipping classes?

Teachers

How many different teachers does [child's name] have?
How does he/she get along with each teacher?
How does he/she get along with the principal and other school staff?
Is there anyone at school who is especially important to him/her?

Homework

How much homework does [child's name] typically have?
Ask about homework for each subject area.

How much time do you expect a student to spend on homework?
How much time does [child's name] spend on homework?
Does [child's name] have any trouble with homework?

(*If yes*) What kind of trouble?
Does he/she get any help with homework at school?

(*If yes*) How does that work out?
Are homework assignments for [child's name] modified in any way?

Note. Reprinted from McConaughy (2004b). Copyright 2004 by S. H. McConaughy. Reprinted by permission.

subjects, relationships with teachers, and homework in the Semistructured Parent Interview, as discussed in Chapter 5, and in child clinical interviews, as discussed in Chapter 3. Even if teachers have not reported concerns about a child's academic performance, it is usually good to ask some of these general questions to a get a picture of school functioning. The parallel formats of the parent, teacher, and child interviews facilitate comparisons between different perspectives on these issues.

Teaching Strategies

Section IV includes questions about different instructional strategies that teachers might use in their classrooms. For each of the seven strategies listed in Table 6.4, interviewers can ask how often teachers or others (e.g., teacher aides) use that approach in their classrooms and how well the child responds to the strategy. Interviewers can check boxes on the interview protocol to indicate the frequency of use (often occurs, sometimes, seldom/never) and teachers' perceptions of how the child responds (responds well, doesn't respond well).

School Interventions for Behavior Problems

School staff can use many types of interventions to address school behavior problems. Section V of the Semistructured Teacher Interview protocol lists 14 interventions shown in Table 6.5. Versions of these approaches have been discussed widely in the educational and psychology literature. Interviewers can use this list to ask teachers whether they think such an intervention might work with a particular child in their classroom or school, and whether they or others are actually using the intervention. The interview protocol provides boxes that you can check to indicate teachers' perceptions of the potential effectiveness of each intervention (will work, might work, won't work) and the acceptability of each intervention (doing now, willing to try, won't try).

TABLE 6.4. Sample Questions about Teaching Strategies

What teaching or instructional strategies do you or other people use in your classroom?

How well does [child's name] respond to this strategy?
Ask the teacher(s) about each strategy and how the child responds to each one that is relevant.

Large-group instruction/teacher lecture
Small-group instruction
One-on-one instruction/individual aide
Independent seatwork
Independent hands-on projects
Peer cooperative learning groups/projects
Peer tutoring

Has [child's name] ever been retained/held back a grade?

(If yes) When? For what reason?
Do you think that retention was appropriate?
How do you think he/she felt about being retained/held back?

Note. Reprinted from McConaughy (2004b). Copyright 2004 by S. H. McConaughy. Reprinted by permission.

TABLE 6.5. Sample Questions about School Interventions for Behavior Problems

Let me ask you about a number of different approaches for dealing with children's school behavior problems.
Which of these do you think might work to address [child's name]'s behavior problem(s)?
Which of these are you already doing or would you be willing to try in your classroom/this school setting?
Ask about each intervention listed below.

Classwide rules/behavioral expectations
Classwide behavior program/token reward system
Individual student behavior plan/contract
Classwide social skills instruction
Individual or small-group social skills instruction
Peer buddy system/peer tutoring
Cooperative learning groups/projects
Individual attention from teacher/teacher aide
In-school suspension
Out-of-school suspension
Self time-out/quiet place to work
Self-monitoring
Special education/IEP
Section 504 plan/accommodations
Other—describe:

Do you want help or support for dealing with [child's name]'s problems in your classroom/your situation?

(If yes) What kind of support would work best for you?

Note. Reprinted from McConaughy (2004b). Copyright 2004 by S. H. McConaughy. Reprinted by permission.

Special Help/Services

Section VI surveys teachers about 13 types of special help or special services, shown in Table 6.6. Interviewers can use this list to ask teachers whether the child is currently receiving any of these services. Interviewers can check boxes on the protocol form to indicate teachers' responses (yes, no, don't know). Interviewers can then ask follow-up questions about the frequency and duration of each current service, and whether the child has received similar services in the past. They can also ask teachers whether they think the types of current services are appropriate ("Do you think this is enough/the right kind of help?") and whether other types of services are available.

The sample questions in Sections IV, V, and VI are more structured than questions in earlier sections of the teacher interview protocol. The lists of teaching strategies, school interventions for behavior problems, and special help or services are intended to reduce time and increase the efficiency of these parts of the teacher interview. However, you should feel free to follow up with more open-ended questions about each of these areas, as time permits. The checklists can also serve as prompts to ask about different strategies, interventions, or services that teachers might not mention spontaneously. If the interview is conducted with more than one teacher at the same time, you can check the appropriate boxes in Sections IV, V, and VI to indicate the general consensus about each question and use space in the right-hand columns of the protocol to write notes about differences in approaches or perceptions.

School-based practitioners can use the Semistructured Teacher Interview as a component of multimethod assessment. They can also use the interview protocol for initial stages of problem identification and problem solving in ongoing behavioral consultation. For behavioral consulta-

TABLE 6.6. Sample Questions about Special Help or Services

Does [child's name] currently receive any special help/special services in school?
Ask the teacher about each type of special service and note his/her comments.

Special education/IEP
Remedial instruction/Title I services
Speech and language services
Adaptive physical education
Section 504 plan/accommodations
Behavioral consultation/behavioral specialist
Individual aide
Guidance services
School psychology services
Psychotherapy/mental health services
Social skills training
School social worker
Gifted and talented program/enrichment
Other—describe:

How often does he/she receive this special help?
How long has he/she received special help?
What kinds of help has he/she received in the past?
Do you think this is enough/the right kind of help?
Are there any other types of services available?

Note. Reprinted from McConaughy (2004b). Copyright 2004 by S. H. McConaughy. Reprinted by permission.

tion, teachers' descriptions of observable priority behaviors in Section II can form the basis for "operational definitions" of target behaviors for direct observations and progress monitoring. Answers to questions in Sections IV, V, and VI can establish which teaching strategies, interventions, and services have already been tried and what approaches are acceptable to teachers. This information, combined with other data, can then be used to develop BIPs that target specific problem behaviors.

CONCLUDING THE TEACHER INTERVIEW

Conclude the interview by thanking teachers for taking time out of their busy schedules to talk about the child. Then review any pertinent confidentiality issues discussed at the beginning of the interview. If you plan to write a report, it is usually good to summarize the type of information that will be included (e.g., teacher-reported problems, the child's current academic performance, suggestions regarding interventions, results of teacher rating scales). You can tell teachers again that you will not quote their exact words or name them personally in written reports, as recommended earlier. Teachers may also appreciate hearing about plans for additional data collection and any future meetings with them and/or parents. You may also want to involve certain teachers in future data collection and progress monitoring. Summarizing the next steps to be taken can often assure teachers that their reports are valuable and that the time they devoted to the interview has not been wasted.

SUMMARY

This chapter discussed the use of semistructured interviews to obtain teachers' perspectives on children's school functioning. Many of the questioning strategies discussed in previous chapters on child and parent interviews also apply to teacher interviews. The Semistructured Teacher Interview (Appendix 6.1) provides a protocol for obtaining information from teachers that can assist in development of school-based interventions. Questions in the first two sections of the teacher interview mirror behavioral interviewing strategies used in the Semistructured Parent Interview (Appendix 5.1). After asking teachers to describe their concerns about the child, interviewers ask questions about specific problems that can become targets for functional behavioral assessment. Other sections of the teacher interview cover the child's academic performance, teachers' instructional strategies, school interventions for behavior problems, and special help or services currently provided to the child. The format of the Semistructured Teacher Interview assumes that practitioners will also use standardized teacher rating scales and other procedures to obtain a multimethod assessment of the child.

Semistructured Teacher Interview

Child's name _____ Age _____ Gender _____
First   Middle   Last

Interviewer's name _____ Date ____ / ____ / ____
First   Middle   Last   Month   Day   Year

Teacher's name _____ Role/class _____

CONFIDENTIALITY AND PURPOSE OF THE INTERVIEW

Thank you for taking your time to meet with me today and for completing the various questionnaires that you received before our meeting. I have reviewed the information that you provided on these forms. In this interview, I would like to hear more about your concerns about [child's name]. Your perspective(s) is important for evaluating [child's name]'s functioning.

    The information you provide will be summarized in a written evaluation report. My usual practice is not to include direct quotations of teachers' comments in written reports. However, I may have to report information to appropriate legal authorities or others (such as parents) if there is reason to suspect child abuse or when the child poses a danger to self or a danger to other persons. In such cases, I may have to quote what you said directly, but I will try to confer with you about that ahead of time.

I. CONCERNS ABOUT THE CHILD	RESPONSES/COMMENTS
What concerns you most about [child's name]? *If the teacher has more than one concern, list each area of concern.*	
When did you first become concerned about this? *If the teacher has more than one concern, note when first concerned for each area of concern.*	
How long has this been a problem? *If the teacher has more than one concern, note duration for each area of concern.*	
If the teacher's main concerns are academic problems, ask questions in Section III first and then return to Section II. If the main concerns are behavioral or emotional problems, continue with Section II.	
II. SCHOOL BEHAVIOR PROBLEMS Does [child's name] currently have behavior problems at school? ☐ Yes ☐ No ☐ Don't know (*If yes*) What kind of behavior problems?	

(continued)

	RESPONSES/COMMENTS

Specific Nature of the Problems

When [child's name] has this behavior problem, what exactly does he/she do? What does he/she say? Give me some examples of this problem.
If there is more than one problem, ask the teacher to describe each one.

How long has he/she been having this problem?

How often does this problem occur now?

Under what circumstances does this problem occur?

Where and when does this problem usually occur?
Ask for specific descriptions of where and when each problem occurs: e.g., classroom, recess, lunch, transition periods, group situations, independent work, morning, afternoon.

Priorities for Interventions

Which of the problems we have discussed are you most concerned about now? Which do you think is the most important to address now?

Antecedents and Consequences of Priority Problem(s)

Let's talk about the problem(s) you think are of most concern. What usually happens before this problem occurs? What seems to set it off?
If more than one area of concern, ask about the top two or three problems.

What usually happens after this problem occurs?
What do you do? What do other people do?

How do you usually deal with this problem in your classroom? How do you react?

Replacement Behaviors

What would be acceptable or alternative behavior related to this problem? What would you like to see [child's name] do instead?

What does [child's name] do well? What do you see as his/her strengths that might help to address this problem(s)?

(continued)

	RESPONSES/COMMENTS

Other Possible Problem Areas

If behavior rating scales (e.g., ASEBA Teacher's Report Form or BASC-2 Teacher Rating Scale) have been completed and scored prior to the interview, list all problem scales with scores in the borderline or clinical ranges (compared to the relevant normative sample). Summarize the results for the teacher. Ask about problem areas that were not discussed as major concerns.

Before our meeting, you completed a questionnaire about [child's name]'s behavior. The questionnaire listed behaviors that can be scored on scales describing different problem areas. Your ratings produced scores indicating severe problems in:

_____

_____

_____

_____

_____

_____

_____

We have already discussed some of these problem areas. What about the problem areas we have not discussed. How much are you concerned about these problems?

Under what circumstances do these problems occur?

What is currently being done to address these problems?

Are there any other areas where you think [child's name] has behavioral or emotional problems?

Do you have concerns about situations outside of school that might affect [child's name]'s behavior or emotional functioning?

(continued)

III. ACADEMIC PERFORMANCE	RESPONSES/COMMENTS

III. ACADEMIC PERFORMANCE

Does [child's name] currently have academic or learning problems?

☐ Yes   ☐ No   ☐ Don't know

(*If yes*) What kind of problems?
Summarize all subject areas in which the teacher reports academic or learning problems.

Why do you think [child's name] is having academic or learning problems now?

How long has he/she had these problems?

Subject Areas/Grades/Activities

What are [child's name]'s best subject areas in school? What does he/she like best?

What are [child's name]'s worst subject areas, if any? What does he/she like least?

What grades has [child's name] received in the most recent marking period?
Ask about each subject area.

Have [child's name]'s grades changed remarkably in any area?

What are his/her extracurricular activities (e.g., sports, clubs, school play, band, choir)?

Does [child's name] have any problems with school attendance/skipping classes?

Teachers

How many teachers does [child's name] have?
How does he/she get along with each teacher?
How does he/she get along with the principal and other school staff?

Is there anyone at school who is especially important to him/her?

Homework

How much homework does [child's name] typically have?
Ask about homework for each subject area.

How much time do you expect a student to spend on homework?
How much time does [child's name] spend on homework?

Does [child's name] have any trouble with homework?
(*If yes*) What kind of trouble?

(continued)

Homework *(cont.)*	**RESPONSES/COMMENTS**

Homework *(cont.)*

Does he/she get any help with homework at school?
(*If yes*) How does this work out?

Does he/she get any help with homework at home? (*If yes*) How does this work out?

Are homework assignments for [child's name] modified in any way?

IV. TEACHING STRATEGIES

What teaching or instructional strategies do you or other people use in your classroom?

How well does [child's name] respond to these strategies?

Ask the teacher(s) about each strategy and how the child responds to each one that is relevant. Check the appropriate boxes to indicate the teacher's responses. If you are interviewing several teachers at once, you can indicate the general consensus among them and write notes regarding any differences about teaching strategies.

Large-group instruction/teacher lecture
☐ Often occurs ☐ Sometimes ☐ Seldom/never
☐ Responds well ☐ Doesn't respond well

Small-group instruction
☐ Often occurs ☐ Sometimes ☐ Seldom/never
☐ Responds well ☐ Doesn't respond well

One-on-one instruction/individual aide
☐ Often occurs ☐ Sometimes ☐ Seldom/never
☐ Responds well ☐ Doesn't respond well

Independent seatwork
☐ Often occurs ☐ Sometimes ☐ Seldom/never
☐ Responds well ☐ Doesn't respond well

Independent hands-on projects
☐ Often occurs ☐ Sometimes ☐ Seldom/never
☐ Responds well ☐ Doesn't respond well

Peer cooperative learning groups/projects
☐ Often occurs ☐ Sometimes ☐ Seldom/never
☐ Responds well ☐ Doesn't respond well

Peer tutoring
☐ Often occurs ☐ Sometimes ☐ Seldom/never
☐ Responds well ☐ Doesn't respond well

Other—describe:

(continued)

Retention

Has [child's name] ever been retained/held back a grade?

☐ Yes ☐ No ☐ Don't know

(If yes) When? For what reason?

Do you think that retention was appropriate?

How do you think he/she felt about being retained/held back?

V. SCHOOL INTERVENTIONS FOR BEHAVIOR PROBLEMS

Let me ask you about a number of different approaches for dealing with children's school behavior problems.

Which of these do you think might work to address [child's name]'s behavior problem(s)?

Which of these are you already doing or would you be willing to try in your classroom/this school setting?

Ask about each intervention listed below. Check the appropriate boxes to indicate the teacher's responses. If you are interviewing several teachers at once, you can indicate the general consensus among them and write notes regarding any differences about services.

Classwide rules/behavioral expectations
☐ Will work ☐ Might work ☐ Won't work
☐ Doing now ☐ Willing to try ☐ Won't try

Classwide behavior program/token reward system
☐ Will work ☐ Might work ☐ Won't work
☐ Doing now ☐ Willing to try ☐ Won't try

Individual student behavior plan/contract
☐ Will work ☐ Might work ☐ Won't work
☐ Doing now ☐ Willing to try ☐ Won't try

Classwide social skills instruction
☐ Will work ☐ Might work ☐ Won't work
☐ Doing now ☐ Willing to try ☐ Won't try

Individual or small-group social skills instruction
☐ Will work ☐ Might work ☐ Won't work
☐ Doing now ☐ Willing to try ☐ Won't try

RESPONSES/COMMENTS

(continued)

162

V. SCHOOL INTERVENTIONS FOR BEHAVIOR PROBLEMS *(cont.)*	RESPONSES/COMMENTS

V. SCHOOL INTERVENTIONS FOR BEHAVIOR PROBLEMS *(cont.)*

Peer buddy system/peer tutoring
☐ Will work ☐ Might work ☐ Won't work
☐ Doing now ☐ Willing to try ☐ Won't try

Cooperative learning groups/projects
☐ Will work ☐ Might work ☐ Won't work
☐ Doing now ☐ Willing to try ☐ Won't try

Individual attention from teacher/teacher aide
☐ Will work ☐ Might work ☐ Won't work
☐ Doing now ☐ Willing to try ☐ Won't try

In-school suspension
☐ Will work ☐ Might work ☐ Won't work
☐ Doing now ☐ Willing to try ☐ Won't try

Out-of-school suspension
☐ Will work ☐ Might work ☐ Won't work
☐ Doing now ☐ Willing to try ☐ Won't try

Self time-out/quiet place to work
☐ Will work ☐ Might work ☐ Won't work
☐ Doing now ☐ Willing to try ☐ Won't try

Self-monitoring
☐ Will work ☐ Might work ☐ Won't work
☐ Doing now ☐ Willing to try ☐ Won't try

Special education/IEP
☐ Will work ☐ Might work ☐ Won't work
☐ Doing now ☐ Willing to try ☐ Won't try

Section 504 plan/accommodations
☐ Will work ☐ Might work ☐ Won't work
☐ Doing now ☐ Willing to try ☐ Won't try

Other-describe:

Do you want help or support for dealing with [child's name]'s problems in your classroom/ your situation?

(If yes) What kind of support would work best for you?

(continued)

VI. SPECIAL HELP/SERVICES

Does [child's name] currently receive any special help/special services in school?

Ask the teacher(s) about each type of special service and note comments.

Special education/IEP
☐ Yes ☐ No ☐ Don't know

Remedial instruction/Title I services
☐ Yes ☐ No ☐ Don't know

Speech and language services
☐ Yes ☐ No ☐ Don't know

Adaptive physical education
☐ Yes ☐ No ☐ Don't know

Section 504 plan/accommodations
☐ Yes ☐ No ☐ Don't know

Behavioral consultation/behavioral specialist
☐ Yes ☐ No ☐ Don't know

Individual aide
☐ Yes ☐ No ☐ Don't know

Guidance services
☐ Yes ☐ No ☐ Don't know

School psychology services
☐ Yes ☐ No ☐ Don't know

Psychotherapy/mental health services
☐ Yes ☐ No ☐ Don't know

Social skills training
☐ Yes ☐ No ☐ Don't know

School social worker
☐ Yes ☐ No ☐ Don't know

Gifted and talented program/enrichment
☐ Yes ☐ No ☐ Don't know

Other—describe:

How often does he/she receive this special help?
How long has he/she received special help?
What kinds of help has he/she received in the past?
Do you think this is enough/the right kind of help?
Are there any other types of services available?
Do you have any other school concerns?

7

Interpreting Clinical Interviews for Assessment and Intervention Planning

Previous chapters have highlighted the value of clinical interviews for assessing children's functioning. In child clinical interviews you can learn children's views of their problems and competencies and at the same time directly observe their behavior, affect, and interaction style. In parent and teacher interviews, you can learn firsthand parents' and teachers' views of children's problems and competencies and what situations or life circumstances affect their functioning. Learning each informant's perspective helps you and others weigh different options for ameliorating problems and boosting competencies. Hearing parents' and teachers' views also helps you evaluate what each party is able and willing to do on the child's behalf. Hearing children's views helps you evaluate their level of awareness of their own competencies and problems and how receptive they might be to different interventions.

RECORDING AND REPORTING INTERVIEW INFORMATION

For traditional semistructured interviewing as well as behavioral interviewing, practitioners have usually relied on written notes (and sometimes audio- or videotaped recordings) to document information. For evaluation and clinical records, practitioners often write reports that summarize information they judge to be important from their interviews. Such anecdotal reports provide qualitative data derived from clinical interviews. Chapters 5 and 6 provided reproducible protocols that practitioners can use to record their notes from interviews with parents (Appendix 5.1) and teachers (Appendix 6.1), which can then form the basis for written reports.

Structured diagnostic interviews typically follow more rigid, standardized protocols for asking questions and recording interviewees' answers regarding symptoms and other criteria for psychiatric diagnoses. The interviewee's responses are then aggregated into "yes" or "no" decisions regarding the presence (or absence) of specific diagnoses. Appendix 5.3 provided a protocol that school-based practitioners can use for recording information from structured diagnostic interviews with parents. They can then decide whether or not to include parents' reports of DSM-IV diagnostic criteria in their written evaluation reports. As indicated in Chapter 5, practitioners who use the structured diagnostic interview should have training in theory and practice for making DSM-IV diagnoses. They should also gather information from other sources to formulate diagnostic conclusions.

Chapters 3 and 4 listed questions for child clinical interviews organized according to the topic areas outlined in Table 3.1. Many of these questions were modeled on questions in the SCICA Protocol (McConaughy & Achenbach, 2001). School-based practitioners can use the tables in Chapters 3 and 4 to guide their child clinical interviews. Another option is to obtain the SCICA Protocol from the ASEBA (www.ASEBA.org).

In addition to obtaining children's self-reports from interviews, you can also observe many different aspects of their functioning: characteristics of dress and motor coordination; behavioral functioning, such as activity level, distractibility, nervous mannerisms; social–emotional functioning, such as range of affect, interaction style, level of insight, and mood state (e.g., anger, anxiety, apathy, unhappiness); and cognitive and communication skills, such as receptive and expressive language, reasoning, and problem-solving (Hughes & Baker, 1990; Merrell, 2003). Recording observations of these characteristics is as important as recording children's responses to questions.

SCICA Rating Forms and Scoring Profile

The SCICA (McConaughy & Achenbach, 2001) provides two structured rating forms that interviewers can use to rate their observations and children's self-reported problems. The SCICA Observation Form contains 120 items for rating observations of children's behavior during the interview. Examples include the following: argues; avoids eye contact; defiant, talks back, or sarcastic; disjointed or tangential conversation; doesn't sit still, restless or hyperactive; limited conversation; sudden changes in mood or feelings; and unhappy, sad, or depressed. The SCICA Self-Report contains 125 items for rating problems that children may report in response to open-ended questions around the various topic areas of the interview. Examples include the following: Reports acts of cruelty, bullying, or meanness to others, including siblings; reports being disobedient at home; reports deliberately harming self or attempting suicide; reports feeling worthless or inferior; reports not being liked by peers; reports getting into physical fights; and reports worrying. There are also two open-ended items for observations or self-reports not covered by the more specific items.

After completing the SCICA, interviewers rate the child on each item of the Observation and Self-Report Forms using a 4-point scale from 0 (no occurrence of the problem) to 3 (definite occurrence with severe intensity or more than 3 minutes duration). The SCICA manual (McConaughy & Achenbach, 2001) provides rules for scoring the items 0, 1, 2, or 3 to describe the interviewer's observations and children's self-reported problems. A training videotape provides additional opportunity for practitioners to learn SCICA scoring procedures. Many of the SCICA observation and self-report items have counterparts on the CBCL and TRF, which facilitates comparisons of interview data with parent and teacher reports about the child.

SCICA interviewer ratings are then scored on a standardized profile of problem scales. The SCICA Profile includes the following five empirically based syndrome scales for problems observed by the interviewer: Anxious, Withdrawn/Depressed, Language/Motor Problems, Attention Problems, and Self-Control Problems. Three additional syndrome scales include problems reported by the child during the interview: Anxious/Depressed, Aggressive/Rule-Breaking, and Somatic Complaints (scored only for ages 12–18). Derived from factor analyses, the syndrome scales comprise groups of problems that statistically co-occur. Additional factor analyses produced an Internalizing grouping comprising the Anxious and Anxious/Depressed scales and an Externalizing grouping comprising the Aggressive/Rule-Breaking, Attention Problems, and Self-Control Problems scales.

In addition to the empirically based scales, the SCICA Profile has six scales for scoring problem items that are consistent with DSM-IV diagnoses: Affective Problems, Anxiety Problems, Somatic Problems, Attention Deficit/Hyperactivity Problems, Oppositional Defiant Problems, and Conduct Problems. The SCICA DSM-oriented scales correspond to similar scales scored from the CBCL, TRF, and YSR (Achenbach & Rescorla, 2001). The SCICA Profile also provides separate scores for Total Observations and Total Self-Reports.

The SCICA Profile can be scored by hand or by computer. The profile provides normalized clinical T-scores and percentiles for ages 6–11 and 12–18 for the eight syndrome scales, Internalizing, Externalizing, Total Observations, Total Self-Reports, and the six DSM-oriented scales. The clinical T-scores indicate how an individual child's score on each scale compares to scores obtained by clinical samples of children in each of the two age groups. By examining the profile of SCICA scale scores, practitioners can identify areas in which a child exhibited severe problems or fewer problems, compared to other clinically referred children. In this way the SCICA Profile enables users to judge the severity of children's problems in relation to an empirical standard, which is not available from other interview formats.

The SCICA Profile is especially useful for making classification or eligibility decisions that require judgments about the severity of problems. An example is determining whether a child meets IDEA criteria for special education services under the category of emotional disturbance (ED). The IDEA definition of ED states that a child must exhibit specific characteristics to "a marked degree." The CBCL, TRF, and YSR scoring profiles provide T-scores derived from normative samples of nonreferred children as an empirical standard for judging deviance or "marked degree." The clinical T-scores from the SCICA, on the other hand, are derived from clinically referred samples. As a result, moderate to high clinical T-scores from the SCICA scoring profile usually indicate more severe problems than similar scores derived from normative samples of nonreferred children. Accordingly, McConaughy and Achenbach (2001) consider SCICA T-scores of 55 or higher (at or above the 69th percentile) to indicate severe problems, in contrast to higher T-score cut points on other ASEBA profiles.

INTEGRATING CLINICAL INTERVIEWS WITH OTHER ASSESSMENT DATA

Although clinical interviews have considerable value for assessment and intervention planning, they should never serve as the sole source of information for such purposes. Instead, information from clinical interviews must be integrated with other assessment data to make judgments about children's functioning and to decide which, if any, services may be required to meet their needs. Accordingly, Table 1.2 in Chapter 1 outlined five axes of multimethod assessment to consider: parent reports, teacher reports, cognitive assessment, physical assessment, and direct assessment of the child.

It is beyond the scope of this book to discuss all aspects of multimethod assessment in detail. Instead, the focus is on how to integrate interview information with other assessment data for decision making and intervention planning. To illustrate this process, the next sections summarize information obtained from multiple sources for the five case examples introduced in previous chapters. The interview and assessment data were derived from research and clinical work with many children, with appropriate changes in case information to protect confidentiality. As indicated earlier, all names are pseudonyms. To illustrate multimethod assessment, each of the five cases includes a child clinical interview, parent and teacher interviews, standardized rating scales, direct observations in the school setting, and cognitive and academic testing. Although the SCICA Profile is included to illustrate quantitative interpretations of child interview data, the anecdotal information is also important for understanding different informants' perspectives and for planning interventions. The SCICA manual (McConaughy & Achenbach, 2001) provides detailed discussion of the SCICA Profiles, along with other assessment data, for three cases (Bruce Garcia, Catherine Holcomb, and Karl Bryant). In addition to the SCICA, the five cases in this chapter also include the CBCL and TRF, and three include the YSR, for purposes of illustration. However, multimethod assessment can incorporate any of the standardized parent and teacher rating scales listed in Tables 5.3 and 6.2. Table 7.1 lists additional examples of standardized self-reports for children old enough to reflect on their own behavior and feelings.

Case Example: Andy Lockwood

As indicated in Chapter 1, 7-year-old Andy Lockwood was referred for evaluation because his mother and teacher were concerned about his slow progress in school, even after repeating first grade. Chapter 3 provided two segments from the child clinical interview with Andy. From these it became clear that Andy was well aware of his academic difficulties. Although he did not seem distressed about repeating first grade, he still thought the work was hard and disliked just about everything in school. He seemed to feel overwhelmed by the amount of work, but liked getting extra help. In another part of the interview, Andy described himself as one of "the kids who are being bad" in school. However, he thought the bad kids were "luckier" than other kids because they got happy faces on a card to help them be good. He said that he only had one more happy face to go to get a treat. However, it was not clear that Andy understood what counted as "good" behavior.

On the SCICA Profile, Andy obtained a score at the 81st percentile on the Aggressive/Rule-Breaking scale, indicating that he reported many more problems of this nature than other clinically referred children. Andy obtained scores at the 79th percentile on the Attention Problems scale and at the 73rd percentile on the Attention Deficit/Hyperactivity Problems scale, reflecting the interviewer's observations of inattention and restlessness during the interview. Andy also scored at the 79th percentile on the Anxious scale, reflecting his lack of confidence, fear of making mistakes, and frequent requests for feedback on academic screening tasks.

In the parent interview Ms. Lockwood reported that Andy was the younger of two children. The parents had divorced when Andy was 2 years old. Andy's father continued to visit with the children every other weekend. Ms. Lockwood, who was college educated, began work as a secre-

TABLE 7.1. Examples of Published Self-Report Scales

Instrument and scales	Items and scales	Normative samples	Publisher
Academic Competence Evaluation Scales—Student Form (ACES; DiPerna & Elliott, 2000)	68 items *Competence/Adaptive Scales* Academic Enablers Total Score, Interpersonal Skills, Engagement, Motivation, Study Skills, Academic Skills Total Score, Reading/Language Arts, Mathematics, Critical Thinking	Combined norms for boys and girls, grades 6–8 and 9–12	Harcourt Assessment, Inc. 19500 Academic Court San Antonio, TX 78204-2498 800-211-8378 www.psychcorpcenter.com
ASEBA[a] Youth Self-Report (YSR; Achenbach & Rescorla, 2001)	14 competence and 105 problem items *Problem Scales* Total Problems, Internalizing, Externalizing, Withdrawn/Depressed, Somatic Complaints, Anxious/Depressed, Social Problems, Thought Problems, Attention Problems, Rule-Breaking Behavior, Aggressive Behavior, Affective Problems, Anxiety Problems, Attention/Deficit Hyperactivity Problems, Oppositional Defiant Problems, Conduct Problems *Competence/Adaptive Scales* Total Competence, Activities, Social	Separate norms for boys and girls, ages 11–18	Research Center for Children, Youth, & Families, Inc. One South Prospect St. Burlington, VT 05401-3456 802-264-6432 www.ASEBA.org
Behavior Assessment System For Children–2 Self-Report of Personality (BASC-2 PRS; Reynolds & Kamphaus, 2004)	139–185 items *Problem Scales* Emotional Symptoms Index, Inattention/Hyperactivity, Internalizing Problems, School Problems (ages 8-21), Attitude to School, Attitude to Teachers, Sensation Seeking, Atypicality, Locus of Control, Social Stress, Anxiety, Depression, Sense of Inadequacy, Somatization, Attention Problems, Hyperactivity, Alcohol Abuse (ages 18–25), School Maladjustment (18–25) *Competence/Adaptive Scales* Personal Adjustment, Relations with Parents, Interpersonal Relations, Self-Esteem, Self-Reliance	Separate norms for boys and girls, ages 8–11, 12–21, and 18–25	American Guidance Service 4201 Woodland Road Circle Pines, MN 55014-1796 800-328-2560 www.agsnet.com
Behavioral and Emotional Rating Scale (2nd edition) Parent Rating Scale (BERS-2; Epstein, 2004)	57 items *Competence/Adaptive Scales* Total Strengths Score, Interpersonal Strengths, School Functioning, Intrapersonal Strengths, Family Strengths, Affective Strengths, Career Strengths	Separate norms for boys and girls, ages 11–18	PRO-ED 8700 Shoal Creek Boulevard Austin, TX 78757-6897 800-879-3202 www.proedinc.com

(continued)

TABLE 7.1. (continued)

Instrument and scales	Items and scales	Normative samples	Publisher
Conners–Wells Adolescent Self-Report Scales (CASS; Conners,1997)	27 items (short form) *Problem Scales* ADHD Index, Conduct Problems, Hyperactivity, Cognitive Problems/Inattention	Separate norms for boys and girls, ages 12–17	MHS P.O. Box 950 North Tonawanda, NY 14120-0950 800-456-3003 www.mhs.com
Millon Adolescent Clinical Inventory (Millon, 1993)	160 items *Problem Scales* 30 scales with 5 dimensions	Separate norms for boys and girls, ages 13–19	Pearson Assessments P.O. Box 1416 Minneapolis, MN 55440 800-627-7271 www.pearsonassessments.com
Minnesota Multiphasic Personality Inventory—Adolescent Version (MMPI-A; Butcher et al., 1992)	478 items *Problem Scales* 7 validity scales, 10 basic clinical scales, 15 content scales	Separate norms for boys and girls, ages 14–18	Pearson Assessments P.O. Box 1416 Minneapolis, MN 55440 800-627-7271 www.pearsonassessments.com
Personality Inventory for Youth (PIY; Lachar & Gruber, 1995)	270 items *Problem Scales* Cognitive Impairment, Impulsivity/Distractibility, Delinquency, Family Dysfunction, Reality Distortion, Somatic Concern, Psychological Discomfort, Social Withdrawal, Social Skills Deficits	Separate norms for boys and girls, ages 9–19	Western Psychological Services 12031 Wilshire Boulevard Los Angeles, CA 90025-1251 800-648-8857 www.wpspublish.com
Social Skills Rating System—Student Form (SSRS-S; Gresham & Elliott, 1990)	34–39 items *Competence/Adaptive Scales* Total Social Skills, Cooperation, Assertion, Empathy, Self-Control	Separate norms for boys and girls, grades 3–6 and 7–12	American Guidance Service 4201 Woodland Road Circle Pines, MN 55014-1796 800-328-2560 www.agsnet.com
Youth's Inventory–4 (YI-4; Gadow & Sprafkin, 1999)	113 items *Problem Scales* 13 DSM-IV Disorders, Inconsistency	Separate norms for boys and girls, ages 12–18	Checkmate Plus P.O. Box 696 Stony Brook, NY 11790-0696 800-779-4292 www.checkmateplus.com

*Note.*ᵃASEBA, Achenbach System of Empirically Based Assessment.

170

tary when Andy entered first grade. Prior to that, she had worked as a substitute teacher, so she thought she had a good idea of what to expect from school.

Ms. Lockwood acknowledged that Andy was easily distracted and had trouble doing schoolwork:

> "Everyday, he brings home worksheets that he hasn't finished in class. Then we have to spend time after dinner getting them done. He complains that they are boring, but I sometimes wonder if he understands what he is supposed to do. When I explain it to him, he gets everything right. But if I'm not sitting right next to him, he starts daydreaming and fooling around and doesn't work. It gets pretty frustrating having to nag him all the time to get things done."

At the end of the last school year, Andy's teacher sent home a pile of worksheets to complete, but Ms. Lockwood decided that all the work was "ridiculous" and told Andy he didn't have to do it. Ms. Lockwood thought that Andy's current teacher didn't like him because she called home frequently complaining about his behavior in school. The teacher seldom had anything nice to say about Andy. Ms. Lockwood said that her older daughter had had similar problems when she was younger, but now was doing fine in fifth grade.

Ms. Lockwood described Andy's early development as normal, although he had some trouble with his fine-motor skills, such as tying shoelaces. He also seemed to depend on others to do things for him. She said that Andy was still a very active child who likes sports and being outdoors. She also said that she had trouble disciplining Andy at times because "he wants to do everything his own way." She reported occasionally resorting to spanking, but mostly she sent him to his room when he disobeyed. She indicated that she would be open to trying a "behavior system" with Andy if someone would help her with it. When she had tried "checklists" in the past, they didn't seem to work very well. When asked about Andy's strengths, Ms. Lockwood said that he seemed very creative; he loved to draw and make things with clay and other crafts materials; he enjoyed building things with Legos; and he had a great sense of humor.

Following the general interview, the school psychologist conducted a brief structured diagnostic interview with Andy's mother. Ms. Lockwood endorsed requisite symptoms and other criteria for a DSM-IV diagnosis of ADHD—Combined Type (314.01). She also reported some oppositional behavior at home.

In her interview with the school psychologist, the teacher reported that Andy had beginning first grade skills because he was a "repeater," but at midyear he was falling behind in reading, language arts, and math. He did better in science and social studies. He seemed to like hands-on projects, but did not like writing assignments. The teacher was frustrated with Andy's inability to keep his mind on academic tasks. "In my class, he's in outer space," she said. "He's a bright boy who is severely sidetracked and seems to be in his own world." When asked to give an example of what she meant, the teacher said, "He's distracted by everything. He does not recognize when he is being spoken to. If I give a direction and then ask him to repeat it, he can't do it."

When asked about circumstances and types of tasks that were difficult, the teacher reported:

> "He has a lot of difficulty finishing his work without one-to-one supervision. He seems to become more easily distracted if the task he is doing is hard for him—like math papers. Some-

times, incentives work for him and other times, they don't. It is very difficult to find something that works for him consistently."

Through further probing, the school psychologist learned that the teacher put "happy faces" or stickers on Andy's papers when he finished them correctly. But often the work was not done on time, so she made Andy stay in during recess to finish it, and then he would not get a happy face. At the end of each week, if he had done his work, Andy could earn a treat from his mother. However, he seldom earned the treats. The teacher sent a note home each Friday summarizing Andy's performance that week. She did not use any formal method for charting his progress or work completion.

When asked about Andy's social relations, the teacher reported that he had difficulty getting along with other children because he acted immature and silly. He seemed to "gravitate" toward other kids who got into trouble. He clowned around in class to get attention and disturbed other kids when they were supposed to be working quietly. When Andy became too disruptive, she sent him to the principal's office. At recess, Andy sometimes got into fights with other kids, particularly one other boy. Andy always said that the fights were not his fault and that the other kid started it by calling him names or teasing.

On the CBCL and TRF, Andy's mother and teacher both scored him in the clinical range (above the 97th percentile) on the Attention Problems and Attention Deficit/Hyperactivity Problems scales, indicating severe problems compared to nonreferred 6- to 11-year-old boys. The teacher's ratings produced scores above the 98th percentile on the TRF Inattention and Hyperactivity–impulsivity subscales. Both informants also scored Andy in the borderline to clinical range on the Social Problems and Aggressive Behavior scales. Andy's mother scored him low on the CBCL School scale, and his teacher scored him low on the TRF Adaptive Functioning scale.

The school psychologist observed Andy several times in class under various instructional conditions. Andy showed a consistent pattern of inattention, distractibility, and low on-task behavior that corroborated the parent and teacher reports. The school psychologist observed that Andy stayed on-task when the teacher gave specific directives (e.g., "Get your work out") and stood by his desk to give him help or let him sit next to her desk. Although Andy frequently raised his hand or approached the teacher to ask for help, he did not always get a response from the her. When the teacher wasn't paying attention to Andy or wasn't physically near him, he was usually off task, staring out the window or looking around the room, talking to other students, or clowning to get other students' attention.

On a standardized intelligence test, Andy scored in the high-average range for verbal and nonverbal performance ability. Although he scored in the low-average range on tests of working memory, there were no significant differences among the subtest scores. Standardized achievement tests also produced scores in the average to high-average range.

Andy's high scores on standardized parent and teacher rating scales and the SCICA Profile, plus information from parent and teacher interviews and classroom observations, all pointed toward a DSM-IV diagnosis of ADHD–Combined Type (314.01). With this information, the school multidisciplinary team referred Andy and his mother to a mental health clinic for further evaluation and treatment for ADHD. Ms. Lockwood agreed to a trial of methylphenidate for Andy. She also agreed to participate in a parent training group at the clinic that focused on behavioral strategies for children with ADHD and oppositional behavior.

At school the multidisciplinary team developed a Section 504 plan for Andy. The interviews and classroom observations were particularly informative for developing classroom accommodations and behavioral interventions. Andy's plan involved several components. First, the teacher and school psychologist created a positive incentive plan targeted on improving on-task behavior and reducing disruptive behavior in class (e.g., clowning and disturbing others during quiet time). The plan divided each school day into smaller periods that made sense to Andy (e.g., morning to recess, recess to lunch, lunch to end of school day). As Andy met behavioral targets for each time period, he earned points toward a menu of rewards at the end of each day. Andy earned extra points when he avoided fights on the playground. The teacher charted Andy's daily progress toward behavioral goals. She also posted a large chart of classroom rules at the front of the room for all students to see.

Second, the teacher agreed to break Andy's assignments into smaller components to reduce his feelings of being overwhelmed by schoolwork. She checked routinely to ensure that Andy understood directions and then praised him for his efforts. Andy also received small-group instruction in reading and math.

Third, the teacher created regular school–home notes (Kelley, 1990) to keep Andy's mother informed of his progress. She sent Ms. Lockwood a copy of Andy's behavior chart at the end of each week, along with notes about his behavior and accomplishments. The teacher also sent home brief homework assignments to reinforce specific skills taught in class (see Power et al., 2001). Clear instructions for homework assignments, plus a home-based reward system, helped to reduce conflicts between Andy and his mother over homework.

Fourth, with the support of the school psychologist, Andy's teacher used curriculum-based measures to monitor and chart his academic progress. With all of the above educational interventions and mental health services in place for the rest of the school year, Andy successfully moved into second grade the following year.

Case Example: Bruce Garcia

Chapters 3 and 4 provided segments of the child clinical interview with 9-year-old Bruce Garcia. There we learned that Bruce had great difficulty in his social interactions with peers. Though Bruce clearly wanted friends, he seemed not to know how to go about making friends. Arguments over rules of a game often deteriorated into fights. Bruce was also the victim of frequent teasing and physical harassment by peers. With limited coping skills, Bruce felt powerless to deal with these problems and turned to others to defend him. Bruce also reported arguments at home with his mother and stepsister, Barbie. He admitted having difficulty controlling his temper, especially when he felt bossed around. Even small things, such as his mother telling him to do his chores, aroused intensely angry feelings in him.

Bruce's self-reported problems produced a score at the 69th percentile on the SCICA Aggressive/Rule-Breaking scale. He scored at the 92nd percentile on the SCICA Language/Motor Problems scale, reflecting the interviewer's observations of difficulties in expressive language, concrete and tangential thinking, as well as fine-motor problems while producing his KFD (shown in Chapter 3). He also scored at the 69th percentile for observed problems on the SCICA Withdrawn/Depressed scale.

In the parent interview Ms. Garcia reported that Bruce was the middle child in a blended family. She had retained custody of Bruce after divorcing his father when Bruce was age 2. She married Mr. Garcia 2 years later, who then adopted Bruce. Bruce's biological father had been diagnosed with schizophrenia and had been hospitalized several times. Ms. Garcia took Bruce to Florida once to visit his father, but no further visits were planned.

Ms. Garcia reported that Bruce was delayed in speech and motor development and seemed socially immature. As a young child, he had displayed odd behaviors, such as rubbing his stomach over and over and rocking and hitting himself, but he no longer did those things at age 9. Ms. Garcia thought Bruce still seemed young for his age and noted that he had difficulty getting along with other kids. He often came home complaining about being teased and picked on at school and sometimes beaten up. He seldom had other kids over to the house to play. Most of the time, Bruce played with Barbie and her friends. Ms. Garcia thought that Bruce got along best with his 14-year-old stepbrother, Sam, who played football with him and looked out for him. She reported some difficulties disciplining Bruce and Barbie at home, but felt that this was not a big problem, and that her husband was very good at backing her up when she needed it. She also felt that Bruce and Mr. Garcia generally got along well, and that Bruce considered Mr. Garcia to be his dad.

As indicated in Chapter 1, Bruce had received speech and language services since age 4 and, at age 9, was undergoing a 3-year reevaluation for special education services. Bruce's third-grade teacher reported that he was performing at grade level in most subjects, though he had trouble expressing his ideas orally and in written assignments. Sometimes his answers to questions were "way off topic." By contrast, math was a special strength and Bruce's favorite subject. He was in the top math group, working on multiplication and division. The teacher concurred with Ms. Garcia's concerns about Bruce's social interactions. She thought that other students viewed him as "weird" and sometimes avoided him. She said that he stuck out in a group because of odd mannerisms. When asked to give examples, she said he sometimes sucked his fingers, rocked and hummed while in his seat, and twirled around on tiptoes when in line. She also thought he was a bit odd in appearance and dress. When he did try to interact with other kids, the teacher said, he often talked about topics that were not of interest to the other kids (e.g., his collections of marbles and football cards).

Bruce's mother and teacher concurred in their ratings of severe problems on the CBCL and TRF Social Problems and Thought Problems scales, producing scores above the 97th percentile for 6- to 11-year-old boys. They also reported attention problems. Though both mother and teacher noted that Bruce sometimes argued, they did not report temper tantrums or severe problems with aggression or rule-breaking behavior. They reported few problems related to anxiety, depression, or withdrawal.

Cognitive testing indicated that Bruce had average ability, which was in sharp contrast to an IQ score in the mildly retarded range he had received at age 4. Testing at age 9, however, showed a significant discrepancy between Bruce's high-average verbal ability and his below-average nonverbal performance. His particular strengths were in verbal reasoning and acquired knowledge, in contrast to weaknesses in visual–spatial reasoning and processing speed. He showed average working memory and attention. Additional testing revealed below-average expressive language skills and poor visual–motor integration.

Achievement tests, on the other hand, indicated above-average math skills and average skills in all other areas, consistent with reports of academic performance from Bruce's teacher. When a special education aide observed Bruce in the classroom, he was on task only 45% of the time, compared to 90% for two randomly selected "control" boys.

Bruce's pattern of problems did not appear to qualify for any specific DSM-IV diagnosis, although he showed some characteristics that might suggest Asperger's Disorder. Although attention problems and some hyperactivity might also suggest ADHD, such a diagnosis would fail to capture his unusual behavior and thought processes. Other possible diagnoses were Pervasive Developmental Disorder or an emerging thought disorder. His biological father's diagnosis of schizophrenia suggested possible genetic vulnerabilities that might account for some of his odd behavior and uneven pattern of cognitive functioning.

The school multidisciplinary team decided that the assessment results justified continuation of speech and language services, particularly focusing on pragmatic and expressive language. In addition, interviews and high scores on standardized rating scales revealed significant problems in peer relations. To address his social problems, Bruce was enrolled in a social skills program with several other children. *Skillstreaming the Elementary School Child* (McGinnis & Goldstein, 1997) is an example of a program that would be especially good for Bruce. Skillstreaming offers lessons in the acquisition of 60 discreet skills that can then be reinforced in the classroom and at home. For each child in the program, parents and teachers complete "skillstreaming checklists" to identify specific deficits that can become targets for instruction. The program includes lessons on classroom survival skills, friendship-making skills, dealing with feelings, alternatives to aggression, and dealing with stress—many of which could be very beneficial for Bruce. Regular consultation between the social skills trainer and Bruce's mother and teacher would also help to generalize specific skills from group sessions to other settings.

Case Example: Catherine Holcomb

Parent, teacher, and child interviews were especially important for understanding the different perspectives on Catherine Holcomb's functioning. The clinical interview with Catherine revealed lingering sadness over the death of her father, even though he had died 4 years ago. In the interview segment in Chapter 4, Catherine told the school psychologist that she often had sad thoughts about her father that intruded into her school day. Catherine described most of her school subjects as "boring," but also admitted to difficulty understanding math problems.

The SCICA Profile produced an elevated score at the 93rd percentile on the Anxious/Depressed scale, indicating that Catherine reported many more problems related to anxiety and depression than other clinically referred children. Elevated scores on the Anxious (73rd percentile), Withdrawn/Depressed (98th percentile), and Affective Problems (98th percentile) scales also indicated that Catherine looked very sad and withdrawn during the interview, as well as manifesting related problems such as self-consciousness, low energy, poor eye contact, and reluctance to talk about feelings.

During the parent interview, Ms. Holcomb acknowledged that Catherine seemed sad and withdrawn, but more often she just seemed "irritable and hard to get along with." Ms. Holcomb said that Catherine argued with her and often had temper tantrums. She also argued and fought with her older brother, though the fights were usually not physical. When Ms. Holcomb tried to "lay down the rules with her," Catherine typically started crying and stomped off to her room. Ms. Holcomb relied mostly on time-outs as punishments, although she did not think they worked very well. She said that she never spanked her kids. When asked more about the family and home situation, Ms. Holcomb reported that her work as an accountant sometimes required long hours at the office. Over the past years, she had relied on several different housekeepers, who also provided child care when she could not be home. Ms. Holcomb described her late husband as a good man who had enjoyed the outdoors. When he was alive, the family often spent time at their summer camp, hiking, canoeing, and picnicking. Ms. Holcomb said that she was "depressed" for the first year or so after her husband had died, but she had not seen a counselor. Instead, she used her work as a way "to move on." She thought that her son Billy was the one who missed his father the most after his death. But now Billy was in high school and involved with friends and sports activities.

Ms. Holcomb and Catherine's fifth-grade teacher both expressed concerns about her poor school performance, which had prompted the referral for evaluation. Ms. Holcomb told the school psychologist that her arguments with Catherine usually centered on homework. She thought that Catherine "was certainly smart enough," but seemed lazy and not interested in schoolwork. "Sometimes it's like pulling teeth just to get her to finish a math paper," she said. Reading assignments also created difficulties, especially when she had to answer questions or write book reports. However, Catherine did seem to enjoy reading books of her own choosing, especially fantasies and mystery stories.

In her interview with the school psychologist, Catherine's teacher described Catherine as "listless and hard to motivate," saying "it was hard to know what was going on with her." The teacher wondered if Catherine had an attention deficit or a learning disability. Catherine often failed to complete assignments, which resulted in poor or failing grades. She sometimes had difficulty understanding directions, but mostly seemed to be daydreaming or not concentrating. When the teacher called on her in class, she often didn't know what was expected and seemed embarrassed. Although Catherine was not disruptive, the teacher had to remind her to do her own work instead of watching what others were doing. She seldom asked for help from the teacher. Catherine left the classroom for 30 minutes of remedial tutoring in math and reading twice a week. When asked about her strengths, the teacher reported that Catherine was good in drawing and seemed to enjoy hands-on activities in art class.

Scores on standardized rating scales supported impressions of withdrawal and depression from interviews. Catherine's mother and teacher rated her in the clinical range on the CBCL and TRF Withdrawn/Depressed and Affective Problems scales, indicating severe problems for 6- to 11-year-old girls. Catherine's teacher also rated her in the clinical range on the TRF Anxious/Depressed scale. Similar to ratings by her mother and teacher, Catherine's self-ratings on the YSR produced high scores for internalizing problems. However, Catherine scored the YSR item "Unhappy, sad, or depressed" as "not true," which was a sharp contrast to her reports of sadness and her sad demeanor in the child clinical interview. In the clinical interview, Catherine also reported that she had not discussed her sad feelings with anyone prior to the interview. Catherine began to open up about her feelings as the interview progressed, which suggested that she might now be amenable to psychotherapy.

In addition to depression and withdrawal, the interviews suggested that Catherine had a very limited social network. In the child clinical interview, Catherine reported that she had no close friends and she seemed not to know how to make friends. For example, she said that she usually played alone at recess because other kids didn't like her and she didn't like the games other kids played. She preferred playing with younger children because they didn't tease her or boss her around. Ms. Holcomb also reported that Catherine had no friends and instead "stuck to herself."

She said that Catherine preferred solitary activities, such as reading books and doing crafts. Although she belonged to Girl Scouts, Catherine seldom attended meetings because she didn't like them. On weekends, she spent most of her time in her room. Catherine's teacher described her as a "loner." She said that at recess, Catherine wandered around the playground by herself or hung around the playground supervisors.

Low scores on the CBCL and TRF competence and adaptive scales indicated limited social involvement and poor school performance, compared to other girls Catherine's age. Catherine's mother and teacher both rated her academic performance as below average. Her teacher rated her very low in terms of how hard she was working, how much she was learning, and how happy she was, compared to other students in the class. The teacher reported that Catherine had failing grades in math, social studies, and science. The teacher also scored Catherine in the borderline range on the TRF Attention Problems scale.

In the context of the parent and teacher reports, it was surprising to learn that Catherine's full-scale IQ on an intelligence test was in the superior range and that she showed no significant deficits among subtest scores. Standardized achievement tests revealed average academic skills in all areas.

Based on information from Catherine's assessment, the school multidisciplinary team concluded that she met IDEA criteria for ED. There was especially strong evidence of the ED characteristic of a "general pervasive mood of unhappiness or depression." The school psychologist also rendered a DSM-IV diagnosis of Dysthymic Disorder (300.4) based on her interpretation of information from the child clinical interview, a structured diagnostic interview with Ms. Holcomb, and other assessment data.

The clinical interviews were especially important in tailoring interventions to meet Catherine's needs. From all perspectives, Catherine appeared to be a good candidate for cognitive-behavioral therapy for anxiety and depression (Merrell, 2001). Accordingly, Catherine began individual psychotherapy with a clinical psychologist who provided school-based mental health services. The psychologist also held occasional joint sessions with Catherine, her mother, and her brother to address relationship problems at home.

The school multidisciplinary team developed an IEP that focused on reducing Catherine's social withdrawal and improving her organizational skills. The school psychologist conducted classroom observations and additional interviews with the teacher to obtain an FBA of Catherine's academic difficulties. Based on the FBA, the team developed a BIP targeted on improving productivity and completion of assignments. The BIP involved a coordinated effort among the classroom teacher, special educator, school psychologist, and Catherine's mother.

Catherine remained in her fifth-grade classroom for most of her school day, with instructional support in math and study skills. Because several other fifth-grade students also had problems in peer relations, the school psychologist provided weekly social skills training to the entire class, focusing on making friends, coping with social problems, and controlling anger. The fifth-grade teacher and school psychologist consulted regularly on social skills that could be reinforced throughout the school day.

Prompted by what she had learned about her relationship with Catherine, Ms. Holcomb decided to seek individual psychotherapy to address her own symptoms of depression. Ms. Holcomb's psychotherapy, coupled with interventions for Catherine, proved to be very helpful in reducing conflicts at home.

Case Example: Karl Bryant

The interview with 12-year-old Karl Bryant in Chapter 3 offered a vivid picture of his aggressive behavior toward other children at school. Unlike Bruce, Karl was more often the perpetrator than the victim of aggression. A sense of self-righteousness and lack of guilt overlaid his descriptions of fighting and cruelty toward peers. In the interview segments in Chapter 4, Karl hinted at conflicts with his parents, although he viewed their discipline as "fair," unlike what happened at school. He seemed to have a positive relationship with his stepfather and respected him as the "boss of the house." After probing from the interviewer, Karl acknowledged arguments with his mother and having been punched and hit by her in the past when he did something wrong. A striking feature of Karl's interview was his strong desire to be treated fairly by adults and his views of what constituted unfair treatment at school.

On the SCICA Profile, Karl's self-reports produced a score at the 97th percentile on the Aggressive/Rule-Breaking scale, indicating severe problems compared to other clinically referred 12- to 18-year-olds. The interviewer's observations of Karl also produced high scores for Attention Problems (79th percentile) and Self-Control Problems (92nd percentile). Karl's openness about his problems during the clinical interview contrasted sharply with his self-ratings on the YSR, which produced scores below clinical cut points on all scales.

In the parent interview Karl's mother, Mrs. Ladd, reported that Karl had had a history of behavior problems from an early age, including temper tantrums, hyperactivity, and aggressive behavior. She said that he had always been difficult to discipline because he insisted on having his own way. When he was 6 years old, the family pediatrician initiated a trial of stimulant medication for hyperactivity. However, Mrs. Ladd discontinued the medication after a year because she felt it was ineffective. When asked about their current discipline strategies, Mrs. Ladd said, "we mostly try to reason with Karl, but this often ends up in long, drawn-out arguments." Since his marriage to Karl's mother, Mr. Ladd had tried to lay down rules at home—for example, when kids had to do homework or chores, when kids could watch TV or use the computer, where Karl could go out at night. When Karl broke the rules, he was sent to his room or grounded. Detentions at school resulted in being grounded for a month. Despite these efforts, Mrs. Ladd reported that "it's a constant struggle to deal with Karl's defiant behavior."

Mrs. Ladd felt that Karl's behavior had deteriorated after agreed-upon visits with his biological father during Christmas and summer vacations. Mrs. Ladd suspected that Mr. Bryant provided very little supervision and instead let Karl do "pretty much whatever he wanted." Mrs. Ladd reported that Mr. Bryant was an alcoholic, as was his own father, and had been physically abusive toward her. Mrs. Ladd said that as a young child, Karl had witnessed several violent episodes between his parents, but he had never been the victim of physical abuse. Karl's parents had divorced when he was 5 years old.

School records indicated that Karl had received several in-school suspensions for aggressive and defiant behavior in the past year. He was also suspended out of school once for smoking on school grounds. Karl's homeroom teacher reported that he was failing three of his sixth-grade subjects, largely due to suspensions and incomplete assignments. The school staff had tried several different behavior plans with Karl, including a point system targeted on homework completion and reducing disruptive behavior in class. Karl occasionally met with the guidance counselor when he got into trouble on the playground. When he got into fights, he was sent to the principal's office and given an in-school suspension. However, the teacher felt that none of these interventions had worked very well. She said:

"Karl wants to please but is often unable to control his temper when things don't go his way. He seeks attention by asking questions constantly and bothering other students. He's very loud in class. He gets into many fights with other kids he doesn't know well and sometimes with his own friends. He seems to have good days and bad days. He really has been trying to improve his behavior, but he has a long way to go. I think he has a hard time with authority figures. He doesn't get along with the principal at all. One good thing is the way he shows great concern for other kids when they have a problem. His energy level is amazing."

Mrs. Ladd and the sixth-grade teacher both rated Karl in the clinical range on the CBCL and TRF Aggressive Behavior scale, and in the borderline to clinical range on the Social Problems scale. Karl's teacher rated him in the borderline clinical range on the Anxious/Depressed, Attention Problems, and Rule-Breaking scales, and Mrs. Ladd rated him in the borderline range for Thought Problems. These high scores indicated severe problems compared to norms for 12- to 18-year-old boys. Mrs. Ladd also rated Karl low on the CBCL Social and School scales. Observations by the school psychologist corroborated the teacher's reports of disruptive and aggressive behavior. The school psychologist also observed that Karl frequently sought the teacher's attention in class.

The teacher's impression that Karl was a "bright boy" was backed by a high-average score for verbal ability on an intelligence test. The intelligence test showed no specific deficits, except a below-average score for auditory attention span. Karl also scored in the average range on standardized achievement tests.

After the school multidisciplinary team examined all the information from multiple sources, they concluded that Karl met IDEA criteria for ED. The aggressive behavior reported in interviews and on standardized rating scales provided strong evidence of the ED characteristic, "inappropriate types of behavior or feelings under normal circumstances." There was also strong evidence of "an inability to build or maintain satisfactory relationships with peers and teachers." The team determined that these behavioral and emotional problems had a direct adverse effect on Karl's school performance, leading to failing grades in spite of his high-average intellectual ability and average academic skills. The pattern of Karl's behavioral problems was also consistent with a DSM-IV diagnosis of Conduct Disorder (312.8), but this was not a reason to deny him special education services for ED (for discussion of this issue, see McConaughy & Skiba, 1993; Skiba & Grizzle, 1991, 1992).

The clinical interviews with Karl and his mother and teacher suggested that he was a good candidate for a school-based behavioral contract. It became obvious that Karl needed clear and consistent rules and consequences to fit his conventional level of moral reasoning. Although the school staff had previously tried a point system with Karl, further probing in the teacher interview revealed that the system was loosely defined and limited only to the homeroom setting. Knowing this, it was certainly worth trying a behavioral contract again, but now including clearly defined behavioral goals that applied across all school settings. Karl's behavioral contract should also include a menu of material and social rewards to provide variety, plus a clear warning system regarding unacceptable behavior, steps for time-out procedures, and opportunities for problem solving about future behavior. It would also be good to include options for salvaging lost points when Karl demonstrated good anger control. Many published resources are available for helping school staff develop school-based behavioral interventions for students such as Karl. Examples include *Responding to Problem Behavior in Schools* (Crone et al., 2004), *The Tough Kid Book* (Rhode, Jenson, & Reavis, 1993), and *Tough Kid Tool Box* (Jenson, Rhode, & Reavis, 1994).

Karl's description of "success plans" in the clinical interview suggested that, under the right conditions (e.g., his perception of being treated fairly), he would probably respond positively to a well-structured behavioral contract. Involving Karl directly in negotiating the terms of the contract would address his desire to be heard and thus increase his level of commitment. To maintain consistency, the contract would need to be a coordinated effort among all school staff who had contact with Karl. Ongoing behavioral consultation between the school psychologist and Karl's teacher would provide a venue for developing such a contract and monitoring Karl's progress. Conjoint behavioral consultation (Sheridan et al., 1996) might be especially appropriate in Karl's case to maintain consistency between home and school.

Interventions for Karl also needed to extend beyond school. Although Karl minimized any family problems, Mrs. Ladd reported great difficulty managing his behavior at home. In addition, Karl's aggressive behavior, poor social coping skills, and association with other kids who got into trouble put him at risk for future antisocial behavior. Addressing these problems required interventions directed at Karl and his parents. One option was to seek individual psychotherapy for Karl, coupled with parent training in behavior management skills. A good example is the Yale Problem-Solving Skills Training (PSST) and the Parent Management Training (PMT) programs described by Kazdin (2003). This evidence-based program involves weekly individual therapy sessions to teach the child a series of problem-solving steps: identifying the problem; generating alternative solutions; evaluating possible solutions; choosing a solution; and evaluating the consequences of the chosen solution. The sessions incorporate a reward system and homework assignments. Parents then meet with a different therapist to learn how to alter their interactions with the child to reduce aggression and to promote prosocial behavior. The behavioral principles in the Yale program can be applied to other clinical settings.

Social skills training would be an alternative option for Karl. Social skills programs usually involve groups of children, but practitioners can also select components of programs to use in individual sessions. One caveat would be to avoid grouping Karl with other antisocial peers, because research has shown that this approach actually increases problems instead of reducing them (Dishion, McCord, & Poulin, 1999). Social skills training for Karl should focus on social problem solving and alternatives to aggression, as done in the PSST program, as well as anger management, perspective taking, and postconventional moral reasoning.

The *Anger Coping and Coping Power Program* (Lockman, Barry, & Pardini, 2003) is an example of one approach that includes separate sessions for children and parents. Parent sessions address social reinforcement and positive attention, the importance of clear house rules, behavioral expectations and monitoring procedures, and effective discipline strategies. Examples of other published social skills programs are *Aggression Replacement Training* (Goldstein, Glick, & Gibbs, 1998), *Skillstreaming the Adolescent* (Goldstein, McKinnis, Sprafkin, Gershaw, & Klein, 1997), and *The Tough Kid Social Skills Book* (Sheridan, 1997). In addition, *The Tough Kid Parent Book* (Jenson, Rhode, & Hepworth, 2003) provides practical strategies for parents that dovetail with *Tough Kid* social skills taught in small-group sessions.

Case Example: Kelsey Watson

As we learned in Chapter 4, Kelsey Watson was admitted to a psychiatric hospital at age 13, where she was diagnosed with Major Depressive Disorder (296.2) and placed on antidepressant medication. At age 14 she was placed in a residential group home in the custody of the state social service agency. She continued to take antidepressant medication and received weekly therapy sessions with a mental health counselor at the group home. When she entered eighth grade in the local school, the school staff referred her for a psychological evaluation to determine if she needed additional school-based services.

It became apparent during the clinical interview with Kelsey that she was experiencing serious emotional and behavioral problems, including depression, suicidal thoughts, alcohol and drug use, and risky sexual activity. Kelsey's openness in discussing her problems was reflected in scores above the 80th percentile on the SCICA Anxious/Depressed and Aggressive/Rule-Breaking scales. Kelsey also appeared nervous and agitated during the interview, as reflected by a score at the 73rd percentile on the SCICA Anxious scale. In addition to the interview, Kelsey completed the YSR and the Reynolds Adolescent Depression Scale—2nd edition (RADS-2; Reynolds, 2002). Kelsey's self-ratings on the YSR produced a clinical range score (above 97th percentile) on the Rule-Breaking scale, which indicated more antisocial behavior than typical of 12- to 18-year-old girls. At the same time, she scored herself in the normal range on other YSR scales, including those measuring anxiety, depression, and withdrawal. She also scored below the clinical cut point on the RADS-2, although she did report suicidal thoughts. These differences between the SCICA versus the YSR and RADS-2 suggested that Kelsey was much more willing to disclose emotional problems in a face-to-face interview than to acknowledge them on self-report questionnaires.

One of the counselors at the group home summarized Kelsey's history and current functioning in a phone interview. The same counselor also completed the CBCL. (Kelsey's mother lived in a different town and refused to provide information for the evaluation.) The counselor reported that Kelsey was still adjusting to her new environment in the group home. Although she followed general routines, she often seemed argumentative and sad. She continued to make comments to the staff about suicide and occasionally cut and picked at her skin, but none of these behaviors appeared to be life threatening. Kelsey had threatened to run away and twice had left the grounds without permission. She also disobeyed "no smoking" rules at the group home. The counselor said that residential staff kept a close watch on Kelsey's behavior and supervised her activity in the community. Although Kelsey was supposed to visit her mother once a week, her mother seldom arranged visits, which upset Kelsey. Although the CBCL produced scores below clinical cut points on all scales, Kelsey scored near the 90th percentile on the Anxious/Depressed and Rule-Breaking scales.

Ratings by two of Kelsey's eighth-grade teachers produced clinical range scores on the TRF Anxious/Depressed, Social Problems, and Rule-Breaking scales. One of the teachers also scored Kelsey in the borderline clinical range on the TRF Withdrawn/Depressed scale. In a joint interview the teachers expressed particular concerns about Kelsey's emotional state and social interactions. They worried that Kelsey seemed fascinated by drugs and sex and talked about her experience with both. Drugs and sex appeared as recurrent themes in her creative writing assignments, and the teachers had overheard her talking with peers about drugs and sex. The teachers also thought that Kelsey was very flirtatious toward boys. The teachers worried that Kelsey tended to gravitate toward fringe groups that got into trouble in the community. Though there was no dress code at the school, Kelsey's typical attire clearly stood out as different from the mainstream kids.

The teachers did not think Kelsey was a "behavior problem" in classes. Though she sometimes whined about certain assignments, she was not disrespectful or disruptive. She generally kept to herself and sometimes seemed sad and in her own world. Although the teachers thought Kelsey had average ability, they felt that she lacked certain basic eighth-grade skills. For example, she had trouble doing math involving fractions or word problems, and she could not organize her ideas for writing assignments. Kelsey also had very poor study skills. When asked about her strengths, the teachers said that Kelsey seemed to be very creative. She also liked doing projects on the computer, which was one way to get her to complete writing assignments.

Consistent with the teachers' impressions, cognitive testing with Kelsey produced scores in the high-average to superior range. Achievement tests produced average scores in reading and written language, but below average scores in math.

The psychological evaluation indicated that Kelsey had a history of persistent emotional and behavioral problems. This made it all the more surprising that she had never received any special education services for ED. In the clinical interview Kelsey reported persistent feelings of sadness that were consistent with her DSM-IV diagnosis of Major Depressive Disorder and her treatment with antidepressant medication. Scores on parent and teacher rating scales indicated high levels of anxiety and depression, compared to normative samples. Given Kelsey's high-average ability and the absence of evidence of LD, the school multidisciplinary team recommended placement in a district special education program for children with ED.

Because Kelsey had previously attempted suicide, it was important to establish in the child clinical interview that she had no current plans for suicide. Nonetheless, her suicidal ideation, coupled with depression and impulsive behavior, placed her at risk for future suicide attempts. The psychologist emphasized this risk in her written evaluation report and recommended careful monitoring of Kelsey's mood and behavior, especially during and immediately following home visits to her mother. The psychologist encouraged Kelsey's current group home therapist to develop a "no suicide" contract with her. The psychologist also recommended close monitoring for any wrist-cutting behavior similar to what Kelsey had reported in the past. (See Chapter 8 for more detailed discussion of assessing suicide risk and self-mutilation.)

The child clinical interview also indicated risk for substance abuse. Kelsey's initial alcohol and drug use most likely involved experimentation with peers, which is not uncommon among adolescents. However, the fact that Kelsey began experimenting with alcohol and marijuana at age 12 was worrisome, and her use of heroin was particularly alarming. Kelsey's regular cigarette smoking, coupled with her continued desire to get high on marijuana, suggested that she was moving beyond experimentation. Given this information, the psychologist recommended a more thorough evaluation of Kelsey's substance use by a local alcohol and drug abuse treatment program. The psychologist also recommended enrollment in a school-based prevention program for alcohol and drug abuse.

In addition, Kelsey's early and continued sexual activity placed her at high risk for teenage pregnancy, as well as HIV and other STDs. Continued association with deviant peers and adults could also place her at risk for sexual abuse, rape, and sexual exploitation, including prostitution. Sex education and learning about safe sex practices would be especially appropriate for Kelsey. Along this line, it was encouraging to learn in the child clinical interview that Kelsey wanted to talk with a gynecologist or Planned Parenthood about safe sex practices.

Finally, Kelsey's association with antisocial fringe groups highlighted the importance of nurturing involvement with nondeviant, prosocial peers. This was one area in which school-based practitioners could be especially helpful. For example, school staff could encourage Kelsey to participate in sports, clubs, and other activities of interest. In the clinical interview Kelsey reported special interests in computers. In fact, she thought it was "cool" to do schoolwork on the computer, and she liked belonging to chat groups. She also enjoyed writing, music, and theater. These were all strengths that could be cultivated in school-based interventions. At the same time, adults would need to monitor Kelsey's use of the Internet to guard against access to dangerous websites, given her suicide risk and past involvement in cult activities.

SUMMARY

Clinical interviews with children, parents, and teachers provide their own windows on children's behavior, emotions, and life circumstances. As indicated in previous chapters, no one data source provides a definitive picture of children's functioning. Instead, practitioners must obtain different perspectives on children and then integrate data across multiple sources. The SCICA utilizes standardized rating scales and a scoring profile to provide a quantitative picture of children's self-reported problems and interviewers' observations. The SCICA Profile facilitates comparisons of interview data with quantitative data from standardized parent and teacher rating scales. In addition, interviews with children, parents, and teachers are rich sources of information that cannot be obtained in other ways, as discussed in Chapters 3–6.

To illustrate how data from multiple sources can be applied to intervention planning, this chapter summarized findings for the five case examples discussed in previous chapters. All five children showed poor school performance, but for different reasons. Multisource data indicated that three children (Catherine Holcomb, Karl Bryant, and Kelsey Watson) were good candidates for special education services for ED. One child (Andy Lockwood) qualified for a Section 504 plan due to ADHD. Another child (Bruce Garcia) received speech and language services. In addition to academic interventions, the interviews were especially useful in tailoring other interventions to meet each child's needs, including behavioral contracts, individual psychotherapy, social skills training, classroom accommodations, and family interventions.

8

Assessing Risk for Suicide

DAVID N. MILLER *and* STEPHANIE H. McCONAUGHY

Suicidal behavior (i.e., ideation, attempts, completion) among children and youth is a problem of national concern. Indeed, the problem is so pervasive that in October of 2004 President George W. Bush signed the nation's first youth suicide prevention bill into law. Suicide currently is the third leading cause of death among children and young adults in the United States, trailing only accidents and homicide. Recent data show that more teenagers and young adults die annually of suicide than from cancer, heart disease, AIDS, birth defects, stroke, and chronic lung disease combined (Centers for Disease Control and Prevention, 2002). The risk for suicidal behavior increases significantly during adolescence, with adolescent boys being at particular risk. Although girls *attempt* suicide at a higher rate than boys, nearly five times more boys than girls in the 15- to 19-year-old age range *commit* suicide (Gould & Kramer, 2001).

Because children and adolescents spend much of their time in schools, school-based practitioners can play a key role in identifying those who may be at risk for suicide (Miller & DuPaul, 1996). It is critically important that school-based practitioners be knowledgeable about a variety of issues regarding suicide risk, including liability and legal issues; limits of confidentiality; possible risk factors, precipitants, and warning signs of suicidal behavior; how to conduct effective suicide risk assessments; and how to distinguish between genuine suicidal behavior and nonsuicidal self-mutilation or deliberate self-harm. This chapter discusses each of these issues and provides practical guidelines for assessing suicide risk.

David N. Miller, PhD, is Assistant Professor in the School Psychology Program at the University at Albany, State University of New York. Prior to his current position, he served as Director of the Pre-doctoral Internship in Professional Psychology at Centennial School of Lehigh University, an alternative day school for students with severe behavior disorders. As a practicing school psychologist, he has extensive experience conducting assessments of children's emotional and behavioral disorders, including suicide risk assessments. His research interests include suicidal behavior and other internalizing problems of children and adolescents.

LIABILITY AND LEGAL ISSUES

School-based practitioners should realize that school districts "have been found liable for not offering suicide prevention programs, providing inadequate supervision of a suicidal student, and failing to notify parents when their children were suicidal" (Lieberman & Davis, 2002, p. 535). Most court cases involving schools have concerned issues of *foreseeability* and *negligence* in student suicides. Historically, districts and school personnel have not been held liable for failing to prevent a student's suicide, per se. However, in several cases, they have been held liable when school personnel were egregiously negligent in their failure to prevent suicide, or when foreseeability of suicide was evident, but an adequate response was not provided. For example, if a student writes or talks about committing suicide, courts have ruled that adults (particularly school psychologists and counselors) should be able to foresee the possible suicide risk. Courts also have ruled that schools and individual school personnel can be found negligent when they fail to notify parents or guardians of students who are known or believed to be suicidal. Similarly, it is considered negligent not to provide close supervision of students considered to be at risk for suicide. Even under conditions in which a particular student denies suicidal intent, if school personnel suspect the student is suicidal, they have a legal obligation to notify parents/caretakers (for details of court cases, see Lieberman & Davis, 2002).

Although courts have recognized that most schools are not equipped to provide extensive treatment or therapy for suicidal students, they have upheld the notion that "school personnel are in a position to make referrals and have a duty to secure assistance from others, with parental involvement, when a child is at risk" (Davis & Sandoval, 1991, p. 176). School-based practitioners should also be aware that successful litigation against schools has occurred in the rare event of a student suicide after the student was either suspended or expelled (Lieberman & Davis, 2002). Later sections of this chapter address issues of confidentiality, duty to warn parents, and immediate protective actions for suicidal students. For additional information on ethical and legal issues, see Jacob and Hartshorne (2003).

RISK FACTORS, PRECIPITANTS, AND WARNING SIGNS

Youth suicide is a complex phenomenon that includes many possible risk factors, as outlined in Table 8.1 (Kalafat & Lazarus, 2002). One of the best predictors of future behavior is past behavior. Accordingly, the single best predictor of a suicide attempt is a history of previous suicide attempts (Miller & DuPaul, 1996). There is also strong evidence that the overwhelming majority (over 90%) of children and adolescents who commit suicide suffered from one or more mental disorder. For example, record reviews on suicide completers indicated that girls most often experienced depression; boys experienced depression, combined with substance abuse and disorders of impulse control, such as Conduct Disorder (Shaffer et al., 1996). Alcohol and substance abuse is especially worrisome because it can increase the likelihood of an impulsive act of suicide. Other research has also suggested that gay and lesbian youth may be especially vulnerable to suicidal ideation and completion (Lieberman & Davis, 2002). Because they view their situation as hopeless, impossible, and/or a sign of weakness, suicidal youth are often unwilling to seek help and feel isolated or cut off from other people. Seeing no way out, they turn to suicide as their last resort. Some may even view suicide as a noble solution to their problems.

TABLE 8.1. Risk Factors for Suicide

Child/adolescent risk factors

Previous suicide attempt

Current suicidal ideation (thoughts), intent, and plan (resolve)

Mental disorders—particularly mood disorders (e.g., Major Depression, Dysthymic Disorder, Bipolar Disorder) and disorders of low-impulse control (e.g., Conduct Disorder)

Personality disorders for ages 18 and older, particularly Borderline Personality Disorder

Co-occurring alcohol and substance abuse disorders

Feelings of hopelessness and helplessness

Impulsive and/or aggressive tendencies

Gay or lesbian sexual orientation

Unwillingness to seek help because of stigma attached to mental and substance abuse disorders and/or suicidal thoughts

Isolation, a feeling of being cut off from other people

Ineffective coping mechanisms and inadequate problem-solving skills

Cultural and/or religious beliefs—for example, the belief that suicide is a noble resolution of a personal dilemma

Family and environmental risk factors

Easy access to lethal methods, especially guns and medications

Exposure to suicide and/or family history of suicide

Influence of significant people—family members, celebrities, peers who have died by suicide—through direct personal contact or inappropriate media representations

Local epidemics of suicide that have a contagious influence

Barriers to accessing mental health treatment

Note. Adapted from Kalafat and Lazarus (2002). Copyright 2002 by the National Association of School Psychologists, Bethesda, MD. Adapted by permission of the publisher.

Family history and environmental factors are also important to consider. Easy access to lethal methods is a key risk factor in most child and adolescent suicides. The presence of firearms in the home, particularly loaded guns, greatly increases the risk for suicide completion, especially for boys. Access to lethal medications (pills) increases the risk, especially for girls. Family history of suicide and personally knowing someone who committed suicide are additional risks. Suicidal youth can also be influenced by suicides of celebrities or other significant people or highly publicized suicides by other youth in the local community. Family problems, such as divorce and strained parent–child relationships, may contribute to suicide risk, though it is important to remember that many youth who experience family problems do not commit suicide. Internet access to websites about suicide and suicide "chat rooms" pose additional risks. In most cases, there are multiple risk factors.

Stressful Events

Risk for suicidal behavior is increased when acute situational crises or stressful life events, such as some type of loss of an interpersonal nature, occur in conjunction with other more chronic risk factors, such as depression, substance abuse, and access to lethal methods (Gould & Kramer,

TABLE 8.2. Stressful Events That May Trigger Suicidal Behavior

Breakup from boyfriend or girlfriend

Disappointment and rejection, such as a dispute with a boyfriend/ girlfriend, failure to get a job, or rejection from college

Bullying or victimization

Getting into trouble with authorities (e.g., school, police); not knowing and being afraid of the consequences of getting into trouble

Death of a loved one or significant other

Conflict with family; family dysfunction

Disappointment with school results; school failure

High demands at school during examination periods

Unwanted pregnancy; abortion

Infection with HIV or other sexually transmitted diseases

Anniversary of a death of a friend or loved one

Separation from friends, girlfriends/boyfriends

Relational, social, work, or financial loss

Severe or terminal physical illnesses

Serious injury that may change the individual's life course

Note. Adapted from Kalafat and Lazarus (2002). Copyright 2002 by the National Association of School Psychologists, Bethesda, MD. Adapted by permission of the publisher.

2001; Lieberman & Davis, 2002). Researchers have identified several stressful events that often precipitate suicidal behavior in youth (Gould & Kramer, 2001; Kalafat & Lazarus, 2002). Although these events may not directly cause suicide, they have the potential to trigger suicidal behavior in vulnerable youth. Table 8.2 lists several of these potential precipitating events. No one particular stressful event is highly predictive of suicide. However, suicide risk rises as the number and emotional intensity of stressful events increase.

Warning Signs for Suicide

It is widely believed that most individuals who are seriously thinking about suicide give signals or display warning signs. Because children and adolescents typically do not refer themselves for treatment, it is critically important to be aware of warning signs of possible suicidal behavior. Table 8.3 lists several common warning signs of youth suicide discussed by other authors (Lieberman & Cowan, 2004; Lieberman & Davis, 2002; Merrell, 2003; Poland & Lieberman, 2002).

Suicide notes should always be taken seriously, as should suicide threats. Sometimes threats are "cries for help" that can be direct ("I want to die," "I am going to kill myself") or indirect ("The world/my family would be better off without me"). Suicidal youth may share clear plans, or hint at plans, to friends and sometimes to adults. They may also show increased interest in guns or other lethal methods and talk about how to gain access to methods. Making final arrangements can include giving away prized possessions, farewell gestures, or putting affairs in order. Sudden changes in behavior might take the form of withdrawing from friends or family, increased sadness or apathy, or a sudden switch from negative feelings to feelings of peacefulness. Changes in habits

TABLE 8.3. Warning Signs for Suicide

Suicide notes

Suicide threats

Suicide plan/method/ access

Making final arrangements

Sudden changes in behavior, friends, or personality

Changes in physical habits and appearance

Preoccupation with death and suicide themes

Increased inability to concentrate or think clearly

Loss of interest in activities that were previously important or pleasurable

Symptoms of depression

Increased heavy use and abuse of alcohol and/or drugs

and appearance can include loss of sleep or sleeping too much, sudden changes in weight, or poor personal hygiene. Preoccupation with death or suicide themes might appear in drawings, journals, poetry, or conversation. Some suicidal youth visit Internet websites that feature themes about death, suicide, or violence, as well as instruction on suicide methods. Symptoms of depression include excessive and prolonged sadness, feelings of hopelessness or helplessness, along with other warning signs listed in the table (e.g., weight gain or loss, loss of pleasure, and sleep problems). Use of alcohol and/or drugs is not only a key risk factor for suicide, but can also be a warning sign when there is an increase in use or abuse.

As indicated earlier, one of the best predictors of suicide is previous suicide attempts. However, no single risk factor, stressful event, or warning sign will predict suicidal behavior with perfect accuracy. Furthermore, some students may exhibit multiple risk factors or warning signs and still not make a suicide attempt. Because suicide is a relatively rare event, it is not possible to predict with a high degree of precision. Fortunately, however, interviews and other assessment procedures, when used appropriately, can help to identify youth at risk for suicidal behavior. The next sections discuss multimethod procedures for assessing suicide risk, with a particular emphasis on the child/adolescent clinical interview.

MULTIMETHOD RISK ASSESSMENT

Interviewing Children and Adolescents

The individual clinical interview of the child or adolescent is the single most important component of a good suicide risk assessment. Because of its importance and the sensitivity of the topic, interviewing youth who may be suicidal can be an extremely stressful and anxiety-provoking experience for both the interviewer and the interviewee. It is important that interviewers not become so intimidated by the process of suicide risk assessment that they become immobilized. Having a standard protocol for the interview can greatly reduce anxiety in a suicide risk assessment. Additionally, gaining experience in conducting suicide risk assessments should boost confidence and decrease discomfort and anxiety.

When you interview a youth about potential suicide, it is important to remain calm and to proceed in a concerned but matter-of-fact manner (Poland, 1995). Barrett (1985) identified three important issues that practitioners must consider to effectively assist suicidal youth: (1) They must not let their attitudes toward death, in general, and suicide, in particular, interfere with their ability to be reasonably comfortable with the topic; (2) they must be careful not to exhibit anxiety or irritation to interviewees; and (3) they must deal with feelings of insecurity or lack of confidence and seek out additional training and support, as needed.

Several structured and semistructured interviews have been developed to focus specifically on child and adolescent suicidal behavior. However, many of these are expensive, difficult to acquire, and vary widely in their reliability and validity (Goldston, 2003). Nevertheless, it is imperative that professionals dealing with potentially suicidal youth have a specific set of questions that will quickly and reliably obtain needed information. Lieberman and Davis (2002) and Poland (1989) provided examples of specific issues to cover in interviews about suicide risk:

- What warning sign(s) initiated the referral?
- Has the youth thought about suicide?
- Has the youth tried to hurt himself/herself before?
- Does the youth have a plan to harm himself/herself now?
- Has the youth told anyone about the suicide plan, and what is the possibility of rescue?
- Has the youth imagined the reaction of others to his/her death?
- Does the youth understand the finality of death?
- Has the youth made any final arrangements?
- What method is the youth planning to use, and does he/she have access to the means?
- What is the youth's support system (e.g., parents, other adults, counselors, friends)?
- What does the youth perceive as deterrents to suicide?

Although all of the above issues are important to address, the most serious indicators of high risk for suicide include previous suicide attempts, clear plans and methods, access to lethal means, and making final arrangements.

Brock and Sandoval's (1996) Student Interview for Suicide Risk Screening (SISRS) is particularly appropriate for school-based practitioners. Their interview, shown in Appendix 8.1, consists of four components: engagement, identification, inquiry, and assessment. The SISRS is appropriate for comprehensive assessments of students who appear at moderate to high risk for suicide, such as students who have experienced an acute crisis or who have given warning signs for suicide. Another useful interviewing tool is the Brief Suicide Risk Assessment Questionnaire (BSRAQ) developed by Miller (2004), presented in Appendix 8.2. The BSRAQ is a brief screening device that practitioners can use to determine whether further assessment of suicide risk is warranted.

Youth who are seriously contemplating suicide typically experience a high degree of subjective distress and emotional upheaval. Even so, many will respond to interview questions openly and honestly if the questions are posed by a caring, respectful, and empathic adult. Poland (1989) provided the following guidelines for the interview process:

- Calmly gather information to assess lethality of method and identify a course of action.
- Use effective listening skills by reflecting feelings, remaining nonjudgmental, and not minimizing the problem.

- Communicate caring, support, and trust, while providing encouragement for coping strategies.
- Emphasize the youth's worth and previous coping skills; be hopeful.
- Gather information about the youth's and family's history, with emphasis on suicide and substance abuse.
- Emphasize alternatives to suicide.
- Do not make any deals to keep the suicidal thoughts or actions a secret. Explain the limits of confidentiality, and why it is in the youth's best interest to inform parents or guardians so everyone can work together to assist him/her.
- Keep notes of your interaction with the youth.
- Do not leave high-risk youth alone.
- Get supportive collaboration from colleagues.
- Be familiar with community resources.
- Outline for the youth the steps that will be taken to help him/her.

Interviewing Teachers and Parents/Caregivers

Research suggests that teachers and parents/caregivers often are unaware of the suicidal behaviors exhibited by children in their care. However, when used in conjunction with child/adolescent interviews, teacher and parent interviews can be helpful, particularly for examining informants' perceptions across multiple environments and contexts. Table 8.4 shows examples of questions for teachers, and Table 8.5 lists questions for parents (Davis & Sandoval, 1991).

Other Assessment Methods

In addition to interviews, several self-report rating scales are available for assessing suicide risk and suicidal behavior. Self-report scales can be useful as initial screening measures to identify youth who should be individually interviewed for a more thorough assessment of suicide risk. One example is the Suicidal Ideation Questionnaire (SIQ; Reynolds, 1988), a school-based screening procedure for identifying adolescents at-risk for suicidal behavior. Reynolds (1991) recommended using the SIQ in a two-step process: (1) All students in a classroom or school are asked to complete the SIQ; and then (2) those students who score at clinically significant levels on the SIQ report measure are individually interviewed by a mental health professional in the school (e.g., school psychologist or counselor). Research has shown that this two-step approach successfully identifies students at-risk for suicide (Shaffer & Craft, 1999). Unfortunately, other studies also suggested that this approach may meet with some resistance among school personnel

---

TABLE 8.4. Questions for Teachers Regarding a Student's Risk for Suicide

Have you noticed any major changes in your student's schoolwork since school started?

Have you noticed any behavioral, emotional, or attitudinal changes?

Has the student experienced any trouble in school? What kind of trouble?

Does the student appear depressed and/or hostile and angry? If so, what clues does the student give?

Has the student either verbally, behaviorally, or symbolically (in an essay or story) threatened suicide or expressed statements associated with self-destruction or death?

TABLE 8.5. Questions for Parents or Caregivers Regarding a Student's Risk for Suicide

Has any serious change occurred in your child's or family's life recently?

(*If yes*) How did your child respond?

Has your child had any accidents or illnesses without a recognizable physical basis?

Has your child experienced a loss recently?

Has your child experienced difficulty in any areas of his/her life?

Has your child been very self-critical, or does he/she seem to think that you or teachers have been very critical lately?

Has your child made any unusual statements to you or others about death or dying? Any unusual questions or jokes about death or dying?

Have there been any changes you've noticed in your child's mood or behavior over the last few months?

Has your child ever threatened or attempted suicide before, or attempted to harm himself/herself in any way?

Have any of your child's friends or family, including yourselves, ever threatened or attempted suicide?

How have these last few months been for you? How have you reacted to your child (e.g., with anger, despair, empathy)?

(Eckert, Miller, DuPaul, & Riley-Tillman, 2003; Miller, Eckert, DuPaul, & White, 1999; Scherff, Eckert, & Miller, 2005). Some school personnel may feel that suicide screening is too intrusive. Others may believe that asking specific questions regarding suicide will lead students who are not suicidal to become suicidal as part of the screening. However, there is no empirical support for the latter belief.

Because currently available rating scales for assessing youth suicidality vary in their reliability and validity, it is important to choose an instrument with sound psychometric properties. The choice of instruments should also be based on the specific needs of the assessor, the purpose for which the instrument will be used, and the outcome the assessor wants to measure (Goldston, 2003). Practitioners who use standardized self-report scales should be aware that there is no "gold standard" with regard to these instruments, and that currently no one instrument (or combination of instruments) can predict with high accuracy who will attempt or commit suicide. Keeping this caveat in mind, Table 8.6 lists examples of commercially available self-report scales that have demonstrated reasonable utility for identifying potentially suicidal youth. In addition to these instruments, other broad-spectrum instruments, such as the ASEBA YSR (Achenbach & Rescorla, 2001) and BASC-2 Self-Report—Child and BASC-2 Self Report—Adolescent (Reynolds & Kamphaus, 2004), contain problem items that may indicate suicidal thoughts and suicide attempts. Goldston (2003) provides a comprehensive description and review of a variety of suicide risk assessment instruments.

TABLE 8.6. Standardized Self-Report Scales for Assessing Suicide Risk

Adolescent Psychopathology Scale (APS; Reynolds, 1998)

Beck Scale for Suicidal Ideation (BSSI; Beck & Steer, 1991)

Children's Depression Inventory (CDI; Kovacs, 1992)

Reynolds Adolescent Depression Scale—2nd edition (RADS-2; Reynolds, 2002)

Reynolds Child Depression Scale (RCDS; Reynolds, 1989)

Suicidal Ideation Questionnaire (SIQ; Reynolds, 1988)

Some practitioners also use projective techniques (e.g., Rorschach, figure drawings, apperception tests) to assess depression and suicide risk. However, because these methods have not demonstrated adequate reliability or validity for identifying suicidal youth, they are not recommended for conducting suicide risk assessments.

Immediate Interventions for Suicidal Students

When students appear at risk for suicide, it is especially important to assess lethality of the intended suicidal methods and then take action to protect them against carrying out their plans. Research has shown that boys more often use firearms and girls more often use medications (pills) or poisons in suicide attempts. As indicated earlier, boys are five times more likely than girls to complete suicide, perhaps because of the immediate lethality of guns. If a suicide assessment indicates moderate to high risk for suicide, school-based practitioners must take immediate protective action.

Breaking Confidentiality

The first step is to inform the youth that you have a duty to report the suicidal thoughts and/or attempts. This requires breaking the confidentiality of the child/adolescent interview. For this reason, it is important always to begin your clinical interviews by stating the limits of confidentiality: that you must inform other people when you suspect that a youth is planning to harm himself/herself; planning to harm someone else; or is being abused, endangered, or harmed by someone else. Chapters 2 and 4 described ways to discuss confidentiality in the beginning of child and adolescent interviews. At the end of the interview, clearly explain what steps need to be taken to provide immediate protection for those at moderate to high risk for suicide. Say who will be informed about the suicide risk. If you can, solicit the youth's cooperation in the steps to be taken. Never leave the suicidal youth alone in an unsupervised or unsecured setting (including the restroom). You may have to involve other school staff to help in the supervision, especially when you need to talk privately with other people on the phone or in person.

Notifying Parents

School-based practitioners must be aware of protocols and policies for crisis interventions, such as reporting suicide risk. Notifying parents (or other legal guardians) is an essential step. In their guidelines for suicide interventions, Poland and Lieberman (2002) posed four important questions to consider regarding parent notification: Are the parents available? Are the parents cooperative? What information do the parents have that might contribute to the assessment of risk? What mental health insurance, if any, does the family possess? (The question about insurance is important for assessing access to mental health services outside of school.)

If parents are available and cooperative, then school-based practitioners must provide information about mental health services available in the community. With parental permission, you can contact the service provider to provide pertinent information and then follow up to make sure that the youth arrived at the service agency. It is essential to obtain written consent from parents to release information to other agencies. If there is imminent danger of suicide, Sattler (1998) recommended that you notify parents immediately, ask them to come to your office to get their child, and advise them to seek admission to an emergency room or hospital for their child.

If a youth is in immediate danger of suicide and the parents are uncooperative or deny the danger, then school-based practitioners may decide to contact local law enforcement or child protection services to take action on the youth's behalf. If the parents are not available, school-based practitioners may have to take action themselves to ensure the safety of a high-risk youth. Usually this action is taken in collaboration with an established school-based crisis team. The team may decide that the level of risk warrants escorting the youth to an emergency room in a hospital, a mental health facility, or other community agency.

If a youth does not want parents notified, try to elicit reasons. Based on information from the suicide risk assessment, the crisis team must then determine whether the youth would be placed in a more dangerous situation by notifying the parents. If this is the case, then it is usually appropriate to notify child protection services or local law enforcement. However, it will still be necessary to notify parents about the youth's suicide risk and to attempt to gain their support for an immediate intervention.

Removing Access to Methods

For any youth with suicide risk, it is essential to "suicide-proof" the home and other home-like environments (e.g., frequently visited homes of friends or relatives). This means eliminating access to lethal methods, such as guns, poisons, medications, knives, and other objects that could be used to inflict self-harm. Potentially lethal medications should be placed in locked cabinets. Guns and other weapons should be kept in locked cabinets, without the youth's access to the key, or removed to a safe place unknown to the youth. If a gun cabinet has a glass window, the guns should be moved to a more secure place. Eliminating access to guns can be especially challenging in some families, especially those who enjoy hunting and other gun sports. Access to the Internet is another environmental risk. Parents of suicidal youth should carefully monitor use of the Internet and be especially watchful of a youth's visits to websites that feature death and morbid themes, have suicidal or violent games, or teach methods for suicide or perpetrating violence.

No-Suicide Contracts

For many suicidal youth, it is a good practice to obtain a promise or contract stating that they will not make any suicide attempts or otherwise try to harm themselves. In the no-suicide contract the youth makes a personal agreement to seek help instead of attempting suicide (for an example of such a contract, see Poland & Lieberman, 2002). The contract can be verbal or written. A written contract may carry more weight with the youth, especially if it is on official stationery. The contract should include names and phone numbers of persons or hotlines to contact if a crisis occurs. It can also outline alternative actions that the youth may take to deal with a crisis situation. Such contracts should always be individualized to fit the youth's issues and circumstances. A youth's refusal to make such a promise or contract can be a warning sign of high risk for suicide, which may require further protective action such as hospitalization.

Documentation

Every school district should have protocols for addressing suicide risk in students. The protocols should require documenting information from the assessment process and documenting the steps taken by various school-based practitioners to address the problem. The interview protocols in

Appendix 8.1 and 8.2 can be used for documentation of the suicide risk assessment. School-based practitioners should also carefully record and date all other actions taken on behalf of the at-risk youth, including notification of parents and referrals and reports to mental health professionals or community and government agencies.

DIFFERENTIATING SUICIDE RISK FROM SELF-MUTILATION/DELIBERATE SELF-HARM

Although firearms and pills are common methods for suicide (Gould & Kramer, 2001), the use of other methods is not unusual. One possible method involves the self-destruction of body tissue, such as the cutting of an artery in an attempt to commit suicide through self-inflicted blood loss. However, some children and adolescents engage in the intentional self-destruction of body tissue without deliberate suicidal intent (Favazza, 1998). These individuals engage in what has been variously described as self-mutilation, deliberate self-harm, or parasuicide, and they are often colloquially referred to as "cutters" (because most children and adolescents who engage in this behavior use knives or other sharp objects to cut themselves). Cutting behavior often appears to provide rapid, but temporary, relief from stress and tension, a sense of security or control, and/or decreases in distressing thoughts or feelings (Favazza, 1998).

Although youth who engage in repetitive self-mutilation (SM) are at increased risk for suicidal behavior (Favazza, 1998), research suggests that SM and suicide attempts are two different types of problems with different etiologies (Ross & Heath, 2002). Making an accurate distinction between actual suicidal behavior and SM is critical, because despite some similarities in appearance, they serve different functions: The individual attempting suicide is trying to end his/her life, whereas the individual engaging in SM is typically trying to maintain it.

Self-mutilation often begins during early adolescence, although it can begin earlier, and may persist for years, or even decades, if not effectively identified and treated. In contrast to suicide completion, SM appears to be more prevalent in girls than in boys, and the number of individuals who engage in SM is likely underestimated and increasing. Additionally, research suggests that it may sometimes, though not always, be precipitated by one or more episodes of sexual or physical abuse (Favazza, 1999; Ross & Heath, 2002).

Because youth who engage in SM are often secretive and reluctant to refer themselves for treatment, identification and assessment of these individuals can be difficult. This problem is further complicated by the lack of standardized assessment instruments for SM. If a youth is suspected of engaging in SM, a comprehensive assessment should include both direct observations/ examinations (e.g., checking for cuts or burn marks and the presence of unusually heavy or unseasonable clothing designed to mask scars) and individual interviews with the youth, parents/caregivers, and school personnel (Miller & DeZolt, 2004). When interviewing the youth, practitioners should directly ask if she/he is engaging in self-mutilation (e.g., "Some kids cut themselves, not because they want to die, but because the cutting makes them feel better in some way. Have you ever done that?"). If the youth reports SM, a suicide risk assessment should immediately be conducted as well. The following areas should also be assessed, as they may have implications for treatment: (1) degree of anger and its expression; (2) degree of self-esteem and self-concept; (3) history of abuse, particularly sexual abuse; (4) possible cognitive distortions; and (5) family tolerance for expression of feelings (Favazza, 1999).

Additionally, you should inquire about the events that precipitate and follow acts of SM, including asking about where acts of SM occur and what the goals, benefits, and consequences of the acts are for the youth engaging in it (Miller & DeZolt, 2004). Conducting an FBA (Watson & Steege, 2003) can also be useful for linking assessment to intervention. An FBA involves gathering information about antecedent conditions, actual behaviors, and consequences of the behaviors to determine the reason or function of SM. For example, the function of SM for one individual might be escape (e.g., releasing mounting anxiety and unbearable tension), whereas for another it might be attention (e.g., a teenage girl who cuts herself to receive attention from a boyfriend). Identical behaviors (e.g., skin cutting) may serve different functions for different individuals and will therefore lead to different interventions (Miller & DeZolt, 2004).

When SM is suspected, assessment may need to be multidisciplinary. For example, although a school psychologist or counselor may be involved in interviewing the youth, a school nurse may be needed to conduct a physical inspection, particularly if the possible SM is not immediately visible.

Interventions for Youth Who Self-Mutilate

If it has been clearly established that an individual engages in SM, parents or caregivers should be contacted. As with treatment for suicidal behavior, school personnel will typically not be directly involved in treatment, but they can provide support by making appropriate referrals and securing assistance from others. Unfortunately, little information is available on effective treatments for youth who engage in SM. For some individuals, behavioral and cognitive strategies such as relaxation techniques, thought stopping, and cognitive therapy may be useful (Miller & DeZolt, 2004). A form of cognitive-behavioral therapy known as dialectical behavior therapy (DBT; Linehan, 1993) has shown some promise (Favazza, 1999). DBT focuses on the faulty problem-solving behaviors, low distress tolerance, and inadequate coping skills that contribute to SM. Cognitive-behavioral procedures may also be combined with pharmacotherapy. Treatment of youth who engage in SM can often be difficult. It requires practitioners "who are compassionate and flexible, and who demonstrate sensitivity to individual needs and a commitment to a multidisciplinary approach to treatment" (Miller & DeZolt, 2004, p. 293).

SUMMARY

Assessing youth at risk for suicidal behavior is one of the most anxiety-inducing, but often necessary, tasks for mental health professionals, including school-based practitioners. Given the critical importance of this problem and its lethal potential, it is imperative that school-based practitioners have the knowledge, skills, and confidence to conduct effective suicide risk assessments. Unfortunately, school-based practitioners may have limited experience with suicide risk assessments; therefore, there is need for improved training and continuing professional development, as well as consultation with colleagues, for this kind of assessment. Conducting a thorough suicide risk assessment is the first step toward providing effective suicide prevention and intervention.

Student Interview for Suicide Risk Screening (SISRS)

Child's name _____
First   Middle   Last

Child's date of birth ____/____/____ Age _____ Gender _____ Grade _____
Month Day   Year

Interviewer's name _____ Date ____/____/_____
Month Day   Year

Engagement

It seems things haven't been going so well for you lately. Your parents and/or teachers have said _____. Most teens/children would find that upsetting.

Have you felt upset, maybe had some sad or angry feelings you've had trouble talking about? Maybe I could help you talk about these feelings and thoughts?

Do you feel like things can get better, or are you worried (afraid, concerned) things will just stay the same or get worse?

Are you feeling unhappy most of the time?

Identification

Other teenagers/children I've talked with have said that when they feel sad and/or angry, they thought for a while that things would be better if they were dead. Have you ever thought that?

Is this feeling of unhappiness so strong that sometimes you wish you were dead?

Do you sometimes feel that you want to take your own life?

How often have you had these thoughts?

(continued)

Inquiry

What has made you feel so awful?

What problems/situations have led you to think this way?

Tell me more about what has led you to see killing yourself as a solution.

What do you think it would feel like to be dead?

How do you think your father and mother feel? What do you think would happen to them if you were dead?

Assessment

A. Current Suicide Plan

Have you thought about how you might make yourself die?

Do you have a plan?

On a scale of 1 to 10, how likely is it that you will kill yourself? When are you planning to, or when do you think you will do this?

Do you have the means with you now, at school or at home?

Where are you planning to kill yourself?

Have you written a note?

Have you put things in order?

(continued)

Student Interview for Suicide Risk Screening *(page 3 of 3)*

B. Prior Behavior

Has any one that you know of killed or attempted to kill themselves? Do you know why?

Have you ever threatened to kill yourself before? When? What stopped you?

Have you ever tried to kill yourself before? How did you attempt to do so?

C. Resources

Is there anyone or anything that would stop you?

Is there someone whom you can talk to about these feelings?

Have you or can you talk to your family or friends about your feelings of suicide?

Summary:

Brief Suicide Risk Assessment Questionnaire

Child's name _____
First   Middle   Last

Child's date of birth ____/____/____ Age _____ Gender _____ Grade _____
Month Day Year

Interviewer's name _____ Date ____/____/_____
Month Day Year

Ask the student about the incident that was reported. (It is critical that students be asked directly about their suicidal thoughts, wishes, plans, etc. A history of suicidal thoughts and/or feelings increases risk, as does a high frequency of such behavior.)

1. Ask if the student has:

   A. A specific plan to commit suicide

   B. A method for doing so (e.g., gun, taking pills, hanging)

   C. The availability of the method (e.g., gun in the home)

   D. A particular date/time scheduled for attempting/committing suicide (i.e., no specific time plan vs. specific plan)

   E. Level of stress the student is currently experiencing (low, moderate, or high stress)

   F. The availability of resources (e.g., help available, extent of support network; family and friends may be available but unwilling to help)

2. Has the student attempted suicide in the past?

3. Is the student in possession of any lethal methods (e.g., guns, pills, knife)? If this student is in possession of a lethal method/weapon, ask him/her to relinquish it.

4. Based on this risk assessment, indicate your rating of the student's probability for engaging in suicidal behavior (circle one).

   Low Risk   Moderate Risk   High Risk

Summary:

9

Assessing Youth Violence and Threats of Violence in Schools

School-Based Risk Assessments

WILLIAM HALIKIAS

In recent years schools and communities have become increasingly worried about the safety of schools and violence from students (Kingery & Coggeshall, 2001; Poland, 1990; Poland & McCormick, 1999). The so-called "school shootings" in towns such as Littleton, Colorado; Pearl, Mississippi; Jonesboro, Arkansas; West Paducah, Kentucky; and Springfield, Oregon, altered perceptions about the presumed threat that children posed to others (Elliott, Hamburg, & Williams, 1998; Ryan-Arredondo et al., 2001; for brevity, the word *child* in this chapter includes adolescents in middle school and high school). The event at Columbine High School in Littleton, Colorado, was one of the most disturbing incidents in this category. On April 20, 1999, two students carefully planned an assault and managed to kill 13 people before committing suicide.

School shootings, as well as the terrorist attacks of September 11, 2001, have probably increased the number of child referrals from schools for risk-of-violence assessments. Compared with other evaluations of children's functioning, the school-based risk assessment (SBRA) is one of the most challenging. Questions about a child's potential for violence pose an array of complex predicaments that go to the heart of the assessment enterprise. These predicaments include traditional problems associated with prediction of future behavior and the assessment of dangerous-

William Halikias, PsyD, is a Senior Associate Faculty member of the Department of Clinical Psychology at the Antioch New England Graduate School. As a licensed practicing psychologist and board-certified diplomate for the American Board of Assessment Psychology, he practices clinical and forensic psychology and consults to schools, courts, and mental health agencies. He teaches advanced seminars in psychology and the law, child and family psychology, and psychological assessment. His research interests include development of scientist-practitioner models of psychological assessment and consultation.

A version of this chapter appeared in Halikias (2004). Copyright 2004 by the American Psychological Association. Adapted by permission.

ness. Of no small consequence to the child and his/her family, SBRAs help decide whether some children remain part of a school community or lose that right. An SBRA is usually a coerced procedure that involves quasi-judicial ramifications similar to the evaluations performed by forensic psychologists. This chapter addresses all school-based practitioners, including school, clinical, and counseling psychologists, who may conduct such evaluations for schools.

The SBRA model flows from a scientist-practitioner orientation (Lambert, 1993; Stricker & Trierweiler, 1995; Stricker, 2002) and draws heavily from a pragmatic philosophy (Fishman, 1999; Rorty, 1982). Pragmatic psychology attempts to integrate historically opposing camps of positivism—the belief that all germane knowledge falls within the bounds of science—and the idiographic tradition in which naturalistic, case-driven, and qualitative information is the focus of inquiry. The scientist-practitioner model also seeks to integrate science with the local culture. This approach focuses on problems a psychologist faces and tries to solve in clinical practice. The scientist-practitioner model and pragmatic psychology help to shape the philosophy of the SBRA toward solution-focused strategies of school violence prevention, based on pertinent and available scientific literature.

SOCIAL CONTEXT OF RISK ASSESSMENTS

The increased calls for SBRA are part of a shift in societal attitudes toward juvenile offenders. Over the past 20 years there has been a movement away from protection and rehabilitation of wayward youth toward punishment and retribution (Halikias, 2000). This movement followed dramatic increases in juvenile crime between 1980 and 1994 (Dahlberg, 1998). The shift from juvenile rehabilitation to retribution was also fueled by retrospective studies of adult criminals with an early offending profile (e.g., Farrington et al., 1990; Piquero & Buka, 2002). Researchers and media commentators (e.g., Powers, 2002) voiced alarm about a seeming plague of child and adolescent predators, and state legislators enacted more punitive measures for young lawbreakers. These various factors merged and helped to undermine the juvenile court's mandate of therapeutic jurisprudence. However, juvenile crime has historically fluctuated, rising or falling without evident causes. Recently, between 1994 and 1999, juvenile crime rates reversed course and abruptly declined. Nevertheless, public and media attention galvanized on the notion that serious child and adolescent lawbreaking was running rampant (for a historical review, see Halikias, 2000).

In reality, school shootings are rare events. However, the vivid nature of reporting them leads people to overestimate the chance that such events will occur. For each incident of a school shooting, the public has had repeated exposure to emotional and graphic images of its perpetrators and victims. In 1999 alone, the major television networks aired 296 stories on school shootings (Stossel, 1999, as cited in Reddy et al., 2001). In contrast to beliefs that such violence is widespread, school remains one of the safest places for a child or adolescent (Burns, Dean, & Jacob-Timm, 2001), and the chance that a person will be murdered at school is less than one in a million (U.S. Department of Education & U.S. Department of Justice, 1999).

Because school shootings are rare events, it is very difficult to accurately identify perpetrators ahead of time. Profiling is one way that has been attempted to weed out violent students (American Psychological Association, 1993). However, profiling efforts suffer from many problems. First, profiling can create very high false-positive rates. That is, many more children may fit the characteristics of the "shooter" profile, whereas only a very few such children may actually carry out a school shooting. Second, profiling relies on stereotypes that are inappropriate when applied to individuals. Third, profiling often includes characteristics or behaviors that occur in many children (i.e., high base-rate phenomena). Examples are the presence of serious behavior problems in general, aggressive behavior, feelings of isolation, feelings of being victimized, etc. Fourth, profiling relies too much on media reports, rather than sound scientific studies, in its speculations about causes of school violence.

Predicting school violence is a dubious undertaking (Mulvey & Cauffman, 2001). For example, predicting that all children referred for SBRAs, even those who bring a weapon to school, will not act violently, would result in a very high accuracy rate but miss the few who will act violently. On the other hand, predicting that every child referred for an SBRA will engage in violence will produce a high false-positive rate. One rule of Bayes's theorem—a formula that calculates probabilities—is that predictive accuracy increases as the base rate approaches 50% (Kamphuis & Finn, 2002). Consider, then, the conundrum of a risk of violence assessment: If 50 people in 1,000 will be violent, the evaluator could predict the null hypothesis—that nobody will be violent—and achieve a 95% accuracy rate. However, that would also produce a 5% inaccuracy rate. When these probabilities get applied to school violence, the evaluator faces seemingly impossible odds.

Furthermore, the assessment of risk for a young person involves more error than assessing violence in adults because children are still moving through developmental stages that make it more difficult to chart their future (Dodge & Pettit, 2003). For example, attempts to predict which delinquents will become chronic offenders later have produced unacceptably high false-positive rates (Wenk, Robinson, & Smith, 1972).

ASSESSING DANGEROUSNESS VERSUS THREATS OF VIOLENCE

One confusing aspect of the SBRA is distinguishing between "dangerousness" versus "threats of violence." The school shootings turned attention to assessing threats of school violence. However, many students referred for SBRAs are more suited for assessments of dangerousness.

Individuals considered to be dangerous often display excessive anger and chronic or intermittent aggression toward others. Many have emotional or conduct problems. These individuals fit the dangerousness assessment model. It considers the risk that a person with a history of aggression will behave that way in the future. Although opining about dangerousness remains controversial, a considerable body of research can guide thinking about risk assessments of dangerousness.

Children referred for evaluations of dangerousness fit the literature on violent juveniles. An important consideration for this group is whether their transgressions occur at a specific phase of development or in a specific context, or whether their behavior is more ongoing or trait-like. Research has shown a strong association between high frequency of offending and increased likelihood of persistent antisocial acts (Loeber, 1988; Tremblay et al., 1999). Conduct problems that begin early in childhood look more invariable than those that begin in adolescence (Lahey & Loeber, 1994). Some children also progress through a series of behaviors that increases or decreases their chances of engaging in chronic criminal behavior (Halikias, 2000; Patterson, Forgatch, Yoerger, & Stoolmiller, 1998). Comorbid factors, including hyperactivity combined with conduct problems (Lynam, 1996), or low socioeconomic status and conduct problems (Nagin &

Tremblay, 2001), exert a compelling influence on the stability of aggression. Life-persistent offenders represent a fraction of adjudicated youth, but they commit the majority of juvenile crimes, including violent offenses (Daleg & Levader, 1998; Moffitt, 1993).

A second group of individuals is more appropriate for violence and threat assessments. The violence assessment model was derived from work of the United States Secret Service (USSS) of the Department of the Treasury, an agency whose mandate includes protecting national leaders, candidates, and visiting heads of state from assassination and assassination attempts (Fein & Vossekuil, 1998). This model focuses on individuals who select a target and plan acts of violence. The USSS data base, called the Exceptional Case Study Project (ECSP), helped define targeted school violence. The ECSP was a study of people who planned and carried out an attack or near-attack on a prominent person in the United States since 1949 (Fein & Vossekuil, 1998). The ECSP used a pragmatic and case-centered approach to delineate the attacker's history, motivation, thoughts, and behavior before the attack or attempted attack. The same strategy was then applied to school shootings under the heading of the Safe School Initiative (SSI; Fein et al., 2002; Vossekuil, Fein, Reddy, Borum, & Modzeleski, 2002).

The SSI data base included 37 school shootings and 41 attackers, ages 11–21, since 1974. All of the subjects were male and all were current students or recent students at the school. The sample showed a mix of racial, ethnic, and sociocultural backgrounds, with 75% white. Behavioral histories ranged from few or no known problems to multiple problems. Surprisingly, few of the attackers had been diagnosed with a mental disorder, and a minority had a known history of substance use or abuse. However, all had deliberate attack plans, often formulated several weeks before the incident. The most frequently used weapons were handguns, rifles, and shotguns. As a group, the attackers knew how to use guns and had access to weapons, usually from home. Most reported that they felt persecuted or bullied. Some had experienced a loss or other life crisis prior to the attack. They often voiced thoughts about the attack to a peer, but rarely to the intended target(s). Many performed certain acts that, at least in retrospect, produced suspicion: verbal or written statements, drawings about killing and death, or attempts to obtain weapons. As an example, Vossekuil, Reddy, Fein, Borum, & Modzeleski (2000) cited one case in which a boy successfully scared peers by telling them he put rat poison in the cheese shakers at a local restaurant.

Planning the attacks became an important source of identity for youngsters in the SSI and adults in the ECSP studies. The plan appeared to evolve over time: Getting the idea; thinking about it; maybe telling another person seriously or in jest; practicing or rehearsing; and then actually executing or trying to execute the plan. Like the ECSP sample, school shooters did not act on a political ideology. Instead, they had more diverse motives, including gaining notoriety, bringing attention to a grievance, and sometimes creating an elaborate justification for their anticipated death. In short, their attack rationale resembled a perceived solution to a seemingly irresolvable conflict.

The SSI sample provided some insights into characteristics of school attackers. However, the sample was limited by its size, consisting of only 41 attackers and 10 interviews. Significant problems exist when people try to extrapolate from such a small sample to the 60 million children in U.S. schools. Important differences also exist between adult assassins in the ECSP group and violent children, including the availability of community supports and the influence of maturation and development on aggression.

In actual clinical practice, it is sometimes hard to distinguish dangerousness from threats of violence. An example of the former is a child who impulsively injured one or more individuals at school. In this hypothetical case, the student had a history of aggression and other conduct problems, became frustrated, and retaliated. After the incident, students and staff were not surprised that the student committed the act. Given the history of problematic behavior, this situation conforms to the dangerousness model of assessment. In the threat assessment model, the Columbine shooters appeared to be a prototype: a pair of highly motivated and organized adolescents who carefully planned an assault for months, and then effectively carried it out. Hindsight bias aside, probably few in that community had viable and reliable information into the students' intentions or capacity to execute this horrific crime. This case conforms to the threat assessment model, first because those students lacked a well-documented history of past violence, and second, because they planned the attack ahead of time.

PREREQUISITES FOR THE SCHOOL-BASED RISK ASSESSMENT

As indicated above, predicting school violence—and violence, in general—is an inherently problematic undertaking. Practitioners should, therefore, avoid a false sense of certainty about their ability to make accurate predictions in these matters, and instead adopt a case-centered and risk-reduction philosophy. A good SBRA is discovery driven and inductive; it tries to individualize the reasons that a child came to the evaluation, and it considers the interventions that might decrease the child's willingness to commit violent acts. In this sense, the SBRA model is a prevention approach that relies on case management strategies to reduce destructive behavior.

Practitioners who conduct SBRAs must have expertise in clinical child psychology and developmental psychopathology (Magrab & Wohlford, 1990; Roberts, et al., 1998). They should have training in child development; interviewing methods with children, adolescents, and parents; intervention and consultation strategies; and ethical and legal issues affecting minors. In addition, they should have knowledge of educational and support systems affecting children and their families. Without this comprehensive training and experience relevant to children, adult-oriented mental health professionals lack the requisite "boundaries of competence" to perform SBRAs (American Psychological Association, 2002, p. 1063).

SBRAs also require knowledge of the ethical dilemmas involved in coerced evaluations (Committee on Ethical Guidelines for Forensic Psychologists, 1991). In the SBRA, parents have the option of denying consent for the evaluation. However, if they deny consent, their child might face such consequences as restricted access to school, alternative educational settings, or possibly being deprived of an education.

Practitioners who conduct SBRAs must understand the legal requirements covering regular versus special education students. For example, students in special education cannot be deprived of an education due to behavior that is directly related to their disability, even if those actions constitute a risk to others (Katsiyannis & Smith, 2003). Under the requirements of the Individuals with Disabilities Education Act (IDEA), the SBRA may be considered a "manifestation determination" for some special education students: an inquiry into whether the student's disability had a relationship to the problematic behavior, or if the disability impaired or diminished the student's sense of the consequences of his/her actions. The evaluation might also occur as part of a functional behavior assessment (FBA). Whereas the manifestation determination explores the relationship between a disability and a behavior, the FBA identifies techniques to manage the behaviors (Knoster, 2000).

When a special education student has been suspended or otherwise excluded from school, IDEA prohibits the exclusion from exceeding 10 days, by which time the school must allow the student to reenter school or provide some alternative program with the requisite special instruction. Thus, when working with special education students around questions concerning their violence potential, the SBRA often needs to be completed in a timely manner.

CORE QUESTIONS OF THE SCHOOL-BASED RISK ASSESSMENT

Practitioners conducting an SBRA need to focus on several critical areas of inquiry. The SBRA questions shape procedures and data collection methods, and are crucial to formulating a child's level of risk of violence. When conducing an SBRA, the evaluator should avoid relying on dichotomous distinctions (e.g., violent vs. not violent) and diagnostic labels (e.g., DSM-IV diagnosis of Conduct Disorder). Instead, the goals are to understand the factors that brought the child to the SBRA and to offer "thick" rather than "thin" descriptions of the child's status (Fishman, 1999). A thick formulation is essentially a narrative that describes individuals, including their ways of constructing meaning, their human interactions, and their context. Thin descriptions tend to be summaries, abstractions, or diagnostic labels that attempt to group people together based on presumed shared traits or features.

Appendix 9.1 provides a reproducible worksheet with core questions to guide the practitioner in conducting an SBRA (Halikias, 2004). By the end of the assessment, evaluators should be able to answer each question or to designate the question as nonapplicable to a particular student. Answering these questions will provide a protocol for conducting a feedback conference with school staff, the child, and parents at the end of the SBRA. The answers also provide a format for formulating conclusions and making recommendations in the written evaluation. Although these core questions are central to the assessment of dangerousness and/or potential threat of violence, evaluators should not use them to make specific predictions about a child's probability to commit a violent act. Instead, the information derived from these questions should be used to develop violence risk-reduction strategies and recommendations for interventions.

CHARACTERISTICS OF CHILDREN REFERRED FOR SCHOOL-BASED RISK ASSESSMENTS

Children referred for SBRAs are a more diverse group than those in the SSI study, which consisted only of male students who had committed, or tried to commit, a school shooting. Thus evaluations based solely on characteristics of the SSI group are likely to be too limited to be of economic or practical value. For the purposes of evaluation, it helps to consider links between the precipitating event, a student's motivation, and the intensity of case-required management strategies. Grouping students into risk groups based on identified motives and actions captures the diversity among students seen in SBRAs. Appendix 9.2 provides a reproducible worksheet for assigning referred children to one or more of five broad groups, according to risk status and case management requirements (Halikias, 2004). Each of these groups is summarized below. Names and details of the case vignettes have been created or altered to protect confidentiality.

Group A (Low Risk) children come to the SBRA with little or no history of psychological problems, but have done something that violated a current school climate of zero tolerance. This may include a child who brought a plastic gun to school or who forgot he/she had a penknife in his/her backpack. Such children generally require a brief and focused assessment and may benefit from low-intensity interventions, such as a conference with the child, a restitution plan, or apology letter. They generally pose little risk for violence and require the least comprehensive and costly assessments and case management plans.

Children in Group B (Low to Medium Risk) are generally nonviolent students who engaged in a thoughtless and sometimes accidental act that worried others. John, a passive and developmentally delayed 14-year-old, watched a horror flick. The movie scared and stimulated him. The combination of poor judgment and his confusion about use of pronouns resulted in his telling a peer how he had killed people. The peer reported John's statements to the principal. Group B children such as John benefit from direction and support and, like Group A children, need less intensive case management plans. This group may benefit from a behavior contract and/or short-term counseling for problem solving, in addition to the case management strategies for Group A.

Children in Group C (Medium Risk) children may or may not come to the SBRA with a history of psychological problems. For them, the critical incident is often a distress signal that reflects inept problem solving. When Frank transferred to the school, students and teachers noticed that he came to classes dressed in military clothing and made references to guns. An isolated and socially awkward teenager, Frank created elaborate and obviously fanciful stories about his exploits, including telling people that he was a Special Operations soldier assigned to that school. His comportment and stories made him the object of ridicule among some students. Once, after being taunted for telling a tall tale, Frank told the student to "watch your back" because he was going home to get his M-16 rifle. Previous inquiry had indicated that Frank's family owned no firearms and that Frank had no experience with the military or guns. A teacher overheard Frank's statement and reported it to the principal.

A developmental crisis or failure often explains Group C students' behavior and their motivation for engaging in threatening actions. These students profit from focused case management interventions to ameliorate the crisis and their inept problem-solving attempts. Interventions might focus on improving degrading aspects of school climate, as well as improving the student's problem-solving skills, anger management, and/or status and self-esteem.

Children in Group D (High Risk—Specific Target) best reflect the subjects from the SSI study. They may or may not come to the evaluation with a known history of social–emotional and/or conduct problems. The hallmark of this group is their ongoing interest in injuring, or having unwelcome contact with, a target. This group also includes children with obsessional fixations and possible delusions about a fantasized attachment figure. People with such obsessions or delusions often pursue and harass another person with the intent to bond with, possess, or damage them (Meloy, 1999). Given that stalking is a crime in all 50 states, Group D students such as these produce a chain of worrisome behaviors.

The most worrisome behavior would be a developed plan of attack. Group D students spend considerable time thinking about and rehearsing an attack. The perceived enormity of this mission lends a sense of purpose to their life. They often conceive the plan because they have experienced a distressing loss, life change, grievance, or harassment. Vossekuil et al. (2000) reported that in the SSI sample, almost 75% of the students had previously threatened to kill themselves, made a suicidal gesture, or tried to commit suicide.

Because so few students actually carry out a calculated attack at school, a bona fide Group D student is unusual. One would not know how many students in this category actually get referred for evaluations—few in the SSI sample had been previously assessed—or how many change their plans because of the attention they received from an evaluation or subsequent case management. Assigning a child to Group D requires credible information about an attack plan and method. When these students get referred to an SBRA, it is usually because they told somebody or did something that brought them to the attention of school authorities.

Richard, age 17, was a small boy who was targeted as effeminate by a group of students at his high school. He also struggled with juvenile diabetes and ongoing grief about the death of his father 2 years ago. Richard called the students who persecuted him "the jocks" and reported incidents that by most standards constituted severe harassment. This mistreatment had begun in Richard's freshman year. In his junior year, Richard's tormentors pasted a photograph of his head onto the photograph of a young girl wearing underwear and posted it throughout the school. Richard and his mother went to the principal and complained about harassment, but the principal took no action.

Richard became increasingly depressed and his grades dropped. He no longer made the honor roll, an important prior source of self-esteem. He began thinking about suicide, at first tentatively, then with increasing commitment to the idea. His deceased father's handgun was accessible in the home, and the father had taught Richard how to use it. Richard set a date for his suicide and wrote a note, which his mother discovered. He had three sessions with a therapist and adamantly denied that he had serious thoughts of killing himself. Richard's mother believed the crisis had past. However, Richard began thinking about shooting his tormentors before killing himself. This fantasy gave him a sense of mission that temporarily improved his feelings of helplessness and depression. He planned the attack for several months. Richard still had access to his father's handgun and ammunition. He planned to carry out the attack at the high school baseball game scheduled in the spring, an event he knew included most of the students he considered tormentors. He rehearsed the attack in his mind, then on paper, and then finally on the baseball field, where he actually "walked through the motions" of the attack. He aroused suspicion when he took photographs of the baseball field. Fortunately, a teacher discovered Richard's written plans for the attack in his desk. The teacher took the plans to the principal, who then requested an SBRA.

When information suggests that a student falls within Group D, school staff and/or the evaluator must consider alerting law enforcement officials. At this point, the practitioner conducting the SBRA takes a back seat to professionals with the authority and training to conduct searches of person and place. Group D students require careful case management plans that address their motivation for violence and teach them alternative problem-solving strategies, along with restricted access to weapons and increased adult supervision.

A subset within Group D would be the "violent true believer" (Meloy, 2004), for whom a combination of homicidal and suicidal desires merge from an ideology or other strongly held conviction. The attack plan of the violent true believer would be labeled "terrorist." A prototype is Timothy McVeigh, who bombed the federal building in Oklahoma City. At this time, there are no reports of a young person in the United States whose ideology formed an underlying motive for targeting a school and carrying out such a horrific and complex attack.

The classification of Group E (High Risk—Chronic Aggression) moves into the realm of chronic aggressive behavior. Groups D and E are similar in that children in both groups are capable of violence. However, the risk for children in Group D is calculated, future oriented, and usually focused on a specific target. Children in Group E, by contrast, have a known history of conduct problems and aggression. For Group E children, the critical incident is part of a larger pattern of inept and aggressive coping strategies. A discipline, special education, or mental health file often accompanies such children to the evaluation. Following the critical incident, these children may find themselves in juvenile court as well as the SBRA. They often require significant case management interventions, sometimes involving alternative education programs.

Sam, age 18, had been identified in second grade as having an "emotional disturbance" and a language-based learning disability. There was a family history of domestic violence and substance abuse. The state child protection service had removed Sam from the home when he was 11 years old, after his mother's boyfriend had attacked him and broken his arm. Sam was reportedly sexually abused by a foster father while in child protective custody.

Sam had received intensive special education and behavioral support from elementary to high school. He had an extensive high school discipline file, including suspensions for physical fights, insubordination, and intimidation of students and faculty. He experienced two arrests: one for stealing, the other for an assault on a student at school. In his senior year Sam heard that a teacher had spoken negatively about him to his girlfriend. He was suspended after he told the teacher that he would slap her if she ever "dissed" him again. At the time of the suspension, Sam was overheard saying he would bring a gun to school and shoot the teacher.

A subset of Group E students display temperamental traits associated with predatory or instrumental aggression. In this group, impulse control deficits and conduct problems often co-occur (Lynam, 1996), along with a seeming absence of remorse for violating the rights of others. These children also tend to lack empathy and use others for personal gain (Frick et al., 2003). Sometimes these children are described as having "juvenile psychopathy," although this label is controversial. Arguments against the validity of the juvenile psychopathy label rest on important differences between youth who act aggressively versus aggression committed in the context of psychopathy (Nagin & Tremblay, 1999). In either case, males with an early history of aggression stand a high chance of becoming life-persistent offenders (Loeber, Farrington, & Waschbusch, 1998; Broidy et al., 2003). Therefore, practitioners conducting SBRAs should always recognize that a long history of conduct problems suggests less likelihood of remission without appropriate interventions.

SCHOOL-BASED RISK ASSESSMENT PROTOCOL AND FORMAT

The SBRA is an organized and deliberate protocol with specific questions, goals, and criteria. It contains several "gates" or "assessment stations" designed to assess risk for violence. The SBRA model is based on a prevention approach, not a predictive one. It is intended to provide relevant recommendations and case management strategies to reduce a student's risk for destructive behavior. The SBRA can be divided into six stages, each with its own tasks and challenges: referral; review and organization of records; parental interview; collateral interviews; interview of the child; and case formulation, findings, and recommendations. Each of these stages is discussed below.

Referral for a School-Based Risk Assessment

The SBRA begins when a school official makes the referral. The first task is to establish the nature and scope of the evaluation and the evaluator's ability to access corroborating information. An SBRA always involves scrutiny of the critical incident, a review of files, an interview with parents and collateral sources, and interviews with the child. If, at the referral stage, the evaluator determines that the school is unable to provide access to this information—for example, the school only wants the evaluator to interview the student—the information derived from the SBRA will be seriously compromised.

Schools seek SBRAs to ensure that a student is not dangerous or a threat for violence. Sometimes the precipitating incident is worrisome (Group D or E); other times the critical incident may be less worrisome (Group A or B). For example, a child who has assaulted a teacher suggests more risk and need for concern than a child who drew a picture of a soldier with a gun. It is important to determine at the start of the SBRA whether a child comes to the evaluation with a history of dangerous and aggressive behavior or has engaged in a relatively discrete and recent act. It is also important to determine whether the child is so overwhelmed that immediate danger to self or other must be assessed. In the latter case the evaluation should be considered a crisis intervention (Catenaccio, 1995; Newgass & Schonfeld, 2000), and the child should be referred to a crisis team or an organization that specializes in assessing imminent danger to self or others.

Given the ethical issues and the risk of professional conduct complaints in SBRAs and other coerced evaluations, practitioners who conduct such evaluations must carefully document their work (Committee on Ethical Guidelines for Forensic Psychologists, 1991). This documentation begins at the referral stage when the practitioner obtains—or collaborates with staff to generate—a written document requesting the evaluation, identifying its purpose, and specifying questions.

After the referral, the evaluator must provide the student and his/her parents with an informed consent document that contains the terms, procedures, goals, possible outcomes, and limits of confidentiality for the evaluation. Appendix 9.3 provides an example of an informed consent form. School-based practitioners will probably have to modify the usual evaluation request form to inform parents about the distinct nature of the SBRA. When the evaluation takes place as part of a special education process, manifestation determination, or FBA, the focus on violence risk assessment should be clearly identified. Then the evaluator should carefully go over the purposes and scope of the evaluation with the parents at or before the first meeting, answering questions and respectfully addressing their concerns or distress about the process.

Documents Related to the Critical Incident and Other Records

Early in the SBRA, and before conducting interviews, evaluators should study the student's records. The most important of these are documents describing the critical incident that provoked the SBRA. For example, examine written threats and then later integrate these into the interviews with the student and others. Review any school-generated reports, such as a discipline file entry, about the critical incident. Also obtain and review the student's academic file, discipline history, and, if they exist, special education and mental health records. In the case of special education records, knowing that a student has a disability may have crucial implications for understanding his/her actions and formulating case management strategies.

In the SBRA it is important to distinguish between *making* a threat and *posing* a threat (Borum, Fein, Vossekuil, & Berglund, 1999; Reddy et al., 2001). This information may appear in the file. Many people make threats but are not violent or dangerous; others, who *are* dangerous, do not make threats. A person who poses a threat usually displays behavior that underlies a motive to damage a target. In cases of credible threats, the would-be attacker often leaves a trail of goal-directed acts. For example, in order to accomplish a serious attack, a person must know details about a target, have access to and skill with specific weapons, avoid detection, consider possible escape routes, and manage security apparatus or personnel. In other words, a matrix of discrete thoughts and behaviors is necessary to accomplish an act as complex as a planned attack.

The student records may consist of an extensive or relatively brief file. In either case, the first step is to organize the history for the SBRA file. One approach is to replicate the student record chronologically, creating an abstract or excerpts from it. To do this, evaluators can enter the date and then a synopsis of a relevant document into a spread sheet or word processor. In organizing the various documents by dates and content, a chronological history will emerge that will aid in understanding the child and assist with interviews and interpretations of findings.

The next step is to cross-check and verify information. The organization of the SBRA file can be augmented later by interviews with collateral sources, parents, and the youth. Information from two or more sources looks more credible than data from only one source. At the end of the SBRA, the evaluator should have gathered information from multiple sources from which to seek convergence and among which to distinguish salient from rarefied findings.

Interviews with Parents

The parental interview is a critical aspect of the SBRA. School psychologists will probably have discussed with colleagues details of the critical incident that provoked the SBRA. However, because of the power dynamics of an SBRA, it is important to speak to parents early in this process. Often parents are upset, resent the school's demands, and/or view the decision to have their child evaluated as capricious. To address these reactions, assure parents that they play a critical role in the evaluation and that their views are respected, and later try to elicit their cooperation with subsequent recommendations. Avoid acting judgmental about the alleged critical incident or the parents' distress about the evaluation. Remaining nonjudgmental increases the chances of joining with parents and collaborating on solutions to their child's problems. Ethical issues such as beneficence, responsibility, fairness, and respect also apply to interviews with parents (American Psychological Association, 2002). In addition, parents are stakeholders in the SBRA, even if they are not the identified client. The multiple constituents in the SBRA (school, child, parents) are not unlike forensic family evaluations that involve many parties and decision makers (Halikias, 1994).

Appendix 9.4 provides a general outline of steps and questions for interviewing parents and children in the SBRA. After obtaining informed consent from parents, begin by addressing the critical incident and parents' understanding of the child's intimidating behavior. This phase involves reviewing details of the child's actions, reports about the incident, and the parents' understanding of the context that led to the child's action. Also ask parents about their child's mental health and his/her developmental and social history, including any history of child abuse or other trauma, an impulse control disorder, a mood or thought disorder, and cognitive limitations.

Evaluators should then review with parents the core "risk-relevant" questions for the SBRA (Appendix 9.4, Section 6). These questions cover the child's interest in targeted violence, extremist groups, or gang affiliation; recent or anticipated loss, such as the death or illness of an attachment figure; a loss of status; parents' worries about their child's ability to harm himself/herself or others; and the child's access to guns or other weapons and his/her ability to use those weapons. Be sure to ask about weapons in the home or in other locations that are accessible to the child. According to Vossekuil et al. (2002), many school shooters obtained firearms from home, even though parents thought those weapons were secure. It is very important to resist the temptation to gloss over questions about weapons or to accept superficial statements that guns are safe. Many locked gun cabinets have breakable glass fronts so that owners can admire their weapons. Parents may report that the guns are locked in a chest—but the key is readily accessible.

Collateral Interviews with Other Informants

Interviews with collateral sources include students, administrators, teachers, therapists, and community members who have relevant knowledge of the referred child. Unless two meetings are scheduled with the child, the collateral interviews should occur prior to interviewing the child. Otherwise, evaluators cannot incorporate reports about the child's threat or destructive behavior into the child interview. Here the school-based practitioner may have more flexibility than a consulting psychologist. For consulting psychologists, it is possible to make the SBRA a day-long event, and in that case, the collateral interviews should always occur before seeing the child.

Students may be the most difficult collateral group to access, but sometimes they are essential people to interview. In the SSI study, attackers rarely advertised their plans to the intended target or targets, but told friends or peers about it (Fein et al., 2002). Students have a unique culture that often excludes adults in the school. They may know before a teacher that a student is in trouble, has been abused, feels bullied, is seeking weapons, or intimidates others. Fein et al. (2002) described a situation in which a planned attack was so well known among students that 24 had gathered at the school to witness it.

If a child has a history of violence, access to other students may not be as critical. Sufficient information may already exist in the student record or may be elicited from adults. It becomes critical to speak to students when they witnessed threatening statements or behavior or experienced intimidation. When interviewing student witnesses is indicated, school administrators must balance privacy rights (Family Education Rights and Privacy Act, 1999) with a mandate to ensure the safety of others (Safe and Drug Free Schools and Communities Act, 1994). For the consulting psychologist, or when policy directs the school psychologist in this area, a school administrator or the evaluator must obtain parental permission to interview other students. In addition, the evaluator should always obtain an informed consent from each student and others interviewed. Collateral sources should be told how the information they report will be used and the limits of privacy in this situation. Fein et al. (2002) also caution that when a student or adult is a possible attack target, they should be interviewed with "special sensitivity" (p. 54). In addition, psychologists have a duty to warn an intended victim or law enforcement officials when reasonable suspicion exists that one person poses a danger to another (*Tarasoff v. Board of Regents of the University of California*, 1976).

From the collateral interviews, SBRA evaluators learn what others think or know about the referred child, including whether other people fear the child. Learning about other people's fears will help to determine whether the referred child should stay at that school or faces an uphill battle to overcome negative attitudes. Learning the context surrounding people's fears is another reason for asking about these feelings. Hearing frightening gossip is different from experiencing intimidation or having firsthand information of an attack scheme. Two examples illustrate reports about such worrisome behavior. In one case a child threatened to stick another student with a pin that he said contained a deadly virus. In another case, a child approached two students and asked them how to obtain guns. In the first example the child intimidated another student. In the second example the child may have revealed his thinking about a planned attack.

Clinical Interview with the Child

The results of various data collection methods prove invaluable when interviewing the child referred for an SBRA. Such investigatory techniques distinguish evaluations, such as SBRAs, from other mental health or educational assessments. For example, therapists have a different mandate from practitioners who evaluate risk. Because therapists only see the child in the clinical setting, they may fail to consider that the child in their office may look different at school. Because therapists act as advocates or support persons, it may be inappropriate to ask them to jeopardize such a relationship by offering opinions about a child's risk level. Crisis intervention is also different from an SBRA because crisis intervention attempts to determine whether a person is a danger to self or others within the next 24–48 hours. This type of evaluation may miss high-functioning children who are not experiencing an acute crisis but who still need interventions to reduce their potential for violence.

Early tasks in the SBRA include (1) helping the child understand the nature of the evaluation, (2) correcting any misunderstandings, and (3) informing him/her about the potential outcomes of the assessment. The next step is to ask the child to recount the reported statement or action that led to the SBRA. Often these children are afraid or guarded in their responses because restrictions may have been imposed on them, there may be police involvement, or they have a clear sense that they are in trouble. Denial or minimization of substantiated facts are common under these circumstances. In this context, children's lies or distortions provide a window into their problem-solving behavior or response style that may generalize beyond the evaluation. Deception is a complex human interaction that includes dimensions of self-deception or deception of others, minimization or denial, and dissimulation attempts that are sophisticated or primitive. For example, a child who attempts to outsmart a psychologist might look quite different from a child who uses distortion to avoid hurting an attachment figure.

The SBRA, although future oriented, is also retrospective when evaluators use it to try to understand past actions that might have led to the critical incident. In this regard the SBRA resembles the mental status at time of offense (MSO) evaluation in criminal cases. Melton, Petrila, Polythress, and Slobogin (1997) use a "spiraling approach" in the MSO interview, going from general to specific questions, collecting more details from the subject. For example, with children, evaluators can designate a point in time before the critical incident and, in a sequential fashion, move toward the incident. Specifically, ask them about their routine on the day of the incident, what they ate for lunch, the people they saw. Such questions help engender cooperation with more pertinent issues, such as, "When did you get the idea to write this threat?" or "What were you thinking before you slapped the principal?" Situational factors, such as alcohol or other drug use, peer influence, the illness or death of a significant other, or a loss of social status, should be explored during this discussion.

Like many forensic assessments, SBRAs seek details. If a student reports that he drank alcohol the night before an assault, the evaluator can inquire about the type and amount of alcohol consumed. If an incident was prompted by a fight with a friend, the evaluator can ask more questions about that relationship. These details help the evaluator to determine the seriousness and motivation for a destructive act, understand if the act was impulsive or planned, determine contributing personal or environmental factors, and consider how to prevent such behavior in the future.

Following Melton et al.'s (1997) MSO strategy, evaluators can move from general to more probing questioning. Be sure to explore inconsistencies in the child's story and encourage the child to address thoughts or feelings that he/she may have been reluctant to discuss. With more direct and threatening questions, it is important to convey understanding and respect, for example, saying, "I know this is hard for you to talk about, but it's important that I understand it." Always try to employ a supportive rather than confrontational style. These approaches are especially important with adolescents who are hypervigilant to feeling manipulated or humiliated, and who withdraw or go on the offensive when upset. The evaluator walks a tightrope with many adolescents, balancing support with direction, acceptance with skepticism, and neutral with probing questions, trying to build and sustain what has been called a "fragile alliance" (Meeks, 1971).

The SBRA does not rely as heavily on tests as do other forms of psychological evaluations. Instead, the SBRA is a more inductive, investigative, and interview-focused process. The SBRA involves a person-centered approach that includes an assessment of mental status, motivation, and person–situation factors. This pragmatic approach is consistent with the literature on adult threat assessments (Megargee, 2002). In addition, valid tests that predict juvenile violence do not exist. Further, time and cost demands often prevent the routine use of tests or relegate them to a post-risk-assessment phase. However, the SBRA is sometimes integrated into a special education assessment. Performing both functions requires expertise in cognitive test instruments, in addition to expertise in risk of violence assessments.

Case Formulation, Findings, and Recommendations

In the final stage of the SBRA, the evaluator establishes not only a child's dangerousness or risk level for violence, but also the circumstances that may increase or decrease the chances of this behavior. Aggression is usually not a random act but dependent on the interaction of circumstance and temperament. In the formulation stage the evaluator answers the core questions relevant to violence potential, listed in Appendix 9.1. These questions concern a child's motivation for the critical incident, what he or she did or said, the fear that he or she engendered, and other important issues pertinent to the SBRA. Answering these questions helps evaluators formulate a "thick" rather than one-dimensional or dichotomous (violent vs. not violent) description of the child.

The answers to the core questions should also lead to reasonable and cost-effective case management strategies. Unlike a predictive approach, case management allows for postassessment control such as observing and monitoring compliance, providing support, and reassessing the child, if necessary, over time (Heilbrun, 1997).

Recommendations and case management fall on a continuum from minimally intrusive to more intrusive, intensive, and costly strategies (see Appendix 9.2). As indicated earlier, for children who pose low to medium risk (Group A or B), a conference between the child and the principal, a restitution plan, or letter of apology might be indicated. A boy who joked about making a bomb could write a letter of apology or provide a service in recognition of his mistake. A Group C child, who poses medium risk, might benefit from support and problem-solving guidance, including having the school administrator consider ways to improve a degrading school climate, individual therapy to manage feelings of helplessness or anger, and opportunities to enhance status or self-esteem.

Given their high risk for violence, Group D children often require careful case management that may include contracting with a child for safety, removing weapons from the home, using therapeutic and anger management techniques, recruiting a supportive juvenile police officer to work with the youth, and addressing grievances or disabilities.

Group E children, who are chronically aggressive, often need comprehensive and sometimes intensive case management strategies. There is a high rate of language-based learning disabilities in this group (Dionne, Tremblay, Boivin, Laplante, & Perusse, 2003). Children in Group E often have family problems and diagnoses of Oppositional Defiant Disorder or Conduct Disorder. Furthermore, they comprise the majority of youth referred to mental health and other treatment centers (Loeber, Burke, Lahey, Winters, & Zera, 2000) and have a higher frequency of placement in special programs for emotionally disturbed students (Dodge & Pettit, 2003). Interventions might include removing weapons from the home and coordinating school, therapeutic, and community-based services. Alternative school programs, day treatment centers, or residential facilities become options when these children have injured others and continue to pose this risk.

The SBRA usually ends with an oral or written report of observations, findings, and recommendations, along with statements regarding any limitations to conclusions. Reports should be free of jargon, so that parents, administrators, and other nonpsychologists will understand the information. The oral or written report should include a caution on the limitations for predicting school violence and a rationale for a case management approach. As an example, evaluators can introduce the conclusion section of the SBRA with the following statement:

"School staff wanted this evaluation to help them understand Sam's threat potential, learn strategies to avert violence, and help assure that Sam and others remain safe. Given the rarity of this type of violence, a threat assessment, especially of calculated and planned school violence, cannot realistically predict such incidents. Rather, this evaluation attempted to identify risk factors for destructive behavior, and it offers recommendations for ways to help decrease the possibility of violence. In this regard, helping Sam to function more effectively holds the greatest promise for reducing destructive or violent behavior."

SUMMARY

The SBRA is a complex and specialized evaluation procedure that requires knowledge about children's development, an appreciation of the literature relevant to SBRAs, an understanding of school systems and special education procedures, and the ability to conduct the required investigatory procedures. The SBRA also requires ability to determine risk potential, along with an understanding of the limitations of this task. Crafting reasonable case management strategies is a key goal of the SBRA in order to mobilize adults on the child's behalf and reduce risk for violence. The SBRA requires collecting and integrating information across multiple informants and data sources (history, interviews, observations, tests, records). The SBRA systematically organizes data, seeking convergent sources and minimizing the error associated with isolated reports.

The majority of children referred for an SBRA will not pose a danger to others; only a small number fit a targeted violence profile or pose this high level of risk. Practitioners who perform SBRAs have the opportunity to reach a diverse group of students with special needs. With few exceptions, referred children benefit more from supportive services and good case management than from stereotyping and punishment.

School-based practitioners should adopt a pragmatic and case-focused approach to SBRAs, given the limitations of accurately predicting school violence. Instead of making "yes" or "no" conclusions about risk for violence, SBRA evaluators can help others understand the reasons for a child's destructive behavior and offer solution-focused recommendations to improve functional skills in school and the larger society.

School-Based Risk Assessment Worksheet

Child's name _____ Date of birth ___/___/___
                First   Middle   Last   Month Day Year

Child's school _____

Informants _____

Evaluator _____ Dates of evaluation _____

Use this worksheet to conduct interviews with the referred child, parents, and collateral sources. When you have completed the school-based risk assessment, record a succinct answer for each question in the space below or write "nonapplicable" (n/a). Use this completed form when you conduct the feedback conference or write the report.

1. What was the motive for the behavior that brought the child to the evaluation?

2. What has the child said, written, or done that involved a risk for violence?

3. Does the child have pertinent information about a target, if one exists (e.g., the person's schedule, activities, home address)?

4. Does the child have an interest in targeted violence or extremist groups? Is there any gang affiliation or membership?

5. Are weapons available to the child, and does he or she know how to use them?

6. Has the child exhibited intimidating behaviors, such as stalking or harassing others?

(continued)

7. What is the child's mental condition and history of mental illness? Does he/she have delusions, hallucinations, or paranoid states?

8. Is there evidence of substance abuse or dependence?

9. Has there been a recent loss, including a loss of status, that produced feelings of despair?

10. If the child shows history of past violence, does the violence appear to be calculated or impulsive?

11. Were the child's past aggressive actions done in concert with others, or were they solitary acts?

12. Were the child's aggressive actions rare, occasional, frequent, or ongoing?

13. Do people in school or the community have fears about the child's potential for violence? Have others experienced intimidation because of the child's behavior?

14. Are there factors that might increase or decrease the risk of future violence? What are these factors?

APPENDIX 9.2
Risk Assessment Groups and Case Management Strategies

Child's name _____ Date of birth ___ / ___ / ___

First   Middle   Last   Month Day Year

Child's school _____

Informants _____

Evaluator _____ Dates of evaluation _____

Use this form to estimate the risk status of the child referred for a school-based risk assessment. Identifying a child's sense of membership in one or more groups can help you estimate his/her level of violence potential and the intensity of postassessment resources needed. There is no precise empirical method for classifying children referred for school-based risk assessments. However, you can use this form to assign a rough estimate of risk for violence, based on the critical incident and the child's motivation for threatening behavior. A child's apparent membership in a group can guide you in making specific recommendations for case management intervention. Consider that some children may fall between groups or may be assigned to more than one group. Check categories, descriptions, and sample recommendations that apply to this particular child.

☐ Group A. Low Risk

Characteristics	*Case Management*
• Often they have done something that violated a zero tolerance policy. • Come to assessment with little or no history of psychological problems. • History and motivation for act make them appear to pose little risk.	• Conference with child • Restitution plan • Apology letter

---

☐ Group B. Low to Medium Risk

Characteristics	*Case Management*
• Nonviolent children who did something thoughtless and/or accidental. • Come to assessment with little or no history of psychological problems. • History and motivation for act make them appear to pose little risk to harm others, but they may be at risk for future behavior that places their status at school in jeopardy.	• Conference with child. • Restitution plan. • Apology letter. • Behavior contract. • Short-term counseling to address problem solving.

(continued)

☐ **Group C. Medium Risk**	
Characteristics	*Case Management*
• Critical incident is a distress signal. • May or may not come to the assessment with a history of psychological problems. • Inept problem-solving and/or social skills.	• Improve problem-solving skills. • Attend to possible problems reflecting a degrading school climate (e.g., sensitivity training for staff; bullying intervention and prevention programs). • Therapy for possible social–emotional problems (e.g., depression, anxiety, recent loss, family problems). • Designate an adult support person at school who will have daily contact with the child. • Provide anger management therapy when indicated. • Seek ways to enhance child's status or self-esteem at school or in the community.
☐ **Group D. High Risk—Specific Target**	
Characteristics	*Case Management*
• Referral and motivation reflect ongoing interest in injuring or having unwelcome contact with a target. • May or may not come to the assessment with a known history of psychological problems. • Evidence exists that they have considered or begun to implement a plan to injure others emotionally or physically. • Threatening behavior often evolved from a crisis (e.g., loss, harassment, suicidal feelings).	• Contract with child for safety. • Recommend that weapons be removed from the home and other locations to which the child has access (e.g., a friend or relative's home). • Notify law enforcement if a child's behavior or plans pose a threat to a target. • Employ family counseling or anger management techniques to address underlying crisis. • Consider if suicide prevention strategies are indicated. • Consider recruiting a supportive juvenile police officer, or other adult in authority, who has sensitivity to the child's problems to work with the child. • If the child returns to school, structure the school day to ensure regular adult check-ins (at a minimum: at the beginning and end of each school day) with the child. • Consider whether additional assessment is indicated (e.g., assessment for special education, mental health services, psychopharmacotherapy). • Address grievances at school.

(continued)

☐ **Group E. High Risk-Chronic Aggression**

Characteristics	*Case Management*
• Come to evaluation with a known history of emotional, developmental, or conduct problems. • Critical incident is part of a larger pattern of problematic behaviors. • Has a discipline, special education, or mental health file. • Verbal and physical aggression look historical, and usually predate the critical incident by 1 or more years.	• Ascertain if child has received appropriate educational services (e.g., a suspected but not diagnosed language disability). • Incorporate vocational/technical curricula into child's school program, if these appear helpful. • Seek opportunities to expose child to extracurricular activities and prosocial experiences (e.g., clubs, sports, work opportunities). • Recommend that weapons be removed from the home or other locations to which the child has access (e.g., a friend's or relative's home). • Recommend needed mental health interventions (e.g., anger management training, substance abuse counseling, psychopharmacotherapy). • Recommend "wraparound" or other cross-discipline teams to help manage child's behavior. • Examine the need for family counseling or home-based family services. • Recommend ways to reduce abusive or chaotic features in the child's life. • If the child injured others and continues to pose this risk, consider alternative school programs, day treatment centers, or residential facilities. • If child returns to school, structure school day to ensure regular adult check-ins (at a minimum: at the beginning and end of each school day) with the child. • Adopt a "zero tolerance" policy around future aggression and threats of aggression. • Use restitution plans and apology letters when the child has injured another person.

Sample Informed Consent for a School-Based Risk Assessment

INFORMED CONSENT FOR RISK ASSESSMENT EVALUATION

Your child, _____, has been referred to me by the _____ School for a risk assessment evaluation. Specifically, this is an assessment of risk for dangerousness following incidents involving your child and the school. This evaluation may consist of interviews, observations, psychological tests, and a review of records. At the end of this evaluation I may write a report and/or conduct a verbal conference detailing my observations, conclusions, and recommendations. The school will pay for this evaluation.

You will allow me to interview school employees or family members, to review records about your child, or to obtain information from other professionals.

Because the school has referred your child to me and is paying for this service, you acknowledge that I will communicate with and send reports to staff at _____ School.

If you decide to withdraw from this evaluation, you may not retroactively revoke consent for me to communicate with the school about information already obtained from you, your child, significant others, or service providers. Once verbal or written reports are given to the school, I have no control over what they do with this information.

Examples of other circumstances when information from this evaluation may or must be shared with others include, but are not limited to, the following:

1) You may sign a release of information giving me permission to speak with, or send information to, another person or organization.
2) If you or your child present as a clear and present danger to self or other, I must release information in order to protect you, your child, or another person from harm.
3) If I have reasonable cause to believe that a child under the age of 18 years is suffering abuse or neglect, I am required by law to report this information to social services.

It is not possible for me to send you psychological test protocols (the test forms) or manuals because this information is protected by rules mandating test security. Should you wish to obtain this information, you agree to employ a licensed psychologist or certified school psychologist with expertise in test and measurement to review and interpret this information for you. I will, of course, provide you with the results and interpretation of psychological tests.

_____   _____
Parent/Guardian Signature   Date

_____   _____
Parent/Guardian Signature   Date

General Outline for SBRA Parent and Child Interviews

1. Present informed consent or, if it has already been read and signed, review this information with the subject or subjects.

2. Answer questions that parents or children have about the evaluation.

3. Determine whether service providers or service organizations exist for the child or parents (e.g., mental health counselors, past psychiatric hospitalizations). Ask parents and, if appropriate, the child to sign releases that allow the evaluator to speak to these sources. Ask about the existence of other important adult relationships that may serve as useful collateral sources (e.g., employer, minister, relative, coach).

4. Ask a general question about how the parents or child understand what it means to be evaluated for a school-based risk assessment. The answer to this question should result in an initial explanation of the reason for referral. Sometimes the response will be short; other times, it may entail a long discussion.

   a. Be certain that you explore with the parents and child what the child said, wrote, or did that others perceived as threatening.

   b. Ask the child to carefully recount his/her activities that lead up to the critical incident, and obtain details about his/her thoughts and behavior around an alleged incident.

5. Present parents or child with documents related to the critical incident (e.g., written threat from the child, discipline log entry, affidavits or police reports, letter from school to parents) and ask for their responses.

6. Review risk-relevant questions:

   a. What contact has the child had with the identified target, and what is the nature of that relationship? How familiar is the child with that person's schedule, activities, and home address?

   b. What movies, books, computer Internet sites, and group affiliations is the child most interested in or involved with? Begin to explore questions relevant to an interest in targeted violence or extremist groups and any possible gang affiliation.

   c. Have the adults and child describe the exact weapon(s) (e.g., rifles, shotguns, handguns, hunting or military knives, bow and arrows, explosive devices or materials) that exist in the home or elsewhere, to which the youth has access. Obtain details about the security system in place with the weapon(s). Establish the youngster's knowledge about, and skill with, these weapons.

   d. Other than the reason for referral, do the parents or child know of incidents when people felt intimidated or harassed by the child, regardless of whether the parents or child thought that reaction justified? Do the parents worry about their child? Do the parents or child know of people who have expressed fear of the child or concern that he/she could injure themselves or others?

(continued)

e. Ask questions that will provide information about the child's mental health or any history of mental illness, including any attempts at therapy or previous psychiatric hospitalization. Ask if the youngster has experienced abuse (physical, emotional, sexual, neglect). Has there ever been suicidal talk, writings, or actions by the child?

f. Establish academic strengths and weaknesses; include information about, or evidence for, learning or cognitive delays.

g. Perform a focused inquiry about substance use and abuse with the youngster, his/her siblings, and the parents.

h. Ask if the child or family has any present or past involvement with a child protection agency, the police, or courts, and the reasons this involvement.

i. Has there been a recent loss that produced feelings of despair? This loss may include a death or severe, prolonged illness of an important attachment figure. Ask if the youth experienced any recent blows to his/her self-esteem. For example, was the child cut from a sports team? Has the child experienced the loss of a romantic or other important relationship?

j. Ask parents and the child to recount all incidents of physical violence on the part of the child, regardless of whether they view such acts as self-defense and justifiable or intended to harm another person. Establish any possible themes that appear to precipitate aggressive acts. The evaluator comes away from this part of the interview with a sense of how the parents and child describe and perceive past aggression: minimal to substantial, impulsive versus planned, intermittent versus chronic, done in concert with others or alone.

7. Obtain a developmental and social history from the parents. This history may begin with a description of the family's environment and lifestyle at the time of conception, move sequentially through the pregnancy, birth, infancy, preschool years, elementary school, and continue to the critical incident that resulted in the school-based risk assessment. Use the document generated from the file review (notes and excerpts from historical documents) to assist the parents with recall or to ask them to explain contradictions between their reports and information in the record. The history ends with a review of the extended family history, with an eye toward relatives suffering mental health problems, substance abuse issues, learning difficulties, or criminal involvement. This appendix cannot cover the complexities and skill required to obtain a good social and developmental history, and it is assumed the clinician comes to the school-based risk assessment with this knowledge and training.

8. Establish the child's strengths and productive interests in and outside of school.

9. At this point the interview with the parents may be near or past the 2-hour mark, or the 1-hour mark with the child. This is an opportunity to take a break, during which time the clinician can compare notes from the interview with the record and reports about the critical incident. Following the break, the clinician focuses more actively on contradictions between self-reports and reports obtained from the file and collateral sources.

10. Ask the parents and child for any additional information they wish to convey. Ask if they have any questions about the interview process and how they felt about being interviewed. Clarify with them what may happen next in this process.

References

Achenbach, T. M. (1986). *The Direct Observation Form of the Child Behavior Checklist* (rev. ed.). Burlington, VT: University of Vermont, Research Center for Children, Youth, and Families.

Achenbach, T. M. (2001). *Youth Self-Report for Ages 11–18*. Burlington, VT: University of Vermont, Research Center for Children, Youth, and Families.

Achenbach, T. M., & McConaughy, S. H. (1997). *Empirically based assessment of child and adolescent psychopathology: Practical applications* (2nd ed.). Newbury Park, CA: Sage.

Achenbach, T. M., McConaughy, S. H., & Howell, C. T. (1987). Child/adolescent behavioral and emotional problems: Implications of cross-informant correlations for situational specificity. *Psychological Bulletin, 101*, 213–232.

Achenbach, T. M., Newhouse, P., & Rescorla, L. A. (2004). *Manual for the ASEBA Older Adult Forms & Profiles*. Burlington, VT: University of Vermont, Research Center for Children, Youth, and Families.

Achenbach, T. M., & Rescorla, L. A. (2000). *Manual for the ASEBA Preschool Forms & Profiles*. Burlington, VT: University of Vermont, Research Center for Children, Youth, and Families.

Achenbach, T. M., & Rescorla, L. A. (2001). *Manual for the ASEBA School Age Forms & Profiles*. Burlington, VT: University of Vermont, Research Center for Children, Youth, and Families.

Achenbach, T. M., & Rescorla, L. A. (2003). *Manual for the ASEBA Adult Forms & Profiles*. Burlington, VT: University of Vermont, Research Center for Children, Youth, & Families.

Ambrosini, P. J. (2000). Historical development and present status of the Schedule for Affective Disorders and Schizophrenia for School-age Children (K-SADS). *Journal of the American Academy of Child and Adolescent Psychiatry, 39*, 49–58.

American Academy of Pediatrics. (2000). Diagnosis and evaluation of the child with Attention Deficit Hyperactivity Disorder (AC0002). *Pediatrics, 105*, 1158–1170.

American Psychiatric Association. (2000). *Diagnostic and statistical manual of mental disorders* (4th ed., text rev.). Washington, DC: Author.

American Psychological Association. (1993). *Violence in youth: Psychologists' response*. Washington, DC: Author.

American Psychological Association. (2002). Ethical principles and code of conduct. *American Psychologist, 57*, 1060–1073.

Americans with Disabilities Act. (1990). 42 U.S.C., §1201 et seq.

Angold, A., & Costello, J. (2000). The Child and Adolescent Psychiatric Assessment (CAPA). *Journal of the American Academy of Child and Adolescent Psychiatry, 39*, 39–48.

Barkley, R. A. (2006). *Attention-deficit hyperactivity disorder: A handbook for diagnosis and treatment* (3rd ed.). New York: Guilford Press.

Barkley, R. A., & Murphy, K. (2006). *Attention-deficit hyperactivity disorder: A clinical workbook* (3rd ed.). New York: Guilford Press.

Barrett, T. (1985). *Youth in crisis: Seeking solutions to self-destructive behavior.* Longmont, CO: Sopris West.

Beaver, R. B., & Busse, R. T. (2000). Informant reports: Conceptual and research bases of interviews with parents and teachers. In E. S. Shapiro & T. R. Kratochwill (Eds.), *Behavioral assessment in schools: Theory, research, and clinical foundations* (2nd ed., pp. 257–287). New York: Guilford Press.

Beck, A., & Steer, R. (1991). *Manual for the Beck Scale for Suicidal Ideation.* San Antonio, TX: Psychological Corporation.

Bergan, J. R., & Kratochwill, T. R. (1990). *Behavioral consultation and therapy.* New York: Plenum Press.

Bierman, K. L. (2004). *Peer rejection: Developmental processes and intervention strategies.* New York: Guilford Press.

Bierman, K. L., Smoot, D. L., & Aumiller, K. (1993). Characteristics of aggressive–rejected, aggressive (nonrejected), and rejected (nonaggressive) boys. *Child Development, 64*, 139–151.

Bierman, K. L., & Welsh, J. A. (1997). Social relationship deficits. In E. J. Mash & L. G. Terdal (Eds.), *Assessment of childhood disorders* (3rd ed., pp. 328–365). New York: Guilford Press.

Borum, R., Fein, R., Vossekuil, B., & Berglund, J. (1999). Threat assessment: Defining an approach for evaluating risk of targeted violence. *Behavioral Sciences and the Law, 17*, 323–337.

Brassard, M. A., Tyler, A., & Kehle, T. (1983). Sexually abused children: Identification and suggestions for intervention. *School Psychology Review, 12*, 93–97.

Brock, S. E., & Sandoval, J. (1997). Suicidal ideation and behaviors. In G. C. Bear, K. M. Minke, & A. Thomas (Eds.), *Children's needs II: Development, problems and alternatives* (pp. 361–374). Bethesda, MD: National Association of School Psychologists.

Broidy, L. M., Nagin, D. S., Tremblay, R. E., Bates, J. E., Brame, B., Dodge, K. A., et al. (2003). Developmental trajectories of childhood disruptive behaviors and adolescent delinquency: A six-site, cross-national study. *Developmental Psychology, 39*, 222–245.

Buck, G. H., Bursuck, W. D., Polloway, E. A., Nelson, J., Jayanthi, M. J., & Whitehouse, F. A. (1996). Homework-related communication problems: Perspectives of special educators. *Journal of Emotional and Behavioral Disorders, 4*, 105–113.

Burns, M. K., Dean, V. J., & Jacob-Timm, S. (2001). Assessment of violence potential among school children: Beyond profiling. *Psychology in the Schools, 38*, 239–247.

Burns, R. C. (1982). *Self-growth in families: Kinetic family drawings (K-F-D) research and application.* New York: Brunner/Mazel.

Busse, R. T., & Beaver, B. R. (2000). Informant report: Parent and teacher interviews. In E. S. Shapiro & T. R. Kratochwill (Eds.), *Conducting school-based assessments of child and adolescent behavior* (pp. 235–273). New York: Guilford Press.

Butcher, J. N., Williams, C. L., Graham, J. R., Archer, R. P., Tellegen, A., Ben-Porath, Y. S., & Kaemmer, B. (1992). *Minnesota Multiphasic Personality Inventory—Adolescent Version. Manual for administration and scoring.* Minneapolis, MN: Pearson Assessments.

Castillo, E. M., Quintana, S. M., & Zamarripa, M. X. (2000). Cultural and linguistic issues. In E. S. Shapiro & T. R. Kratochwill (Eds.), *Conducting school-based assessments of child and adolescent behavior* (pp. 274–308). New York: Guilford Press.

Catenaccio, R. (1995). Crisis intervention with suicidal adolescents: A view from the emergency room. In J. K. Zimmerman & G. M. Asnis (Eds.), *Treatment approaches with suicidal adolescents* (pp. 71–90). Oxford, UK: Wiley.

Centers for Disease Control and Prevention. (2002). *Web-based injury statistics query and reporting system.* www.cdc.gov/ncipc/factsheets/suifacts.htm

Child Abuse Prevention and Treatment Act. (1974). Public Law 93-247; 42 U.S.C. §5106 et seq.

Coie, J. D. (1990). Toward a theory of peer rejection. In S. R. Asher & J. D. Coie (Eds.), *Peer rejection in childhood* (pp. 365–401). Cambridge, UK: Cambridge University Press.

Coie, J. D., Dodge, K. A., & Kupersmidt, J. B. (1990). Peer group behavior and social status. In S. R. Asher & J. D. Coie (Eds.), *Peer rejection in childhood* (pp. 17–59). Cambridge, UK: Cambridge University Press.

Coie, J. D., & Kupersmidt, J. B. (1983). A behavior analysis of emerging social status in boys' groups. *Child Development, 54,* 1400–1416.

Committee on Ethical Guidelines for Forensic Psychologists. (1991). Specialty guidelines for forensic psychologists. *Law and Human Behavior, 15,* 655–665.

Confidentiality of Alcohol and Drug Abuse Patient Records. (1987, June 9). 52 Fed. Reg. 21796, 21797.

Conners, K. C. (1997). *Conners Rating Scales—Revised Technical Manual.* North Tonawanda, NY: MHS.

Cooper, H., Lindsay, J. J., Nye, B., & Greathouse, S. (1998). Relationships among attitudes about homework, amount of homework assigned and completed, and student achievement. *Journal of Educational Psychology, 90*(1), 70–83.

Crick, N. R., & Dodge, K. (1994). A review and reformulation of social information-processing mechanisms in children's social adjustment. *Psychological Bulletin, 115,* 74–101.

Crone, D. A., Horner, R. H., & Hawken, L. S. (2004). *Responding to problem behavior in schools.* New York: Guilford Press.

Dahlberg, L. L. (1998). Youth violence in the United States: Major trends, risk factors, and prevention approaches. *American Journal of Preventive Medicine, 14,* 259–272.

Daleg, A., & Levader, S. (1998). Twelve thousand crimes by 75 boys: A 20–year follow-up study of childhood hyperactivity. *Journal of Forensic Psychiatry, 9,* 39–57.

Daniel, S., Power, T. J., Karustis, J. L., & Leff, S. S. (1999, November). *Parent-mediated homework intervention for children with ADHD: Its impact on parent–child relationships and parenting stress.* Poster session presented at the annual meeting of the Association for Advancement of Behavior Therapy, Toronto, Ontario, Canada.

Davis, J. M., & Sandoval, J. (1991). *Suicidal youth: School-based intervention and prevention.* San Francisco: Jossey-Bass.

Dionne, G., Tremblay, R., Boivin, M., Laplante, D., & Perusse, A. (2003). Physical aggression and expressed vocabulary in 19–month-old twins. *Developmental Psychology, 39,* 261–273.

Diperna, J. C., & Elliott, S. N. (2000). *Academic Competence Evaluation Scales.* San Antonio, TX: Psychological Corporation.

Dishion, T. J., McCord, J., & Poulin, F. (1999). When interventions harm: Peer groups and problem behavior. *American Psychologist, 54*(9), 775–764.

Dodge, K. A., & Pettit, G. S. (2003). A biopsychosocial model of the development of chronic conduct problems in adolescence. *Developmental Psychology, 39,* 349–371.

Doll, B. (1996). Prevalence of psychiatric disorders in children and youth: An agenda for advocacy by school psychology. *School Psychology Quarterly, 11,* 20–47.

Drach, K. M., Wientzen, J., & Ricci, L. R. (2001). The diagnostic utility of sexual behavior problems in diagnosing sexual abuse in a forensic child abuse evaluation clinic. *Child Abuse and Neglect, 25,* 489–503.

DuPaul, G. J., & Stoner, G. (2003). *ADHD in the schools* (2nd ed.) New York: Guilford Press.

Eckert, T. L., Miller, D. N., DuPaul, G. J., & Riley-Tillman, T. C. (2003). Adolescent suicide prevention: School psychologists' acceptability of school-based programs. *School Psychology Review, 32,* 57–76.

Elliott, D. S., Hamburg, B. A., & Williams, K. R. (1998). Violence in American schools: An overview. In D. Elliott, B. Hamburg, & K. Williams (Eds.), *Violence in American schools* (pp. 3–28). Cambridge, UK: Cambridge University Press.

Elliott, S. N., DiPerna, J. C., & Shapiro, E. (2001). *Academic Intervention Monitoring System guidebook.* San Antonio, TX: Psychological Corporation.

Epstein, M. H. (2004). *Behavioral and Emotional Rating Scale: A strength based approach to assessment* (2nd ed.). Austin, TX: PRO-ED.

Family Education Rights and Privacy Act. (1974). Public Law 93-830. 20 U.S.C. §1232 et seq. (1999).

Farrington, D. P., Loeber, R., Elliott, D. S., Hawkins, J. D., Kandel, D., Klein, M., et al. (1990). Advancing knowledge about the onset of delinquency and crime. In B. Lahey & A. Kazdin (Eds.), *Advances in clinical and child psychology* (Vol. 13, pp. 231–342). NY: Plenum Press.

Favazza, A. (1998). The coming age of self-mutilation. *The Journal of Nervous and Mental Disease, 186,* 259–268.

Favazza, A. (1999). Self-mutilation. In D. G. Jacobs (Ed.), *The Harvard Medical School guide to suicide assessment and intervention* (pp. 125–145). San Francisco: Jossey-Bass.

Fein, R. A., & Vossekuil, B. (1998). *Protective intelligence and threat investigations: A guide for state and local law enforcement officials.* Washington, DC: U.S. Department of Justice. www.treas.gov/usss/ntac/ntac_pi_guide_state

Fein, R. A., Vossekuil, B., Pollack, W. S., Borum, R., Mozeleski, W., & Reddy, M. (2002). *Threat assessment in schools: A guide to managing threatening situations and to creating safe school climates.* Washington, DC: U.S. Secret Service & U.S. Department of Education.

Finkelhor, D. (1988). The trauma of sexual abuse: Two models. In G. Wyatt & G. Powell (Eds.), *Lasting effects of child sexual abuse* (pp. 61–82). Newbury Park, CA: Sage.

Fisher, T. A. (2003). Conducting functional behavioral assessments and designing behavior intervention plans for youth with emotional/behavioral disorders. In M. Breen & C. Fiedler (Eds.), *Behavioral approach to the assessment of youth with emotional/behavioral disorders: A handbook for school-based practitioners* (2nd ed., pp. 73–121). Austin, TX: PRO-ED.

Fishman, D. B. (1999). *The case for pragmatic psychology.* New York: New York University Press.

Foster, S. L., & Robin, A. L. (1997). Family conflict and communication in adolescence. In E. J. Mash & L. G. Terdal (Eds.), *Assessment of childhood disorders* (3rd ed., pp. 627–682). New York: Guilford Press.

Frick, P. J., Cornell, A. H., Bodin, S. D., Dane, H. E., Barry, C. T., & Loney, B. R. (2003). Callous unemotional traits and developmental pathways to severe conduct problems. *Developmental Psychology, 39,* 246–260.

Friedrich, W. N., & Grambsch, P. (1992). Child Sexual Behavior Inventory: Normative and clinical comparisons. *Psychological Assessment, 4,* 303–311.

Gadow, K. D., & Sprafkin, J. (1998). *Adolescent Symptom Inventory–4 norms manual.* Stony Brook, NY: Checkmate Plus.

Gadow, K. D., & Sprafkin, J. (1999). *Youth's Inventory–4 manual.* Stony Brook, NY: Checkmate Plus.

Gadow, K. D., & Sprafkin, J. (2000). *Early Childhood Inventory–4 norms manual.* Stony Brook, NY: Checkmate Plus.

Gadow, K. D., & Sprafkin, J. (2002). *Child Symptom Inventory–4 screening and norms manual.* Stony Brook, NY: Checkmate Plus.

Garbarino, J., & Scott, F. M. (1989). *What children can tell us.* San Francisco: Jossey-Bass.

Goldstein, A. P., Glick, B., & Gibbs, J. (1998). *Aggression replacement training* (rev. ed.). Champaign, IL: Research Press.

Goldstein, A. P., McKinnis, E., Sprafkin, R. P., Gershaw, N. J., & Klein, P. (1997). *Skillstreaming the adolescent* (rev. ed.). Champaign, IL: Research Press.

Goldston, D. B. (2003). *Measuring suicidal behavior and risk in children and adolescents.* Washington, DC: American Psychological Association.

Goleman, D. (1995). *Emotional intelligence.* New York: Bantam Books.

Gould, M. S., & Kramer, R. A. (2001). Youth suicide prevention. *Suicide and Life-Threatening Behavior, 31*(Suppl.), 6–31.

Greenspan, S. I. (1981). *The clinical interview of the child.* New York: McGraw-Hill.

Gresham, E. M., & Elliott, S. N. (1990). *Social Skills Rating System manual.* Circle Pines, MN: American Guidance Service.

Gresham, F. M., & Gansle, K. A. (1992). Misguided assumptions of the DSM-III–R: Implications for school psychological practice. *School Psychology Quarterly, 7,* 79–95.

Gudeman, R. (2003). Federal privacy protection for substance abuse treatment records: Protecting adolescents. *Youth Law News, Journal of the National Center for Youth Law Reprint.* www.youthlaw.org

Halikias, W. (1994). Forensic family evaluations: A comprehensive model for professional practice. *Journal of Clinical Psychology, 50,* 951–964.

Halikias, W. (2000). Forensic evaluations of adolescents: Psychosocial and clinical considerations. *Adolescence, 35,* 467–484.

Halikias, W. (2005). School-based risk assessment: A conceptual framework and model for professional practice. *Professional Psychology: Research and Practice, 35,* 598–607.

Hartmann, D. P., Roper, B. L., & Bradford, D. C. (1979). Some relationships between behavioral and traditional assessment. *Journal of Behavioral Assessment, 1,* 3–21.

Heilbrun, K. (1997). Prediction versus management models relevant to risk assessment: The importance of legal decision-making context. *Law and Human Behavior, 21,* 447–359.

Henggeler, S. W., & Lee, T. (2003). Multisystemic treatment of serious clinical problems. In A. E. Kazdin & J. R. Weisz (Eds.), *Evidence-based psychotherapies for children and adolescents* (pp. 301–322). New York: Guilford Press.

Henker, B., Whalen, C. K., & O'Neil, R. (1995). Worldly and workaday worries: Contemporary concerns of children and young adolescents. *Journal of Abnormal Child Psychology, 23,* 685–702.

Horton, C. B., & Cruise, T. K. (2001). *Child abuse and neglect: The school's response.* New York: Guilford Press.

Hughes, J., & Baker, D. B. (1990). *The clinical child interview.* New York: Guilford Press.

Individuals with Disabilities Education Act. (1990). Public Law 101-476. 20 U.S.C. §1401 et seq. (Reauthorized July 1997). Public Law 105-17. 20 U.S.C. §1400 et seq. (Reauthorized December 2004). Public Law 108-446.

Individuals with Disabilities Education Act Amendments. (1997). Public Law 105-17, 20 U.S.C. Chapter 33, §1414 et seq.

Institute for Youth Development. (1999). *Age of risk behavior debut: Trends and implications.* Washington, DC: Author. www.youthdevelopment.org/download/debut/pdf

Jacob, S. (2002). Best practices in utilizing professional ethics. In A. Thomas & J. Grimes (Eds.), *Best practices in school psychology–IV* (pp. 77–90). Washington, DC: National Association of School Psychologists.

Jacob, S., & Hartshorne, T. S. (2003). *Ethics and law for school psychologists* (4th ed.). Hoboken, NJ: Wiley.

Jenson, W. R., Rhode, G., & Hepworth, M. N. (2003). *The tough kid parent book.* Longmont, CO: Sopris West.

Jenson, W. R., Rhode, G., & Reavis, H. K. (1994). *The tough kid tool box.* Longmont, CO: Sopris West.

Johnston, L. D., O'Malley, P. M., Bachman, J. G., & Schulenberg, J. E. (2004). *Monitoring the future national results on adolescent drug use: Overview of key findings, 2003* (NIH Publication No. 04–5506). Bethesda, MD: National Institute on Drug Abuse. www.monitoringthefuture.org

Kalafat, J., & Lazarus, P. J. (2002). Suicide prevention in schools. In S. E. Brock, P. J. Lazarus, & S. R. Jimerson (Eds.), *Best practices in school crisis prevention and intervention* (pp. 211–223). Bethesda, MD: National Association of School Psychologists.

Kamphuis, J. H., & Finn, S. E. (2002). Incorporating base rate information in daily clinical decision making. In J. E. Butcher (Ed.), *Clinical personality assessment: Practical approaches* (2nd ed., pp. 257–268). New York: Oxford University Press.

Katsiyannis, K., & Smith, C. R. (2003). Disciplining students with disabilities: Legal trends and the issue of interim alternative education settings. *Behavioral Disorders, 28,* 410–418.

Kay, P., Fitzgerald, M., & McConaughy, S. H. (2001). Building effective parent–teacher partnerships. In R. Algozzine & P. Kay (Eds.), *Preventing problem behaviors: A handbook of successful prevention practices* (pp. 104–125). Thousand Oaks, CA: Corwin Press.

Kazdin, A. E. (2003). Problem-solving skills training and parent management training for conduct disorder. In A. E. Kazdin & J. R. Weisz (Eds.), *Evidence-based psychotherapies for children and adolescents* (pp. 241–262). New York: Guilford Press.

Keith, T. Z., & DeGraff, M. (1997). Homework. In G. G. Bear, K. M. Minke, & A. Thomas (Eds.), *Children's needs: II. Development, problems, and alternatives* (pp. 477–487). Bethesda, MD: National Association of School Psychologists.

Kelley, M. L. (1990). *School–home notes: Promoting children's classroom success.* New York: Guilford Press.

Kingery, P. M., & Coggeshall, M. B. (2001). Surveillance of school violence, injury, and disciplinary actions. *Psychology in the Schools, 38,* 117–126.

Knoff, H. (2002). Best practices in personality assessment. In A. Thomas & J. Grimes (Eds.), *Best practices in school psychology–IV* (pp. 1281–1302). Bethesda, MD: National Association of School Psychologists.

Knoster, T. P. (2000). Understanding the difference and relationship between functional behavioral assessments and manifestation determinations. *Journal of Positive Behavior Interventions, 2,* 53–58.

Kohlberg, L. (1976). Moral stages and moralization: The cognitive developmental approach. In T. Lickona (Ed.), *Moral development and moral behavior* (pp. 31–53). New York: Holt, Rinehart, & Winston.

Kovacs, M. (1992). *Children's Depression Inventory manual.* North Tonawanda, NY: MHS.

Kratochwill, T. R., Elliott, S. N., & Callan-Stoiber, K. (2002). Best practices in problem-solving consultation. In A. Thomas & J. Grimes (Eds.), *Best practices in school psychology–IV* (pp. 583–608). Bethesda, MD: National Association of School Psychologists.

Kratochwill, T. R., & Shapiro, E. S. (2000). Conceptual foundations of behavioral assessment in schools. In E. S. Shapiro & T. R. Kratochwill (Eds.), *Behavioral assessment in schools* (2nd ed.): *Theory, research, and clinical foundations* (pp. 3–15). New York: Guilford Press.

Lachar, D., & Gruber, C. P. (1995). *Personality Inventory for Youth.* Los Angeles: Western Psychological Services.

La Greca, A. M. (1990). *Through the eyes of the child.* Boston: Allyn & Bacon.

Lahey, B. B., & Loeber, R. (1994). Framework for a developmental model of oppositional defiant disorder and conduct disorder. In D. K. Routh (Ed.), *Disruptive behavior disorders in childhood* (pp. 139–180). New York: Plenum Press.

Lambert, N. M. (1993). Historical perspective on school psychology as a scientist–practitioner specialization in school psychology. *Journal of School Psychology, 31,* 163–193.

Lee, J. F., & Pruitt, K. W. (1979). Homework assignments: Classroom games or teaching tools? *Clearinghouse, 53,* 31–35.

Lieberman, R., & Cowan, K. C. (2004). *Save a friend: Tips for teens to prevent suicide.* Bethesda, MD: National Association of School Psychologists.

Lieberman, R., & Davis, J. (2002). Suicide intervention. In S. E. Brock, P. J. Lazarus, & S. R. Jimerson (Eds.), *Best practices in school crisis prevention and intervention* (pp. 531–551). Bethesda, MD: National Association of School Psychologists.

Linehan, M. M. (1993). *Cognitive-behavioral treatment of borderline personality disorder.* New York: Guilford Press.

Lockman, J. E., Barry, T. D., & Pardini, D. A. (2003). Anger control training for aggressive youth. In A. E. Kazdin & J. R. Weisz (Eds.), *Evidence-based psychotherapies for children and adolescents* (pp. 263–281). New York: Guilford Press.

Loeber, R. (1988). Natural histories of conduct problems, delinquency, and associated substance use: Evidence for developmental progressions. In B. B. Lahey & A. E. Casdin (Eds.), *Advances in clinical child psychopathology* (Vol. 2, pp. 73–124). New York: Plenum Press.

Loeber, R., Burke, J. D., Lahey, B. B., Winters, A., & Zera, M. (2000). Oppositional Defiant and Conduct Disorder: A review of the past 10 years, Part I. *Journal of the American Academy of Child and Adolescent Psychiatry, 39,* 1468–1484.

Loeber, R., Farrington, D. P., & Waschbusch, D. A. (1998). Serious and violent juvenile offenders. In R. Loeber & D. P. Farrington (Eds.), *Risk factors and successful interventions* (pp. 13–29). Thousand Oaks, CA: Sage.

Lynam, D. R. (1996). Early identification of chronic offenders: Who is the fledgling psychopath? *Psychological Bulletin, 120,* 209–234.

Magrab, P. R., & Wohlford, P. (Eds.). (1990). *Improving psychological services for children and adolescents with severe mental disorders: Clinical training in psychology.* Washington, DC: American Psychological Association.

Mash, E. J., & Terdal, L. G. (1997). Assessment of child and family disturbance: A behavioral-systems approach. In E. J. Mash & L. G. Terdal (Eds.), *Assessment of childhood disorders* (3rd ed., pp. 3–68). New York: Guilford Press.

McClellan, J., McCurry, C., Ronnei, M., Adams, J., Eisner, A., & Storck, M. (1996). Age of onset of sexual abuse: Relationship to sexually inappropriate behaviors. *Journal of the American Academy of Child and Adolescent Psychiatry, 34,* 1375–1383.

McComas, J. J., Hoch, H., & Mace, F. C. (2000). Functional analysis. In E. S. Shapiro & T. R. Kratochwill (Eds.), *Conducting school-based assessments of child and adolescent behavior* (pp. 78–120). New York: Guilford Press.

McConaughy, S. H. (2000a). Self-report: Child clinical interviews. In E. S. Shapiro & T. R. Kratochwill (Eds.), *Conducting school-based assessments of child and adolescent behavior* (pp. 170–202). New York: Guilford Press.

McConaughy, S. H. (2000b). Self-reports: Theory and practice in interviewing children. In E. S. Shapiro & T. R. Kratochwill (Eds.), *Behavioral assessment in schools* (2nd ed.): *Theory, research, and clinical foundations* (pp. 323–352). New York: Guilford Press.

McConaughy, S. H. (2003). Interviewing children, parents, and teachers. In M. Breen & C. Fiedler (Eds.), *Behavioral approach to the assessment of youth with emotional/behavioral disorders: A handbook for school-based practitioners* (2nd ed., pp. 123–169). Austin, TX: PRO-ED.

McConaughy, S. H. (2004a). *Semistructured Parent Interview.* Burlington, VT: University of Vermont, Research Center for Children, Youth, and Families.

McConaughy, S. H. (2004b). *Semistructured Teacher Interview.* Burlington, VT: University of Vermont, Research Center for Children, Youth, and Families.

McConaughy, S. H., & Achenbach, T. M. (1994). *Manual for the Semistructured Clinical Interview for Children and Adolescents.* Burlington, VT: University of Vermont, Research Center for Children, Youth, and Families.

McConaughy, S. H., & Achenbach, T. M. (2001). *Manual for the Semistructured Clinical Interview for Children and Adolescents* (2nd ed.). Burlington, VT: University of Vermont, Research Center for Children, Youth, and Families.

McConaughy, S. H., & Achenbach, T. M. (2004a). *Child and Family Information Form.* Burlington, VT: University of Vermont, Research Center for Children, Youth, and Families.

McConaughy, S. H., & Achenbach, T. M. (2004b). *Manual for the Test Observation Form for Ages 2–18.* Burlington, VT: University of Vermont, Research Center for Children, Youth, and Families.

McConaughy, S. H., Fitzhenry-Coor, I., & Howell, D. C. (1983). Developmental differences in story schemata. In K. Nelson (Ed.), *Children's language* (Vol. 4, pp. 385–421). New York: Erlbaum.

McConaughy, S. H., Kay, P. J., & Fitzgerald, M. (2000). The Achieving Behaving Caring Project for preventing ED: Two-year outcomes. *Journal of Emotional and Behavioral Disorders, 7,* 224–239.

McConaughy, S. H., & Ritter, D. R. (2002). Best practices in multidimensional assessment of emotional and behavioral disorders. In A. Thomas & J. Grimes (Eds.), *Best practices in school psychology–IV* (pp. 1303–1320). Bethesda, MD: National Association of School Psychologists.

McConaughy, S. H., & Skiba, R. (1993). Comorbidity of externalizing and internalizing problems. *School Psychology Review, 22,* 421–436.

McGinnis, E., & Goldstein, A. P. (1997). *Skillstreaming the elementary school child* (rev. ed.). Champaign, IL: Research Press.

McMahon, R. J., & Estes, A. M. (1997). Conduct problems. In E. J. Mash & L. G. Terdal (Eds.), *Assessment of childhood disorders* (3rd ed., pp. 130–193). New York: Guilford Press.

McMahon, R. J., & Forehand, R. L. (2003). *Helping the noncompliant child: Family-based treatment for oppositional behavior.* New York: Guilford Press.

Meeks, J. E. (1971). *The fragile alliance.* Malibar, FL: Krieger.

Megargee, E. I. (2002). Assessing the risk of aggression and violence. In J. Butcher (Ed.), *Clinical personality assessment: Practical approaches* (2nd ed., pp. 435–451). New York: Oxford University Press.

Meloy, J. R. (1999). Stalking: An old behavior, a new crime. *Psychiatric Clinics of North America, 22,* 85–99.

Meloy, J. R. (2004). Indirect personality assessment of the violent true believer. *Journal of Personality Assessment, 82,* 138–146.

Melton, G. B., Petrila, J., Polythress, N. G., & Slobogin, C. (1997). *Psychological evaluations for the courts: A handbook for mental health professionals and lawyers* (2nd ed.) New York: Guilford Press.

Merrell, K. W. (2001). *Helping children overcome depression and anxiety: A practical guide.* New York: Guilford Press.

Merrell, K. W. (2002a). *Preschool and Kindergarten Behavioral Scales—Second Edition.* Austin, TX: PRO-ED.

Merrell, K. W. (2002b). *School Social Behavior Scales—Second Edition.* Eugene, OR: Assessment–Intervention Resources.

Merrell, K. W. (2003). *Behavioral, social, and emotional assessment of children and adolescents.* Mahwah, NJ: Erlbaum.

Merrell, K. W., & Caldarella, P. (2002). *Home and Community Social Behavior Scales.* Eugene, OR: Assessment–Intervention Resources.

Miller, D. N. (2004). *Centennial School of Lehigh University suicide risk assessment questionnaire.* Unpublished manuscript, Lehigh University, Bethlehem, PA.

Miller, D. N., & DeZolt, D. M. (2004). Self-mutilation. In T. S. Watson & C. H. Skinner (Eds.), *Comprehensive encyclopedia of school psychology* (pp. 291–293). New York: Kluwer.

Miller, D. N., & DuPaul, G. J. (1996). School-based prevention of adolescent suicide: Issues, obstacles, and recommendations for practice. *Journal of Emotional and Behavioral Disorders, 4,* 221–230.

Miller, D. N., Eckert, T. L., DuPaul, G. J., & White, G. P. (1999). Adolescent suicide prevention: Acceptability of school-based programs among secondary school principals. *Suicide and Life-Threatening Behavior, 29,* 72–85.

Millon, T. (1993). *Millon Adolescent Clinical Inventory.* Minneapolis, MN: Pearson Assessments.

Moffit, T. E. (1993). Adolescence-limited and life-course persistent antisocial behavior: A developmental taxonomy. *Psychological Review, 100,* 674–701.

Mulvey, E. P., & Cauffman, E. (2001). The inherent limits of predicting school violence. *American Psychologist, 56,* 797–802.

Muris, P., Meesters, C., Merckelbach, H., Sermon, A., & Zwakhalen, S. (1998). Worry in normal children. *Journal of the American Academy of Child and Adolescent Psychiatry, 37,* 703–710.

Nagin, D. S., & Tremblay, R. (1999). Trajectories of boys' physical aggression and hyperactivity on the path to physically violent and nonviolent juvenile delinquency. *Child Development, 70,* 1181–1196.

Nagin, D. S., & Tremblay, R. (2001). Parental and early childhood predictors of persistent physical aggression in boys from kindergarten to high school. *Archives of General Psychiatry, 58,* 389–394.

Naglieri, J. A., LeBuff, P. A., & Pfeiffer, S. L. (1993). *Devereux Behavior Rating Scales School Form.* San Antonio, TX: Psychological Corporation.

Nastasi, B. K. (Ed.). (1998). Mini-series: Mental health programming in schools and communities. *School Psychology Review, 27*(2).

National Association of School Psychologists. (1992). *Professional conduct manual.* Bethesda, MD: Author.

National Association of School Psychologists. (2003a). *Position statement on student grade retention and social promotion.* Bethesda, MD: Author.

National Association of School Psychologists. (2003b). *Position statement on mental health services in the schools.* Bethesda, MD: Author.

Nelson, R., Roberts, M. L., & Smith, D. J. (1998). *Conducting functional behavioral assessments: A practical guide.* Longmont, CO: Sopris West.

Newgass, S., & Schonfeld, D. J. (2000). School crisis intervention, crisis prevention, and crisis response. In A. R. Roberts (Ed.), *Crisis intervention handbook: Assessment, treatment, and research* (2nd ed., pp. 209–228). London: Oxford University Press.

Nuttall, I. V., Li, C., Sanchez, W., Nuttall, R. L., & Mathisen, L. (2003). Assessing culturally and linguistically different children with emotional and behavioral problems. In M. Breen & C. Fiedler (Eds.), *Behavioral approach to the assessment of youth with emotional/behavioral disorders: A handbook for schoolbased practitioners* (2nd ed., pp. 463–496). Austin, TX: PRO-ED.

Parker, J. G., & Asher, S. R. (1993). Beyond group acceptance: Friendship adjustment and friendship quality as distinct dimensions of children's peer adjustment. In D. Perlman & W. H. Jones (Eds.), *Advances in personal relationships* (Vol. 4, pp. 261–294). London: Kingsley.

Parker, J. G., Rubin, K. H., Price, J. M., & DeRosier, M. E. (1995). Peer relationships, child development, and adjustment: A developmental psychopathology perspective. In D. Cicchetti & D. Cohen (Eds.), *Developmental psychopathology: Vol. 2. Risk, disorder and adaptation* (pp. 96–161). New York: Wiley.

Patterson, G. R. (1986). Performance models for antisocial boys. *American Psychologist, 41,* 432–444.

Patterson, G. R., Forgatch, M. S., Yoerger, K. L., & Stoolmiller, M. (1998). Variables that initiate and maintain an early-onset trajectory for juvenile offending. *Development and Psychopathology, 10,* 531–547.

Piaget, J. (1983). Piaget's theory. In P. H. Mussen (Ed.), *Handbook of child psychology* (Vol. 1, pp. 703–732). New York: Wiley.

Piquero, A. R., & Buka, S. L. (2002). Linking juvenile and adult patterns of criminal activity in the providence cohort of the National Collaborative Perinatal Project. *Journal of Criminal Justice, 30,* 259–272.

Poland, S. (1989). *Suicide intervention in the schools.* New York: Guilford Press.

Poland, S. (1990). The role of school crisis intervention teams to prevent and reduce school violence and trauma. *School Psychology Review, 23,* 175–189.

Poland, S. (1995). Best practices in suicide intervention. In A. Thomas & J. Grimes (Eds.), *Best practices in school psychology–III* (pp. 155–166). Bethesda, MD: National Association of School Psychologists.

Poland, S., & Lieberman, R. (2002). Best practices in suicide prevention. In A. Thomas & J. Grimes (Eds.), *Best practices in school psychology–IV* (pp. 1151–1165). Bethesda, MD: National Association of School Psychologists.

Poland, S., & McCormick, J. S. (1999). *Coping with crisis: Lessons learned.* Longmont, CO: Sopris West.

Power, T. J., Karustis, J. L., & Habboushe, D. F. (2001). *Homework success for children with ADHD.* New York: Guilford Press.

Powers, R. (2002, March). The apocalypse of adolescence. *Atlantic Monthly, 289,* 58–74.

Prout, H. T. (1983). School psychologists and social–emotional assessment techniques: Patterns in training and use. *School Psychology Review, 12,* 377–383.

Public Health Services Act. (1987). 42 U.S.C. §201 et seq.

Reddy, M., Borum, R., Berglund, J., Vossekuil, B., Fein, R., & Modzeleski, W. (2001). Evaluating risk for targeted violence in schools: Comparing risk assessment, threat assessment, and other approaches. *Psychology in the Schools, 38,* 157–172.

Rehabilitation Act. (1973). Section 504. 29 U.S.C. §794 et seq.

Reich, W. (2000). Diagnostic Interview for Children and Adolescents. *Journal of the American Academy of Child and Adolescent Psychiatry, 39,* 59–66.

Reich, W., Welner, Z., Herjanic, B., & MHS Staff. (1999). *Diagnostic Interview for Children and Adolescents–IV.* North Tonawanda, NY: Multi-Health Systems.

Reynolds, C. R., & Kamphaus, R. W. (2004). *Behavior Assessment System for Children (2nd ed.) manual.* Circle Pines, MN: American Guidance Service.

Reynolds, W. M. (1988). *Suicidal Ideation Questionnaire manual.* Odessa, FL: Psychological Assessment Resources.

Reynolds, W. M. (1989). *Reynolds Child Depression Scale manual.* Odessa, FL: Psychological Assessment Resources.

Reynolds, W. M. (1991). A school-based procedure for the identification of adolescents at risk for suicidal behaviors. *Family Community Health, 14,* 64–75.

Reynolds, W. M. (1998). *Adolescent Psychopathology Scale psychometric and technical manual.* Odessa, FL: Psychological Assessment Resources.

Reynolds, W. M. (2002). *Reynolds Adolescent Depression Scale manual* (2nd ed.). Odessa, FL: Psychological Assessment Resources.

Reynolds, W. M., & Mazza, J. J. (1994). Suicide and suicidal behaviors in children and adolescents. In W. M. Reynolds & H. F. Johnston (Eds.), *Handbook of depression in children and adolescents* (pp. 525–580). New York: Plenum.

Rhode, G., Jenson, W. R., & Reavis, H. K. (1993). *The tough kid book: Practical classroom management strategies.* Longmont, CO: Sopris West.

Rhodes, R. L., Ochoa, S. H., & Ortiz, S. O. (2005). *Assessing culturally and linguistically diverse students: A practical guide.* New York: Guilford Press.

Roberts, M. C., Erickson, M. T., La Greca, A. M., Russ, S. W., Vargas, L. A., Carlson, C. I., et al. (1998). A model for training psychologists to provide services for children and adolescents. *Professional Psychology: Research and Practice, 29,* 293–299.

Rorty, R. (1982). *Consequences of pragmatism.* Minneapolis: University of Minneapolis Press.

Ross, S., & Heath, N. (2002). A study of the frequency of self-mutilation in a community sample of adolescents. *Journal of Youth and Adolescence, 31,* 67–77.

Rubin, K. H., & Stewart, S. L. (1996). Social withdrawal. In E. J. Mash & R. A. Barkley (Eds.), *Child psychopathology* (pp. 277–310). New York: Guilford Press.

Ryan-Arredonno, K., Renouf, K., Egyed, C., Doxely, M., Dobbins, M., Sanchez, S., et al. (2001). Threats of violence in schools: The Dallas Independent School District's response. *Psychology in the Schools, 38,* 185–196.

Safe and Drug Free Schools and Community Act. (1994). 20 U.S.C. § 7101 et seq.

Saigh, P. A. (1992). Structured clinical interviews and the inferential process. *Journal of School Psychology, 30,* 141–149.

Sattler, J. M. (1998). *Clinical and forensic interviewing of children and families.* San Diego: Author.

Scherff, A., Eckert, T. L., & Miller, D. N. (2005). Youth suicide prevention: A survey of public school superintendents' acceptability of school-based programs. *Suicide and Life-Threatening Behavior, 35,* 154–169.

Shaffer, D., & Craft, L. (1999). Methods of adolescent suicide prevention. *Journal of Clinical Psychiatry, 60,* 70–74.

Shaffer, D., Fisher, P., Lucas, C. P., Dulcan, M., & Schwab-Stone, M. E. (2000). NIMH Diagnostic Interview Schedule for Children Version—Version IV (NIMH DISC-IV): Description, differences from previous versions and reliability of some common diagnoses. *Journal of the American Academy of Child and Adolescent Psychiatry, 39,* 28–38.

Shaffer, D., Gould, M. S., Fisher, P., Trautment, P., Moreau, D., Kleinman, M., & Flory, M. (1996). Psychiatric diagnosis in child and adolescent suicide. *Archives of General Psychiatry, 53,* 339–348.

Shapiro, E. S. (2004). *Academic skills problems: Direct assessment and intervention* (3rd ed.). New York: Guilford Press.

Shapiro, E. S., & Kratochwill, T. R. (Eds.). (2000). Introduction: Conducting a multidimensional behavioral assessment. In E. S. Shapiro & T. R. Kratochwill (Eds.), *Conducting school-based assessments of child and adolescent behavior* (pp. 1–20). New York: Guilford Press.

Sheridan, S. M. (1997). *The tough kid social skills book.* Longmont, CO: Sopris West.

Sheridan, S. M., Kratochwill, T. R., & Bergan, J. R. (1996). *Conjoint behavioral consultation: A procedural manual.* New York: Plenum Press.

Skiba, R., & Grizzle, K. (1991). The social maladjustment exclusion: Issues of definition and assessment. *School Psychology Review, 20,* 577–595.

Skiba, R., & Grizzle, K. (1992). Qualifications vs. logic and data: Excluding conduct disorders from the SED definition. *School Psychology Review, 21,* 23–28.

Slater, B. R., & Gallagher, M. M. (1989). Outside the realm of psychotherapy: Consultation for interventions with sexualized children. *School Psychology Review, 18,* 400–411.

Stanger, C. (2003). Behavioral assessment: An overview. In M. J. Breen & C. R. Fiedler (Eds.), *Behavioral approach to assessment of youth with emotional/behavioral disorders: A handbook for school-based practitioners* (pp. 3–20). Austin, TX: PRO-ED.

Stossel, J. (1999, October 22). Give me a break: Media coverage of school shootings is up though violence in schools is down. *20/20.* New York: ABC News.

Stricker, G. (2002). What is a scientist–practitioner anyway? *Journal of Clinical Psychology, 58,* 1277–1283.

Stricker, G., & Trierweiler, S. J. (1995). The local clinical scientist: A bridge between science and practice. *American Psychologist, 12,* 995–1002.

Sugai, G., Horner, R. H., Dunlap, G., Heinman, M., Lewis, T. L., et al. (1999). *Applying positive behavioral support and functional behavioral assessment in schools.* Washington, DC: OSEP Center on Positive Behavioral Interventions and Support. www.pbis.org/english/Center_Products.htm

Tarasoff v. Board of Regents of the University of California, 551 P. 2d 334 (Cal. Sup. Ct. 1976).

Tremblay, R. E., Japel, C., Perusse, D., Boivin, M., Zocolillo, M., Montplaisir, J., et al. (1999). The search for the age of "onset" of physical aggression: Rousseau and Bandura revisited. *Criminal Behavior and Mental Health, 9,* 8–23.

U.S. Census Bureau. (2003). *Current population reports.* Washington, DC: U.S. Department of Commerce. www.census.gov

U.S. Department of Education. (2002). *Twenty-fourth annual report to Congress on the implementation of the Individuals with Disabilities Education Act.* (2002). Washington, DC: Author. www.ed.gov/print/about/reports/annual/osep/2002/execsumm.htlm

U.S. Department of Education and United States Department of Justice. (1999). *1999 annual report on school safety.* Washington, DC: Author.

U.S. Department of Health and Human Services. (2002). *Child maltreatment 2002: Reports from the states to the National Center on Child Abuse and Neglect.* Washington, DC: U.S. Government Printing Office. www.acf.hhs.gov/programs/cb/publications/cmreports.htm

Vasey, M. W., & Daleiden, E. (1994). Worry in childhood. In G. Davey & F. Tallis (Eds.), *Worrying: Perspectives on theory, assessment, and treatment* (pp. 185–207). New York: Wiley.

Vevier, E., & Tharinger, D. J. (1986). Child sexual abuse: A review and intervention framework for the school psychologist. *Journal of School Psychology, 24,* 293–311.

Vossekuil, B., Fein, R., Reddy, M., Borum, R., & Modzeleski, W. (2002). *The final report and findings of the safe school initiative: Implications for the prevention of school attacks in the United States.* Washington, DC: U.S. Secret Service and U.S. Department of Education.

Vossekuil, B., Reddy, M., Fein, R., Borum, R., & Modzeleski, W. (2000). *Safe school initiative: An interim report on the prevention of targeted violence in schools.* Washington, DC: U. S. Secret Service, National Threat Assessment Center. www.treas.gov/usss/ntac/ntac_ssi_report

Watkins, C. E., Campbell, V. L., Nieberding, R., & Hallmark, R. (1995). Contemporary practice of psychological assessment by clinical psychologists. *Professional Psychology Research and Practice, 26,* 54–60.

Watson, T. S., & Steege, M. W. (2003). *Conducting school-based functional behavioral assessments: A practitioner's guide.* New York: Guilford Press.

Wenk, E. A., Robinson, J. O., & Smith, G. W. (1972). Can violence be predicted? *Crime and Delinquency, 18,* 393–402.

Wissow, L. S. (1995). Child abuse and neglect. *New England Journal of Medicine, 332,* 1425–1431.

Wolfe, D. A., & McEachran, A. (1997). Child physical abuse and neglect. In E. J. Mash & L. G.Terdal (Eds.), *Assessment of childhood disorders* (3rd ed., pp. 523–568). New York: Guilford Press.

Wolfe, V. V., & Birt, J. (1997). Child sexual abuse. In E. J. Mash & L. G. Terdal (Eds.), *Assessment of childhood disorders* (3rd ed., pp. 569–623). New York: Guilford Press.

Ysseldyke, J., & Christenson, S. (1993). *The Instructional Environment System–II.* Longmont, CO: Sopris West.

Zins, J. E., & Erchul, W. P. (2002). Best practices in school consultation. In A. Thomas & J. Grimes (Eds.), *Best practices in school psychology–IV* (pp. 625–643). Bethesda, MD: National Association of School Psychologists.

Index